Diseases of the Brain

Guest Editor

WILLIAM B. THOMAS, DVM, MS

VETERINARY CLINICS OF NORTH AMERICA: SMALL ANIMAL PRACTICE

www.vetsmall.theclinics.com

January 2010 • Volume 40 • Number 1

SAUNDERS an imprint of ELSEVIER, Inc.

W.B. SAUNDERS COMPANY
A Division of Elsevier Inc.

1600 John F. Kennedy Blvd. ● Suite 1800 ● Philadelphia, PA 19103-2899

http://www.vetsmall.theclinics.com

VETERINARY CLINICS OF NORTH AMERICA: SMALL ANIMAL PRACTICE Volume 40, Number 1
January 2010 ISSN 0195-5616, ISBN-13: 978-1-4377-1886-7

Editor: John Vassallo; j.vassallo@elsevier.com
Developmental Editor: Donald Mumford

Veterinary Clinics of North America: Small Animal Practice (ISSN 0195-5616) is published bimonthly (For Post Office use only: volume 40 issue 1 of 6) by Elsevier Inc., 360 Park Avenue South, New York, NY 10010-1710. Months of issue are January, March, May, July, September, and November. Application to mail at periodicals postage rates is pending at New York, NY and at additional mailing offices. Subscription prices are $245.00 per year (domestic individuals), $388.00 per year (domestic institutions), $122.00 per year (domestic students/ residents), $324.00 per year (Canadian individuals), $477.00 per year (Canadian institutions), $360.00 per year (international individuals), $477.00 per year (international institutions), and $177.00 per year (international and Canadian students/residents). To receive student/resident rate, orders must be accompanied by name of affiliated institution, date of term, and the *signature* of program/residency coordinator on institution letterhead. Orders will be billed at individual rate until proof of status is received. Foreign air speed delivery is included in all *Clinics* subscription prices. All prices are subject to change without notice. **POSTMASTER:** Send address changes to *Veterinary Clinics of North America: Small Animal Practice*, Elsevier Health Sciences Division, Subscription Customer Service, 3251 Riverport Lane, Maryland Heights, MO 63043. Customer Service (orders, claims, online, change of address): Elsevier Periodicals Customer Service, Elsevier Health Sciences Division Subscription Customer Service 3251 Riverport Lane Maryland Heights, MO 63043. Tel: 1-800-654-2452 (U.S. and Canada); 314-447-8871 (outside U.S. and Canada). Fax: 314-447-8029. E-mail: journalscustomerservice-usa@elsevier.com (for print support); journalsonlinesupport-usa@elsevier.com (for online support).

Reprints. For copies of 100 or more of articles in this publication, please contact the Commercial Reprints Department, Elsevier Inc., 360 Park Avenue South, New York, NY 10010-1710. Tel.: 212-633-3812; Fax: 212-462-1935; E-mail: reprints@elsevier.com.

Veterinary Clinics of North America: Small Animal Practice is also published in Japanese by Inter Zoo Publishing Co., Ltd., Aoyama Crystal-Bldg 5F, 3-5-12 Kitaaoyama, Minato-ku, Tokyo 107-0061, Japan.

Veterinary Clinics of North America: Small Animal Practice is covered in *Current Contents/Agriculture, Biology and Environmental Sciences, Science Citation Index, ASCA, MEDLINE/PubMed (Index Medicus), Excerpta Medica,* and *BIOSIS.*

Printed and bound in the United Kingdom
Transferred to Digital Print 2011

Contributors

GUEST EDITOR

WILLIAM B. THOMAS, DVM, MS
Diplomate, American College of Veterinary Internal Medicine (Neurology); Professor, Neurology and Neurosurgery, Department of Small Animal Clinical Sciences, College of Veterinary Medicine, University of Tennessee, Knoxville, Tennessee

AUTHORS

WILLIAM H. ADAMS, DVM
Diplomate, American College of Veterinary Radiology (Radiology and Radiation Oncology); Associate Professor of Radiology and Radiation Oncology, Department of Small Animal Clinical Sciences, University of Tennessee College of Veterinary Medicine, Knoxville, Tennessee

SOFIA CERDA-GONZALEZ, DVM
Diplomate, American College of Veterinary Internal Medicine (Neurology); Assistant Professor of Neurology, Neurosurgery, Department of Clinical Sciences, Cornell University College of Veterinary Medicine, Ithaca, New York

CURTIS W. DEWEY, DVM, MS
Diplomate American College of Veterinary Internal Medicine (Neurology); Diplomate, American College of Veterinary Surgeons; Associate Professor of Neurology, Neurosurgery, Department of Clinical Sciences, Cornell University College of Veterinary Medicine, Ithaca, New York

MARTI G. DRUM, DVM, PhD, CCRP
Clinical Assistant Professor, Department of Small Animal Clinical Sciences, University of Tennessee, Knoxville, Tennessee

LAURENT S. GAROSI, DVM, MRCVS
Diplomate, European College of Veterinary Neurology; RCVS recognized specialist in Veterinary Neurology, Head of Neurology, Davies Veterinary Specialists, Manor farm Business Park, Higham Gobion, England, United Kingdom

SILKE HECHT, Dr Med Vet
Diplomate, American College Veterinary Radiology; Diplomate, European College of Veterinary Diagnostic Imaging; Assistant Professor of Radiology, Department of Small Animal Clinical Sciences, University of Tennessee College of Veterinary Medicine, Knoxville, Tennessee

JOHN H. ROSSMEISL Jr, DVM, MS
Diplomate, American College of Veterinary Internal Medicine (Small Animal Internal Medicine and Neurology); Associate Professor, Neurology and Neurosurgery, Department of Small Animal Clinical Sciences, Virginia-Maryland Regional College of Veterinary Medicine, Virginia Tech, Blacksburg, Virginia

SCOTT J. SCHATZBERG, DVM, PhD
Diplomate, American College of Veterinary Internal Medicine (Neurology); Assistant Professor of Neurology, Department of Small Animal Medicine and Surgery, College of Veterinary Medicine, University of Georgia, Athens, Georgia

WILLIAM B. THOMAS, DVM, MS
Diplomate, American College of Veterinary Internal Medicine (Neurology); Professor, Neurology and Neurosurgery, Department of Small Animal Clinical Sciences, College of Veterinary Medicine, University of Tennessee, Knoxville, Tennessee

Contents

The initial evaluation of patients with brain disease is focused on determining the neuroanatomic diagnosis and the etiologic diagnosis. This evaluation is based on obtaining a careful history and performing a neurologic examination. Based on these results, the clinician recommends further diagnostic tests to confirm the diagnosis. By following this orderly process of clinical reasoning, it is usually possible to determine the cause of the patient's brain disease, which provides a prognosis and allows specific therapy.

Magnetic resonance imaging (MRI) is increasingly being used in the diagnosis of central nervous system disorders in veterinary patients and is quickly becoming the imaging modality of choice in evaluation of brain and intracranial disease. This article provides an overview of the basic principles of MRI, a description of sequences and their applications in brain imaging, and an approach to interpretation of brain MRI. A detailed discussion of imaging findings in general intracranial disorders including hydrocephalus, vasogenic edema, brain herniation, and seizure-associated changes, and the MR diagnosis of congenital brain disorders is provided. MRI evaluation of acquired brain disorders is described in a second companion article.

Magnetic resonance imaging (MRI) has revolutionized brain imaging in veterinary medicine, making possible improved characterization of intracranial pathologic processes. This article focuses on MRI features of acquired brain disorders, including infectious inflammatory, noninfectious inflammatory, cerebrovascular, metabolic, nutritional, toxic, degenerative, traumatic, and neoplastic causes. Congenital intracranial disorders are covered in a companion article.

Cerebrovascular disease is defined as any abnormality of the brain resulting from a pathologic process affecting its blood supply. Stroke or cerebrovascular accident (CVA) is the most common clinical manifestation of cerebrovascular disease, and can be broadly divided into ischemic stroke and hemorrhagic stroke. Ischemic stroke results from occlusion of a cerebral blood vessel by a thrombus or embolism, depriving the brain of oxygen and glucose, whereas hemorrhagic stroke results from rupture of a blood vessel wall within the brain parenchyma or subarachnoid space. Previously considered uncommon, CVA is being recognized with greater frequency in veterinary medicine since magnetic resonance imaging has become more readily available. Once the diagnosis of ischemic or hemorrhagic stroke is confirmed, potential underlying causes should be sought after and treated accordingly.

The vestibular system is the major sensory (special proprioceptive) system that, along with the general proprioceptive and visual systems, maintains balance. Clinical signs of vestibular disease include asymmetric ataxia, head tilt, and pathologic nystagmus. Neuroanatomic localization of observed vestibular signs to either the peripheral or central components of the vestibular system is paramount to the management of the patient with vestibular dysfunction, as the etiology, diagnostic approaches, and prognoses are dependent on the neuroanatomic diagnosis. This article reviews functional vestibular neuroanatomy as well as the diagnosis and treatment of common causes of small animal vestibular disease.

Granulomatous meningoencephalomyelitis (GME), necrotizing meningoencephalitis (NME), and necrotizing leukoencephalitis (NLE) are common inflammatory conditions of the canine central nervous system (CNS). While each disease has unique histopathological features, these canine disorders collectively seem to be aberrant immune responses directed against the CNS. A review of the neurologic signs and general neurodiagnostic approach to canine meningoencephalitis (ME) is followed by an overview of the specific clinical and neuropathological features of GME, NME, and NLE. The etiopathogenesis of each disorder is explored, including potential genetic, immunologic, and environmental factors, along with the current and prospective immunomodulatory therapies for ME.

Craniocervical junction disorders are most frequently seen in toy and small-breed dogs. They can present a diagnostic challenge, as multiple anomalies can be present concurrently and share similar clinical manifestations. Some, such as Chiari-like malformations, may be present in asymptomatic dogs. A thorough evaluation of the entire craniocervical junction, frequently using more than 1 imaging modality, is necessary before making treatment decisions.

Hydrocephalus is distension of the ventricular system of the brain related to inadequate passage of cerebrospinal fluid from its point of production within the ventricular system to its point of absorption into the systemic circulation. Developmental disorders are the most common causes of hydrocephalus, but there are other causes as well. Diagnosis is based on the clinical features and on brain imaging to assess ventricular size and to identify any specific causes. Medical therapy can provide temporary relief but definitive treatment usually involves placement of a ventriculoperitoneal shunt. This article discusses the pathophysiology and management of hydrocephalus.

Idiopathic epilepsy is the most common brain disease in dogs and also occurs in cats. Optimal management entails an accurate diagnosis and appropriate drug therapy. In dogs, either phenobarbital or bromide is appropriate as initial therapy. Phenobarbital is the drug of choice for cats. Several other drugs including zonisamide and levetiracetam have the advantage of fewer side effects and are being increasingly used in veterinary medicine. Treatment is successful in most cases, allowing the pet and client to enjoy a good quality of life.

Rehabilitation therapy is a key component of recovery from neurologic disease. Each patient requires a rehabilitation protocol designed specifically for the patient's neurologic condition, owner expectations and level of participation, and expertise of the veterinary team. Initial therapy for nonambualtory patients may include standing exercises, range of motion, pain control, toe pinch exercise, aquatic exercise, and basic nursing care. Sling assisted walking with foot protection, cavaletti rails, and physioroll balancing are used commonly for ambulatory patients. As recovery progresses, stair climbing, carrying or pulling weights, resistance band walking, swimming against resistance, and exercises specific to the home environment are added. Modalities such as electrical stimulation, ultrasound, cryotherapy, and heat therapy are useful adjuncts but do not take the place of active exercise.

FORTHCOMING ISSUES

RECENT ISSUES

RELATED INTEREST
Veterinary Clinics of North America: Exotic Animal Practice
September 2007 (Vol. 10, No. 3)
Neuroanatomy and Neurodiagnostics
Lisa A. Tell, DVM, Dipl. ABVP—Avian, and Marguerite F. Knipe, DVM, Dipl. ACVIM,
Guest Editors

THE CLINICS ARE NOW AVAILABLE ONLINE!
Access your subscription at:
www.theclinics.com

Preface

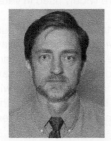

William B. Thomas, DVM, MS
Guest Editor

...all the most acute, most powerful, and most deadly diseases, and those which are most difficult to be understood by the inexperienced, fall upon the brain.
—*Hippocrates (circa 400 BC)*

Few practitioners look forward to seeing a patient with brain disease. As Hippocrates recognized more than 2000 years ago, diseases of the brain are often perplexing and almost always serious. Seizures, blindness, inability to walk, and coma are bad enough, but brain disease can also disturb the one quality that clients treasure the most—their pet's personality.

Fortunately, the ability to diagnose and treat many of these devastating diseases is rapidly advancing. Clients see their relatives and friends getting MRIs, newer antiseizure drugs, and neurosurgery and want the same level of care for their pets. The goal of this issue is to review recent advances in the diagnosis and treatment of some of the more common brain diseases.

The first article discusses the general diagnostic approach to patients with brain disease, focusing on history and neurologic examination. Nothing has improved the ability to diagnose brain disease more than MRI, and Silke Hecht and William Adams thoroughly discuss the use of this imaging modality in two articles. Many veterinarians were taught that dogs and cats do not get strokes, but now it is known that vascular disease is an important cause of brain disease in patients. Laurent Garosi has authored an excellent review of this topic. John Rossmeisl's article on vestibular disease is a clear and practical review of this common group of diseases. Encephalitis is one of the most frustrating diseases encountered. One of the leading researchers in this area, Scott Schatzberg, reviews this topic in an article that will be valuable to general practitioners and specialists alike. Chiari-like malformation and related disorders have emerged as major diseases in small breed dogs, and Sofia Cerda-Gonzalez and Curtis Dewey discuss up-to-date diagnosis and treatment of this important condition. The management of hydrocephalus is reviewed, including the use of ventriculoperitoneal

Vet Clin Small Anim 40 (2010) ix–x
doi:10.1016/j.cvsm.2009.09.010
0195-5616/09/$ – see front matter © 2010 Elsevier Inc. All rights reserved.
vetsmall.theclinics.com

shunts. The article on idiopathic epilepsy discusses the diagnosis and medical treatment of this common condition. Finally, Marti Drum covers physical rehabilitation of neurologic patients, a treatment modality that is becoming more widely used in veterinary medicine.

I would like to thank the authors for their time and expertise. They are all busy clinicians, teachers, and researchers, and finding the time to write an article is always a challenge. I also thank John Vassallo and the staff at Elsevier for their help and patience in the preparation of this issue. I am also grateful for the residents I have worked with, Avril Arendse, Christina Wolf, Joe Mankin, and Curtis Probst, who have taught me so much and helped choose the topics for this issue. I hope that this information will be valuable to clinicians in their treatment of pets with these diseases.

William B. Thomas, DVM, MS
Department of Small Animal Clinical Sciences
College of Veterinary Medicine
University of Tennessee
C247 Veterinary Teaching Hospital
2407 River Drive
Knoxville, TN 37996-4544, USA

E-mail address:
wthomas@utk.edu

Evaluation of Veterinary Patients with Brain Disease

William B. Thomas, DVM, MS

KEYWORDS

• Neurologic examination • History • Diagnosis
• Brain disease

Veterinarians sometimes seem to believe that the neurologic examination is a mystifying process best undertaken only by specialists. The truth is that the initial evaluation of patients with neurologic disease is based on an orderly process of clinical reasoning that involves the same powers of observation that clinicians use daily in other patients. However, as with any clinical skill, performing and interpreting a neurologic examination does require practice. Clinicians are encouraged to occasionally perform a neurologic examination on patients without neurologic disease to become familiar with normal findings and stay proficient in the procedure. With a little practice and basic understanding of the principles, there is no reason why a general practitioner cannot feel comfortable in the initial evaluation of patients with brain disease.

The evaluation of patients with brain disease involves 2 critical questions: "Where is it?" and "What is it?" The first question refers to the anatomic diagnosis, the second to the etiologic diagnosis. Initially, the anatomic diagnosis usually takes precedence over the etiologic diagnosis. When an etiologic diagnosis is elusive, an anatomic diagnosis allows the veterinarian to focus diagnostic tests on the appropriate region of the nervous system. Once the disease is localized, the cause can be determined, based on the clinical features of the various diseases.

This article describes a practical approach to neurologic history and examination. It also briefly discusses some of the diagnostic procedures used to confirm a diagnosis in patients with brain disease, such as analysis of spinal fluid, computed tomography (CT), and magnetic resonance imaging (MRI). Although these procedures are not widely available in most general practices, it is helpful for all clinicians to have a basic understanding of these advanced procedures for cases for which referral is appropriate.

HISTORY

The history is the most essential part of the evaluation. After taking the history, the astute clinician has formulated an appropriate differential list, if not the actual

Department of Small Animal Clinical Sciences, College of Veterinary Medicine, University of Tennessee, 2407 River Drive, Knoxville, TN 37996-4544, USA
E-mail address: wthomas@utk.edu

Vet Clin Small Anim 40 (2010) 1–19
doi:10.1016/j.cvsm.2009.09.002   vetsmall.theclinics.com
0195-5616/09/$ – see front matter © 2010 Elsevier Inc. All rights reserved.

diagnosis. However, many diagnostic errors are due to incomplete or inaccurate histories. Obtaining the history arguably requires greater skill and experience than doing an examination. Consequently, it is important to allot ample time for this part of the evaluation.

A standardized form is useful for history taking, but clinicians should consider the client's specific concerns, and never limit questions to a stereotyped list. When eliciting the history, patience, kindness, and a manner that conveys interest and compassion are essential. The veterinarian should meet the client on a common ground of language and vocabulary. By following these principles, an accurate history is obtained, the clinician develops empathy for the client and patient, and the client develops confidence in the veterinarian.

Signalment

The history starts with the signalment, including the patient's age, breed, and sex, which may provide clues to the diagnosis. For example, congenital or developmental diseases occur most often in the young, whereas neoplasia and degenerative disorders are more common in older patients. Some diseases occur only in a particular sex, for example hypocalcemia associated with lactation.

Chief Concern

The chief concern is the reason the client is presenting the pet to the veterinarian. In most cases, this is a sign, or group of signs, that the client has noticed. The client is encouraged to give a complete account of the pet's illness. Initially, the clinician should interrupt as little as possible, and only to lead the story in the proper direction and to obtain clarification of statements that seem vague or incomplete. Rarely, however, is the client's spontaneous narrative complete. Therefore, the clinician must augment the client's account with specific questions.

The precise meaning that the client attaches to certain words must be determined. For example, some clients use the term "seizure" to refer to an attack of syncope, cataplexy, vestibular dysfunction, or behavior related to pain, instead of a true epileptic seizure. Such ambiguity must be clarified early to avoid wasting time exploring an unlikely diagnosis. It is also important to identify objective observations noticed by clients, rather than their conclusions. An example is "pain". Pain is a subjective sensation; a client cannot observe pain. Rather, they observe certain signs that they may interpret as indications of pain. Examples include crying when the patient is touched, decreased activity, carrying of a limb, or limited neck movement. If a client says the pet is painful, ask about the specific abnormalities that led to this conclusion.

The onset and course of the illness helps identify the etiologic diagnosis. Trauma, vascular disorders, seizures, and syncope have an acute onset. Diseases that progress over several days include inflammatory and metabolic disorders, and some tumors. Degenerative diseases, and some tumors, have an insidious, slowly progressive course. Remissions and exacerbations are characteristic of seizures, syncope, and some metabolic disorders.

Factors that precipitated, exacerbate, or improve the signs are important. For example, feeding often makes hepatic encephalopathy worse. Exercise can precipitate syncope or myasthenia gravis. Prior or current therapy is important, as is the result of such treatment, which includes prescribed treatments and nonprescription drugs or remedies. Realize that clients are often tempted to retrospectively identify a cause for their pet's illness even though such events may be coincidental or even the result of the illness rather than the cause. For instance, once a patient develops brain disease, a client can often recollect a minor traumatic event such as the pet bumping its head while playing. In a patient with ataxia, did the fall off a step cause the ataxia or did the animal fall because it was ataxic? Some conditions will improve spontaneously, so it can be difficult to know whether any improvement is due to any treatment or just the natural history of the disease.

After the chief concern is characterized, clients find it helpful to have their concerns summarized and itemized. This reassures the client that the veterinarian has heard and understood the history, and allows the clinician to determine whether there are other concerns that were not mentioned.

Environment and Family History

Exposure to trauma or toxins has obvious implications. Lead poisoning can be particularly difficult to identify, because the client is often unaware of the source of exposure. Instead, ask about the age of the building and any construction or remodeling. If available, a family history of related disorders is sometimes helpful in identifying genetic disorders, such as epilepsy.

PHYSICAL EXAMINATION

Although the neurologic examination is usually considered separate from the physical examination, in practice much of the neurologic examination can be integrated with the physical examination. The physical examination may identify a systemic disease affecting the nervous system. Examples include fever associated with meningoencephalitis, otitis in a patient with vestibular dysfunction, lymphadenopathy associated with systemic blastomycosis, and a heart murmur in a patient with cerebrovascular disease.

NEUROLOGIC EXAMINATION

The neurologic examination begins the moment the veterinarian first sees the patient. If possible, observe the patient moving freely in the examination area while taking the history. Many animals are more relaxed after they are allowed to spend a few minutes investigating their environment. The neurologic examination, probably more than any other examination, requires the cooperation of the patient. Although a patient can be sedated if necessary to allow examination of many body systems, such sedation will usually preclude an accurate examination of the nervous system. Therefore, anything the clinician can do to foster cooperation on the part of the patient is worthwhile. In anxious patients, gentle petting is useful and helps establish a pleasant tone of the examination. Start with procedures least likely to upset the patient, and delay disagreeable or painful tests until the end of the examination. For example, starting the examination of a grumpy rottweiler by pinching toes to check deep pain perception is likely to put an abrupt end to any further examination.

As mentioned earlier, integrating the neurologic examination with the physical examination is an efficient approach. Start with an assessment of mental status, behavior, and posture while obtaining the history. Next, test cranial nerves while examining the head. Palpate the head, spine, and major muscle groups. Then assess the gait and postural reactions and observe any involuntary movements. Finally, check spinal reflexes and evaluate the sensory system.[1-3]

The thoroughness of the examination is governed by the history, especially the presenting concern. Modify the examination according to the condition of the patient. For instance, it could be dangerous to evaluate postural reactions, such as hopping and wheelbarrowing, in a nonambulatory patient that had been struck by a car and potentially had an unstable vertebral injury. Some parts of the examination cannot be carried out in a comatose or sedated patient.

Mental Status and Behavior

Normal consciousness implies wakefulness and awareness of the environment, and is assessed by observing for appropriate or inappropriate response to the environment (**Table 1**). Lethargy can be caused by systemic illness or brain disease. Delirium and dementia usually indicate forebrain dysfunction. Obtundation, stupor, or coma is usually due to a brain stem lesion or severe, diffuse disease of the forebrain.

Abnormal behavior is identified by comparing the patient's behavior to expected behavior for animals of a similar breed and age. Normal behavior varies with the individual, and the hospital environment will often influence the patient's behavior. Therefore, the client is often able to bring subtle changes in behavior to the veterinarian's attention. Common behavior abnormalities in patients with brain disease include disruptions in the pet's normal sleep-wake cycle, restlessness, aimless pacing or wandering, getting stuck in corners, a tendency to turn and circle to one side, decreased or abnormal interaction with the family, and cognitive dysfunction such as loss of house training or inability to follow commands. In some cases, the client is not able to describe any specific abnormalities other than a vague sense that the pet is not behaving normally. If the client is convinced that this is a change in the pet, this should be considered a significant finding even if the veterinarian is unable to detect abnormalities that are more specific.

Posture

The posture should be upright with the head held straight. Head tilt, in which one ear is held lower than the other, usually indicates vestibular dysfunction. Head tilt must be differentiated from head turn or torticollis. With head turn, the head is held level (one ear is not lower than the other) but the nose is turned right or left. Animals with forebrain lesions may tend to turn their heads and circle in one direction. Torticollis is abnormal curving or twisting of the neck, and can occur with cervical lesions. Ventral flexion of the neck is most commonly seen in cats with neuromuscular weakness, although it can also occur with neck pain.

Table 1 Assessment of consciousness	
Status	**Signs**
Normal	Alert, responds appropriately to environment
Lethargy	Little spontaneous activity, lies quietly or sleeps in the absence of stimuli, will interact with the environment when stimulated, although quality and quantity of interaction are depressed
Obtundation	Appears asleep in the absence of stimulation, can be briefly aroused to minimal interaction
Stupor	Requires vigorous stimulation to provoke arousal, and responds with movement or vocalization but no appropriate interaction
Coma	Unconscious, cannot be aroused even with vigorous or painful stimuli
Dementia	Normal level of consciousness but loss of higher, intellectual function, with impaired interaction
Delirium	Dramatic disruption of higher, intellectual function with inappropriate response to the environment

Recumbent animals may exhibit several abnormal postures. Decerebrate rigidity is characterized by extension of all limbs and opisthotonus (dorsiflexion of the head and neck). This posture is usually caused by a brain stem lesion, and affected patients typically have decreased consciousness. Decerebellate rigidity is less common, occurs with acute cerebellar lesions, and is characterized by opisthotonus, thoracic limb extension, and flexion of the hips or extension of the pelvic limbs. In contrast to decerebrate rigidity, patients with decerebellate posture have normal consciousness. Schiff-Sherrington posture consists of extension of the thoracic limbs with paralysis of the pelvic limbs, and is associated with a lesion affecting the thoracic or lumbar spinal segments. Although the thoracic limbs have increased extensor tone, they are otherwise normal, with intact voluntary movement and postural reactions.

Cranial Nerve Examination

The cranial nerves are evaluated in a sequential fashion, starting with olfaction and ending with tongue movement.[1–3]

Cranial nerve I (olfactory)
Testing of olfaction is only performed if the chief concern is loss of smell. This concern is most common in hunting dogs and police or military detector dogs. The olfactory nerve is tested with a small morsel of canned food. After ascertaining patency of the nostrils, cover the patient's eyes and present the food beneath the nose, observing for normal sniffing behavior. Irritating substances, such as ammonia or isopropyl alcohol, should not be used, because they stimulate trigeminal nerve endings in the nasal passages and produce false results. Many dogs presented for loss of smell actually have some other disorder (eg, musculoskeletal disease) that is interfering with the dog's ability to work, and the client assumes that the inability to work is due to loss of smell. True loss of smell (anosmia) is uncommonly recognized and is usually caused by nasal disease, such as distemper or parainfluenza, rather than brain disease.

Cranial nerve II (ophthalmic)
The alert patient should show visual following and a menace response bilaterally. Assess visual following by dropping cotton balls or moving a toy or ball in front of the patient and observing whether the patient's eyes and head follow the object. To test the menace response, move your hand toward the patient's eye in a threatening manner, observing for a blink response. By covering the contralateral eye, you can test the nasal (medial) and temporal (lateral) visual fields of each eye. The facial nerve controls closure of the eyelid, so, if the menace response is absent, make sure that facial nerve function is normal (see later discussion). Funduscopic examination is an important component of a complete neurologic examination. Evaluate the margins, color, and shape of the optic disk, and examine the vessels and peripheral region of the retina for lesions such as chorioretinitis and hemorrhage.

Note pupil size and any anisocoria. There should be a direct and consensual pupillary light reflex (PLR) in each eye. Pupil size at rest depends on the amount of room light, sympathetic tone, and integrity of the iris. Many patients are anxious during examination, and therefore have high sympathetic tone. When testing the PLR it is important to use a bright light, such as a transilluminator, to overcome sympathetic tone. Incomplete PLRs in a patient with no other abnormalities and normal vision is usually due to a light that is not bright enough, or by iris abnormalities, such as iris atrophy. Loss of vision with a dilated, unresponsive pupil occurs with a lesion of the retina or optic nerve/chiasm/tract. Blindness with normal pupils indicates a lesion of the forebrain; diencephalon, optic radiation, or occipital cortex.

Cranial nerves III, IV, and VI (occulomotor, trochlear, and abducens)

These nerves are considered together because they subserve eye movements. The third nerve also mediates pupillary constriction, which is evaluated by the PLR. Strabismus may be obvious, or it can be detected by shining a light on the cornea. When the eyes are aligned, the light reflection is on the same area in each eye. Observe spontaneous eye movements when the patient looks about. Move the patient's head from side to side and up and down to induce physiologic nystagmus. To test the corneal reflex, touch the cornea with a cotton-tipped applicator moistened with saline. Corneal sensation depends on the ophthalmic branch of the trigeminal nerve. The normal response is a retraction of the globe, mediated by the abducens nerve.

Anisocoria is a difference in resting pupil size. The first step is to determine which pupil is abnormal. Determine whether the larger pupil will constrict with light (PLR). Find out whether the small pupil will dilate in the dark. Close the eyelid for a moment, then open the eye and observe whether the pupil starts to constrict. Causes of an abnormally large pupil with normal vision include iris atrophy, parasympatholytic drugs such as atropine, dysautonomia, and lesions of the occulomotor nerve or its nucleus in the brainstem. Causes of an abnormally small pupil include uveitis, painful corneal conditions such as corneal ulcer, parasympathomimetic drugs, and a lesion of the sympathetic innervation to the eye (Horner syndrome). Other signs of Horner syndrome are a droopy upper eyelid, elevated third eyelid, and enophthalmos.

Cranial nerve V (trigeminal)

The trigeminal nerve provides sensory innervation to the face and motor innervation to the muscles of mastication. The temporalis and masseter muscles are visualized and palpated to detect any swelling, atrophy, or asymmetry. If there is bilateral weakness, the patient may not be able to close the mouth. Test for sensation over the distribution of the 3 branches (ophthalmic, maxillary, and mandibular). Touching the medial canthus of the eye elicits a blink response (palpebral reflex), testing the ophthalmic branch. Eyelid closure depends on motor innervation by the facial nerve. Touching or pinching the upper lip, lateral to the canine tooth, tests the maxillary branch. A normal response is a wrinkling of the face and a blink, which also depends on motor supply by the facial nerve. Some animals also turn or withdraw their heads, indicating a conscious response mediated at the level of the forebrain. The mandibular branch is tested similarly by touching or pinching the lower lip, lateral to the canine tooth.[4]

Cranial nerve VII (facial)

The facial nerve's principal role is motor innervation to the muscles of facial expression. This nerve also innervates the salivary and lacrimal glands. Begin by observing the patient's face for asymmetric eyelid closure, a widened palpebral fissure, spontaneous blinking, or a drooping ear. The ability to blink is tested by eliciting the palpebral reflex. The facial nerve also mediates tearing, which is evaluated with Schirmer test strips.

Cranial nerve VIII (vestibulochochlear)

The vestibulochochlear nerve is involved in hearing and vestibular function. Alert patients should orient their heads and ears toward a loud or unexpected noise, such as a squeaky toy, whistle, or cell phone ringing. Unilateral, or incomplete, deafness is difficult to detect by this crude test. However, the client may notice signs of subtle hearing loss. For example, the animal may sleep soundly or not respond readily to being called. Signs of vestibular dysfunction include head tilt, abnormal nystagmus, and an ataxic, broad-based stance.

Cranial nerves IX and X (glossopharyngeal and vagus)

Because of the intimate relationship between the glossopharyngeal and vagus nerves, they are considered here together. They supply motor and sensory innervation to the pharynx. In addition, the vagus nerve controls laryngeal function. Test these nerves by touching the left or right side of the caudal pharyngeal wall with an applicator stick, and observing elevation of the palate and contraction of the pharyngeal muscles (gag reflex). An asymmetric response is more significant than a bilateral loss of the gag reflex, because this reflex is difficult to elicit in some normal animals. The client is asked about any dysphagia, regurgitation, voice change, or inspiratory stridor. In some cases, it helps to watch the patient drink water and eat soft and hard food.

Cranial nerve XI (spinal accessory)

The spinal accessory nerve supplies motor innervation to the trapezius muscle. A lesion in this nerve results in atrophy of the trapezius muscle. However, this is difficult to detect in most patients, and lesions restricted to this nerve are rare, or at least rarely recognized.

Cranial nerve XII (hypoglossal)

The hypoglossal nerve innervates the muscles of the tongue. The tongue is inspected for atrophy, asymmetry, or deviation. Animals usually lick their noses immediately after the gag reflex is tested. Patients with unilateral loss of innervation may be able to lick only 1 side of the nose, with the tongue usually deviating toward the side of the lesion when actively protruded. Watching the patient drink water also helps assess tongue function.

Palpation

Gentle palpation helps detect swelling, atrophy, or changes in surface temperature. Deep palpation and manipulation detect painful regions. If crying, whimpering, or muscle tensing occur on palpation, more vigorous maneuvers, such as manipulation, are unnecessary and may be dangerous in patients with unstable fractures or luxations.

Head

Palpate the head at the same time that the cranial nerves are examined. Check the calvarium for masses, defects, or persistent fontanelles. After palpating the muscles of mastication, gently open the mouth to detect pain or reduced range of motion of the temporomandibular joints. Retropulse the globe by gently pressing on the closed eyelids to detect pain or a retrobulbar mass.

Spine

Palpate the spine to detect any curvature, displacement, masses, swelling, paraspinal muscle atrophy, or pain, starting caudally and progressing cranially. When palpating the thoracolumbar spine, lightly place 1 hand on the abdomen to detect any tensing of the abdominal muscles, which is a common response to mild spinal pain. The spinous processes, articular processes, and transverse processes or ribs are palpated separately. If palpation is not painful, the spine can be gently manipulated by applying ventral and lateral pressure to extend and flex the spine, respectively. Cervical pain is often manifested by tensing of the cervical muscles and twitching of the ears during palpation or manipulation. If palpation does not induce pain, gently extend and flex the head with one hand while placing the other hand on the cervical muscles to detect muscle tensing.

Muscles

The muscles are initially palpated with the patient standing, noting any change in size or contour. Atrophy is characterized by loss of muscle bulk, which is most apparent when the muscle is compared with its contralateral counterpart. Deeper palpation is used to detect any muscle pain.

Gait

The ability to stand and move requires intact motor and proprioceptive systems. Lesions of the motor system affect the upper motor neuron (UMN) or the lower motor neuron (LMN). This scheme is strictly physiologic, not anatomic, particularly in the case of the UMN, which is functionally composed of a series of neurons extending from their origin in different regions of the brain to their termination on the LMN in the brainstem or spinal cord. Proprioception detects the position or movement of body parts. Receptors sensitive to movement and stretch are located in muscles, tendons, and joints. This information is conveyed by peripheral nerves to the spinal cord, which integrates local reflexes involved in posture and movement. Propriocep-tive information also travels through ascending spinal tracts to the brain stem, cere-bellum, and forebrain, which integrate coordinated movement.

A nonslick surface, such as carpet, grass, or pavement is used to assess gait. Observe the gait from the side, front, and rear. The patient, if able, should be walked, trotted, turned in circles, and walked up and down a short flight of stairs. Allowing the animal to move freely in a confined area is helpful in detecting any tendency to turn or circle to 1 side, which may be missed if the gait is only evaluated with the patient on a leash.

Each foot should come off the ground crisply with no scraping or dragging, clear the ground evenly, and land smoothly without slapping the ground. Walking the patient on concrete or carpet is often helpful in detecting any scuffing of a limb, because the paw can often be heard dragging over the surface. Pay particular atten-tion to stride length; each stride should cover approximately the same distance. Walking the patient up and down stairs, or over an obstacle such as a curb, often helps in identifying subtle weakness, especially in dogs that are too large to hop. Gait abnormalities can be broadly categorized as ataxia, weakness, lameness, or abnormal movements.

Ataxia is an inability to perform normal, coordinated motor activity that is not caused by weakness, musculoskeletal abnormality, or abnormal movements such as tremor or myoclonus. The 3 types of ataxia are sensory, cerebellar, and vestibular.

Sensory ataxia is caused by a lesion affecting the general proprioceptive pathways in the peripheral nerve, dorsal root, spinal cord, brain stem, and forebrain. There is loss of the sense of limb and body position. This loss causes clumsiness and incoordina-tion, resulting in a wide-based stance and a swaying gait. Because proprioceptive pathways are intimately associated with motor pathways, sensory ataxia is often com-pounded by weakness. Mild ataxia is often more evident when the patient is walking instead of trotting.

Cerebellar ataxia is caused by cerebellar disease, and is characterized by errors in the rate and range of movement, especially hypermetria, an overreaching, high-step-ping gait. The head and trunk usually sway erratically from side to side.

Unilateral vestibular dysfunction causes vestibular ataxia, characterized by leaning and falling to 1 side. Other signs of vestibular disease, such as head tilt and abnormal nystagmus, may be evident. With bilateral vestibular dysfunction, the patient main-tains a crouched position, is reluctant to move, and exhibits wide side-to-side head movements.

Weakness is a deficiency in the generation of the gait or the ability to support weight. This deficiency can be manifested as a decreased rate or range of motion, increased fatigability, or inability to perform certain motor acts. Paralysis is a complete loss of motor function, whereas paresis indicates a partial loss of motor function. The 2 types of weakness are UMN and LMN.

UMN weakness is characterized by paresis or paralysis, normal or exaggerated myotatic reflexes, and spasticity. Mild UMN paresis is evident as a delay in the onset of protraction (the swing phase) and an increased stride length. Spasticity is an increase in muscle tone due to hyperexcitable myotatic reflexes. Muscle tone is the velocity-dependent resistance of muscle to passive stretch, and is maintained by intrinsic muscle stiffness and the myotatic reflex. Descending UMN pathways normally attenuate this reflex. Lesions of the UMN pathway cause changes in the excitability of motor neurons, interneuronal connections, and local reflex pathways that, over time, lead to hyperexcitable myotatic reflexes and spasticity. The onset of spasticity varies from days to months after the lesion. Spasticity predominates in the antigravity (extensor) muscles, and results in a stilted gait characterized by decreased limb flexion during protraction. This condition is in contrast to hypermetria, in which there is an increase in limb flexion during protraction.

The LMN is the final common pathway to the effector muscle. Any lesion disrupting the LMN from its origin in the brain stem or spinal cord, throughout its course as a nerve root and peripheral nerve, up to and including the neuromuscular junction and muscle, may cause paresis or paralysis, decreased or absent muscle stretch reflexes, decreased muscle tone (hypotonia), and early and severe muscle atrophy. Depending on severity, LMN weakness is characterized by a short-strided gait that may mimic lameness, tendency to collapse, trembling, "bunny hopping," and ventral neck flexion.

Lameness is usually due to pain. The patient tries to bear weight briefly and gingerly on the affected limb, and then quickly and forcefully plants the contralateral limb to relieve the pain. As a result, the stride of the painful limb is often shortened. When a single limb is severely painful, it is often carried. These symptoms are in contrast with those of a paretic limb, which is often dragged. Patients with bilateral limb pain, such as with hip disease or ruptured cruciate ligaments, may not walk at all or have short-strided, stilted gaits, which can mimic neurologic disease. Supporting the patient and evaluating proprioceptive positioning will often resolve this confusion. Likewise, some neurologic disorders cause lameness suggestive of orthopedic disease. For example, attenuation of a nerve root or spinal nerve by intervertebral disk extrusion or nerve sheath tumor often results in lameness of the limb innervated by the damaged nerve.

Abnormal Movements

There are several patterns of abnormal, involuntary movement seen with neurologic disease. Some of these are evident on examination. Others are so intermittent that the clinician must rely on the client's description. In some cases it is helpful to have the client videotape the episode. A tremor is a rhythmic, oscillatory movement of a body part. Tremor can be localized to 1 region of the body, or can be generalized. A terminal tremor, or intention tremor, occurs as the body part nears a target during goal-oriented movement. This condition is most evident as a head tremor when the patient attempts to sniff an object, eat, or drink. Such tremors are commonly seen with cerebellar disorders. A postural tremor occurs as the limb or head is maintained against gravity. A generalized postural tremor is seen in dogs with steroid-responsive tremor syndrome, certain intoxications, and metabolic disturbances (mycotoxins, metaldehyde, hypocalcemia), and congenital myelin disorders. A common, poorly understood tremor syndrome occurs in English bulldogs, boxers, Doberman pinschers, and occasionally other breeds. It is characterized by spontaneous episodes of tremor restricted to the head. During an episode, patients are otherwise normal, conscious, and responsive.

Myotonia is prolonged contraction or delayed relaxation of a muscle after voluntary or stimulated contraction, seen with congenital and acquired muscle diseases. Myoclonus is a brief, shocklike contraction of skeletal muscle. Physiologic myoclonus occurs in healthy animals, and typically causes no disability. Familiar examples are hiccoughs (brief contractions of the diaphragm), muscle jerks during sleep, and the normal startle response (eyelid blink and brief contraction of the head, neck, and limb muscles in response to a sudden, unexpected stimulus such as a loud noise). Encephalomyelitis caused by canine distemper virus is the most common cause of abnormal myoclonus in dogs. In older literature, this movement is called chorea, but chorea is a more complex, nonrepetitive, irregularly timed movement, not the brief, simple muscle jerk of myoclonus. The muscle contractions are most obvious at rest, and can persist during sleep, or even general anesthesia, usually occurring rhythmically every 1 to 3 seconds. In a few cases, the myoclonus is generalized but more commonly it is restricted to a muscle or a group of muscles innervated by adjacent regions of the spinal cord or brainstem. Limb or jaw muscles are commonly involved, but any skeletal muscle can be affected, including the tongue and extraocular muscles. Other inflammatory diseases of the nervous system can also cause myoclonus in dogs, including granulomatous meningoencephalomyelitis, bacterial encephalitis, protozoal encephalitis, and steroid-responsive meningitis-arteritis.[5]

Dyskinesia is a general term for various forms of abnormal movement. Paroxysmal dyskinesia is characterized by episodes of abnormal movements arising out of a background of normal movement and behavior. These movements include (1) dystonia: sustained muscle contractions resulting in twisting and abnormal posture of the face, trunk, or limbs; (2) atheosis: slow, writhing movements that tend to flow into one another; and (3) chorea: rapid, arrhythmic, brief movements of the face, trunk, or limbs. Paroxysmal dyskinesia can occur as a congenital condition, an acquired idiopathic disorder, or as a reversible side effect of certain drugs, such as metoclopramide or phenobarbital.[6–8]

Postural Reactions

Postural reactions assess the same pathways involved in gait, namely the proprioceptive and motor systems. Their main value is detecting subtle deficits or inconspicuous asymmetry that may not be obvious during observation of gait. Postural reactions are also useful in discriminating between orthopedic and neurologic disorders.

Proprioceptive positioning is tested with the patient standing on a nonslippery surface. The paw is turned over so that the dorsal surface is in contact with the ground. The patient should immediately return the foot to a normal position. Support the animal to avoid body tilt, which would stimulate a vestibular mediated response. Supporting most of the patient's weight is also helpful in those animals reluctant to bear weight because of a painful limb. Another test of proprioceptive positioning is to place a towel or piece of paper under 1 limb of a standing patient and slowly pull the towel or paper laterally. The patient should return the limb to a normal position. This test evaluates proprioception in the proximal region of the limb. If properly supported, most patients with orthopedic disease will have normal proprioceptive positioning. On the other hand, proprioceptive pathways are often compromised early in the course of neurologic disease, so defects in proprioceptive positioning may be detected before there are obvious signs of weakness. Proprioceptive positioning is often referred to as conscious proprioception (CP). In human patients, this is evaluated by having patients close their eyes and communicate whether the examiner is moving a body part, such as a finger, up or down. Because veterinarians cannot directly communicate with their patients, they rely on the patient to replace the limb in a normal position. In addition to the reliance on motor function, it is not known whether this is a conscious response, so it is inaccurate to consider this a test of CP as in human patients.

Hopping reactions are tested by holding the patient so that all of the patient's weight is supported by 1 limb. Move the animal forward or laterally. Normal animals will hop on the limb while keeping the foot under their body for support. Each limb is tested individually, and responses on the left and right are compared. This test is sensitive for subtle weakness or asymmetry. Hypermetria is often evident as an exaggerated limb movement.

The placing response is most practical for smaller animals that can be held. It is particularly useful in cats, which often resent having their feet handled during proprioceptive positioning. The nonvisual (tactile) test is performed first. Cover the patient's eyes, pick the animal up, and move it toward the edge of a table. When the paw touches the table, the animal should immediately place the limb forward to rest the paw on the table surface. The thoracic and pelvic limbs are tested, and the left and right sides are compared. Some pets accustomed to being held may not respond normally. This problem can usually be overcome by holding the animal away from the examiner's body. The resulting insecurity will often convince the animal to make an effort to stand on the table.

Visual placing is tested similarly, except the patient's eyes are not covered. The normal response is to place the paws on the surface as the table is approached, before the paws contact the table. This test may detect visual deficiencies. Each eye can be assessed individually by covering the contralateral eye, and the temporal and nasal visual fields can be evaluated by approaching the table from the side of the patient.

Hemiwalking and wheelbarrowing can be performed if other postural reactions are equivocal, or in large dogs when eliciting the hopping response is physically difficult for the examiner. For hemiwalking, the clinician holds up the limbs on 1 side of the body and moves the patient laterally. The normal reaction is as described for the hopping response. Wheelbarrowing in the thoracic limbs is done by supporting the patient under the abdomen so that the pelvic limbs do not touch the ground, and moving the patient forward. Normal animals will walk with symmetric, alternate movements of the thoracic limbs. The pelvic limbs can be tested similarly by supporting the patient under the thorax and moving the patient backwards.

Muscle Tone

With the patient in lateral recumbency, the limb muscles are gently palpated and put through passive range-of-motion maneuvers. Hypotonia is a loss of normal muscular tone resulting in decreased resistance to passive movement; its presence usually indicates a lesion affecting the LMN. Increased muscle tone (spasticity) suggests a UMN lesion.

Spinal Reflexes

Spinal reflexes assess the integrity of the sensory and motor components of the reflex arc and the influence of descending UMN motor pathways (**Table 2**).

Accurate evaluation of muscle stretch reflexes requires proper technique. The reflex is best elicited by using a rubber-tipped reflex hammer with a weighted head so that a brisk, accurately placed stimulus is applied. Use of other instruments, such as scissors, is not recommended because these do not provide a consistent stimulus and seem less professional to the client. The patient should be as relaxed as possible, although this can be difficult when patients are fearful or in pain. Having an assistant

Table 2
Important spinal reflexes

Reflex	Elicited by	Response	Nerve(s)	Segmental Level
Extensor carpi radialis	Tapping muscle	Extension of carpus	Radial	C7–T1
Thoracic limb flexion	Pinching digit	Flexion of limb	Axillary, musculo-cutaneous, median, ulnar, radial	C6–T1
Patellar	Tapping patellar ligament	Extension of stifle	Femoral	L4–6
Pelvic limb flexion	Pinching digit	Flexion of limb	Sciatic	L6–S1
Perineal	Touching perineum	Contraction of anal sphincter, flexion of tail	Pudendel	S1–3

distract the patient by gentle petting and soothing talk is often helpful. Assessing muscle tone first, by passively moving the limb, also helps relax the patient. For an optimal response to occur, the muscle must be passively maintained in a state of appropriate tension, with plenty of room for contraction. Usually, a position midway between maximum and minimum tension is best.

Myotatic reflexes are graded with regard to force of contraction, speed of contraction, and length or range of motion, using the following scale: 0, absent; 1, present but reduced; 2, normal; 3, exaggerated; 4, markedly exaggerated with clonus. Clonus is repetitive flexion and extension of the joint in response to a single stimulus.

Weak or absent reflexes can occur with:

1. A lesion affecting any part of the reflex arc, including the peripheral nerve, nerve roots, spinal segments, neuromuscular junction, and muscle. Other signs of weakness are usually apparent.
2. Severe rigidity or muscle contraction that limits joint movement, such as fibrosis of a joint or muscle. Absent muscle-stretch reflexes can also be seen in normal animals that are excited or unable to relax. In these patients, other signs of LMN weakness are absent.
3. The state of spinal "shock," which can occur immediately after severe spinal cord injury. This state is characterized by paralysis, areflexia, and loss of sensation caudal to the level of injury. In dogs and cats, spinal shock is short lived, with reflexes returning within about 30 minutes.

Causes of exaggerated reflexes are:

1. A lesion in the UMN pathways cranial to the spinal segment involved in the reflex. Other signs of UMN disease, such as paresis or paralysis, are also evident. Exaggerated reflexes are more common with chronic than with acute UMN lesions.
2. Patients being excited or anxious. In this case, other signs of a UMN lesion are absent. Never diagnose a UMN lesion in a patient with exaggerated reflexes but normal gait and postural reactions.
3. A lesion of the L6 to S1 spinal segments or sciatic nerve can cause an exaggerated patellar reflex (pseudohyperreflexia). This condition is due to decreased tone in the

muscles that flex the stifle and normally dampen stifle extension when the patellar reflex is elicited. Such lesions also cause other abnormalities, such as a decreased flexor reflex.

The most reliable myotatic reflex in the pelvic limbs is the patellar reflex. With the patient in lateral recumbency, place one hand under the thigh to support the limb with the stifle in a partially flexed position. With the other hand, briskly strike the patellar ligament with a reflex hammer. The normal response is a single, quick extension of the stifle. A weak or absent reflex indicates a lesion of the femoral nerve or the L4 to L6 spinal segments. A lesion in the UMN system cranial to the L4 spinal segment may cause a normal or exaggerated reflex. It is important to realize that any UMN lesion severe enough to cause an exaggerated reflex will usually cause some degree of weakness. An exaggerated reflex in the face of normal gait and postural reactions is usually due to examiner error or a tense, excited patient.

The most reliable muscle stretch reflex in the thoracic limb is the extensor carpi radialis reflex. Support the limb under the elbow with the elbow and carpal joint partially flexed. Strike the extensor carpi radialis muscle just distal to the elbow. The normal response is slight extension of the carpus. A weak or absent reflex suggests a lesion of the radial nerve or the C7 to T1 spinal segments, provided there are other signs of weakness. A UMN lesion cranial to C7 spinal segment may cause a normal or exaggerated reflex.

Other myotatic reflexes have been described, and including the gastrocnemius, cranial tibial, biceps, and triceps reflexes. The author considers these reflexes to be unreliable in dogs and cats, and to serve little, if any, useful purpose.

To test the flexor (withdrawal) reflex in the pelvic limb, the patient is maintained in lateral recumbency with the uppermost pelvic limb extended. Gently pinch a toe with the fingers. The normal response is flexion of the hip, stifle, and hock, which is a reflex mediated in the spinal cord. Therefore, a flexor reflex does not mean the patient is aware of the stimulus. It is crucial for the veterinarian to understand the difference between reflex flexion of the limb and conscious perception of the stimulus. The conscious perception of pain is also evaluated at the same time as the flexor reflex; this is discussed in the section on sensory testing. When testing the flexor reflex, the contralateral limb should be observed for extension. Extension of the opposite limb, called a crossed extensor reflex, is abnormal and indicates a UMN lesion cranial to the L4 spinal segment.

The flexor reflex in the thoracic limb is tested in a similar manner. A weak or absent reflex indicates a lesion of the C6 to T1 spinal segments or related nerves (axillary, musculocutaneous, median, and ulnar nerves). A crossed extensor reflex in the thoracic limbs indicates a lesion cranial to the C6 spinal segment.

The perineal reflex is elicited by lightly touching or stroking the perineum with an applicator stick. The left and right sides are tested. Normal response is contraction of the anal sphincter and flexion of the tail. A weak or absent reflex indicates a lesion affecting the S1 to S3 spinal segments or pudendal nerve.

To elicit the cutaneous trunci (panniculus) reflex, use a hemostat to gently squeeze the skin just lateral to the spine. The opposite side is tested similarly. Start over the lumbosacral region and proceed cranially, 1 vertebral level at a time, until the reflex is elicited. The normal response is a bilateral contraction of the cutaneous trunci muscle, resulting in a twitch of the skin over the thorax and abdomen. This reflex is present in the thoracolumbar region, and is absent in the neck and sacral regions. The LMN for this reflex is the lateral thoracic nerve, originating in the C8 to T2 segments and coursing through the brachial plexus. A lesion affecting the thoracolumbar region of the spinal cord may cause a loss of this reflex when the skin caudal to the level of the lesion is stimulated. Pinching the skin cranial to the lesion results in a normal response. A lesion affecting the brachial plexus may cause a loss of the ipsilateral cutaneous trunci reflex with a normal response on the other side, regardless of the level at which the skin is stimulated. This reflex cannot be elicited in some normal animals. Therefore, a total loss of the cutaneous trunci reflex, without deficits in gait and posture, is not clinically significant.

Sensory Testing

Cutaneous sensation includes touch, superficial pain, heat, cold, and vibratory senses. However, in animals, only superficial pain can be reliably tested. Superficial pain, also called fast pain, is sharp, acute, well-localized pain, most commonly originating in the skin. Deep pain, also called slow pain, is felt as burning, aching, poorly localized pain originating from deeper structures. Superficial and deep pain are transmitted through different pathways in the peripheral and central nervous systems. The purpose of testing pain perception is to detect and map out any areas of sensory loss. This testing aids anatomic localization and determination of prognosis. Altered states of consciousness and certain drugs, such as analgesics and sedatives, may alter results and have to be considered when testing sensation.

Superficial pain

Specific cutaneous areas are chosen for testing, based on the anatomy of the cutaneous nerves. A 2-step pinch technique is used for stimulation.[4] With a hemostat, lift and grasp a small fold of skin at the test site. When the patient is quiet, gradually increase the force of the pinch until a response is elicited. This 2-step technique avoids stimulation of adjacent areas and ensures that only the skin at the test site is stimulated. Two types of response may be seen: (1) a reflex flexion of the limb or skin twitch, indicating that the sensory neurons and spinal segments are intact; (2) a behavioral response, such as crying or biting, which indicates that the ascending pain pathways in the spinal cord and brain stem to the forebrain are intact.

Deep pain

The pathways that carry deep pain sensation are more resistant to damage than other pathways, including those responsible for proprioception, motor function, and superficial pain. Therefore, testing deep pain perception is necessary only if superficial pain is absent. When there is no response to pinching with the fingers, use a hemostat to compress the digits or tail. The degree of compression is gradually increased until a response is elicited. Withdrawal of the limb indicates only an intact reflex arc (peripheral nerve and spinal segments). A behavioral response, such as turning the head or vocalization, indicates conscious perception. This response requires the peripheral nerve, spinal segments, and the ascending pathways for deep pain perception in the spinal cord, brain stem, and forebrain. The clinician must not confuse reflex withdrawal with conscious perception.

NEUROANATOMIC DIAGNOSIS

Based on the history and examination, the veterinarian decides whether the patient suffers from a neurologic disease, and, if so, localizes the lesion within the nervous system. This localization can rarely be done based on a single finding. Instead, accurate anatomic diagnosis requires consideration of all findings, including normal and abnormal results. Neurologic deficits depend primarily on the location of the lesion, rather than the cause of the lesion. Certain combinations of neurologic deficits are recognized as characteristic of lesions in specific locations.

Forebrain

Clinically, the forebrain includes the cerebral cortex and white matter, basal nuclei, and diencephalon (thalamus). Epileptic seizures and abnormal behavior are highly suggestive of forebrain disease. Unilateral forebrain lesions may cause circling, usually toward the side of the lesion. Blindness in the contralateral visual field with normal PLRs, and decreased conscious perception of pain on the contralateral side of the body, including the face, are possible. The gait is usually normal, although there may be postural reaction deficits in the contralateral limbs. Spinal reflexes are usually normal, but may be exaggerated.

Brain Stem

The brain stem includes the midbrain, pons, and medulla. Severe brain stem lesions can cause stupor or coma, tetraplegia with decerebrate rigidity, and cardiac and respiratory abnormalities, including apnea and cardiac arrest. Ipsilateral deficits in the function of cranial nerves III to XII are possible. Gait deficits vary from mild, ipsilateral hemiparesis to tetraplegia with normal to exaggerated spinal reflexes.

Cerebellum

Lesions of the cerebellum usually cause ataxia and hypermetria of all limbs without weakness. Proprioceptive positioning is usually normal. Intention tremor and vestibular dysfunction can also occur. Some patients have absent menace responses with no other signs of visual deficits. Severe, acute cerebellar lesions can induce decerebellate rigidity.

Spinal Cord

The most common signs of spinal cord dysfunction are weakness caudal to the lesion, and spinal pain. Lesions affecting the C1 to C5 spinal segments can cause tetraparesis/tetraplegia or ipsilateral hemiparesis/hemiplegia with normal or exaggerated reflexes. In contrast to forebrain and brain stem lesions, mentation and cranial nerves are normal, although an ipsilateral Horner syndrome is possible. Lesions affecting primarily the center of the cord can cause weakness of the thoracic limbs with minimal deficits in the pelvic limbs (central cord syndrome). Severe lesions can cause respiratory paresis or apnea; this happens before deep pain perception is lost. Many cervical lesions cause neck pain, although some brain lesions also cause neck pain.

Lesions affecting the C6 to T2 spinal segments may result in tetraparesis/tetraplegia or ipsilateral hemiparesis/hemiplegia. The thoracic limbs exhibit weak or absent spinal reflexes with hypotonia and rapid muscle atrophy. Spinal reflexes in the pelvic limbs are normal or exaggerated. An ipsilateral Horner syndrome is also possible.

Lesions compromising the T3 to L3 spinal segments may cause varying degrees of weakness in the pelvic limbs with normal thoracic limbs. Reflexes in the pelvic limbs are normal or exaggerated. Acute lesions affecting this region may cause a Schiff-Sherrington posture. The panniculus reflex may be absent caudal to the lesion, and, in severe cases, conscious perception of deep pain is absent caudal to the lesion.

Lesions affecting the L4 to S3 spinal segments cause LMN weakness in the pelvic limbs. The patellar, flexor, and perineal reflexes may be weak or absent with hypotonia. With lesions of 1 or more week's duration, there may be atrophy of the muscles of the pelvic limbs. Severe lesions will cause a loss of deep pain perception in the pelvic limbs and tail.

Peripheral Nerve

Most peripheral nerve lesions cause motor and sensory deficits. There is weakness with decreased postural reactions, decreased muscle tone, and weak or absent spinal reflexes. Cranial nerves may be affected. Superficial and deep pain sensation may be absent. Polyneuropathies usually cause deficits in all limbs, and cranial nerves can be affected. With mononeuropathies, deficits are restricted to regions innervated by the affected nerve.

Muscle

Muscle disorders are often characterized by weakness, fatigability, and stiff, stilted gait. A postural tremor is possible. Palpation may reveal muscle atrophy or pain. A few myopathies cause enlargement of affected muscles due to hypertrophy, swelling, or infiltration with fat or other tissue. Proprioception and other sensations are preserved. Spinal reflexes are usually normal, but may be weak.

Signs of Impending Brain Catastrophe

Patients with progressive brain lesions such as tumor, hemorrhage, edema, or encephalitis can develop increases in intracranial pressure. Initially, the intracranial mass displaces cerebrospinal fluid (CSF) and blood in the veins and venous sinuses such that intracranial pressure remains normal. Progression of the mass can eventually exceed these compensatory mechanisms, and intracranial pressure starts to increase. This can lead to compromised blood flow to the brain or herniation of brain tissue, which can be life threatening. In patients with suspected intracranial masses, frequent examinations are important to detect any signs of increased intracranial pressure, which could have catastrophic consequences. Suggestive signs include tachypnea or abnormal breathing, bradycardia, dilation of 1 or both pupils, deteriorations in consciousness, and decerebrate posturing. Development of any of these signs indicates the need for prompt treatment (eg, mannitol administration, sedation, ventilatory support) to lower intracranial pressure.

ETIOLOGIC DIAGNOSIS

The final step is determining the cause of the lesion. This determination is usually based on careful analysis of the history and selective use of ancillary diagnostic tests. The following is a general outline of the categories of brain disease and their pertinent clinical features.

Patients with congenital or developmental defects usually have nonprogressive or slowly progressive signs early in life. In some cases, there is a history of similar problems in littermates or other family members. Degenerative disorders usually occur in middle-aged or older patients, except in the rare cases of inherited metabolic defects. The onset is typically insidious, and signs progress slowly. Metabolic disorders can affect patients of any age, and cause progressive or paroxysmal signs. Diffuse signs or bilaterally symmetric deficits referable to the forebrain are most common.

Brain tumors are more common in older animals, but neoplasia should never be excluded based on young age alone. Signs are often insidious in onset, except when heralded by seizures, and progress over weeks to months. However, early, subtle signs may be missed, and affected patients may not be presented until the tumor has become large, at which time the signs can progress distressingly fast. Neurologic deficits usually suggest a focal brain lesion.

There are few clinical features unique to inflammatory disorders of the brain. Patients of any age can be affected, and the onset of signs can vary from several days to several months. A common misconception is that animals with inflammatory diseases of the nervous system are usually systemically ill, but many affected patients have no other signs of illness, such as fever.[5] Although the presence of multifocal neurologic signs is considered a hallmark of this category of disease, two-thirds of dogs with inflammatory disease of the nervous system have neurologic deficits referable to a single, focal lesion.[5]

Traumatic brain injury presents with a sudden onset of signs that usually improve with time, unless fatal. However, signs can worsen during the first few days if there is progressive hemorrhage or brain edema. The cause is usually obvious from the history and examination, although the diagnosis may be less clear if the history is inadequate.

Intoxication usually causes an acute onset of signs referable to a generalized or symmetric forebrain lesion. A history of exposure, or at least access to potential toxins, is usually the key to identification. A notable exception is lead poisoning, which can present with a chronic course and no known exposure. The onset of vascular disorders is usually acute, followed by a static phase, and then improvement if the patient survives. Deficits are usually referable to a focal, often asymmetric, lesion.

Diagnostic Tests for Brain Disease

The initial evaluation usually allows the clinician to identify the location of the lesion and in some cases even the etiologic diagnosis. However, often the diagnostic possibilities can be reduced to only 2 or 3. Based on this list of differential diagnoses, the clinician recommends appropriate laboratory examinations to confirm or exclude the possibilities. It is important not to overlook a disease for which there is effective treatment. Each of the treatable causes of the patient's signs must be carefully considered until excluded by clinical and laboratory data. An accurate diagnosis enables the veterinarian to recommend proper treatment, and is helpful in predicting prognosis.

Laboratory evaluation consisting of serum chemistry, electrolytes, complete blood count, and urinalysis is most useful in identifying or ruling out metabolic disorders such as hypoglycemia, hypocalcemia, and polycythemia. Blood ammonia and serum bile acids are helpful in the diagnosis of hepatic encephalopathy. Chest radiographs are indicated in patients with suspected brain neoplasia to identify any primary or metastatic lung tumors.

Skull radiographs are not usually helpful in the diagnosis of brain disease. Exceptions include lytic or proliferative skull tumors and diseases of the paranasal sinuses and middle ear. Skull fractures can often be identified on radiographs, although these findings usually do not affect treatment.

CT was one of the most important developments in brain imaging. For the first time, direct visualization of the brain became possible. Although MRI has surpassed CT in displaying normal and abnormal brain anatomy, CT remains valuable for several reasons. Most importantly, CT is more widely available and less expensive. Monitoring of unstable patients is easier in the CT environment and CT is faster, so it is often preferred as the initial evaluation of unstable animals. Patients with certain implants, such as pacemakers, are not candidates for MRI. CT is excellent in the evaluation of ventricular size, acute intracranial hemorrhage, detecting intracranial calcification, skull fractures, and imaging of the paranasal sinuses and middle ear. Although contrast-enhanced CT is useful in detecting many tumors and granulomas, it is less sensitive than MRI. Other disadvantages of CT include the potential need for iodinated contrast material to visualize brain lesions, beam-hardening artifacts that limit evaluation of the caudal fossa, and difficulty obtaining imaging in planes other than the axial or dorsal.

MRI affords imaging in multiple planes. For example, sagittal images are important in the evaluation of cerebellar herniation and Chiari I-type malformation. MRI is sensitive to subtle changes in tissue signal and is superior to CT in evaluation of neoplasms, inflammatory diseases, and vascular lesions. Meningeal disease is better evaluated by MRI and can be missed on CT, owing to volume averaging with the skull. Based on these advantages, if it is available, MRI is the initial imaging procedure of choice for most patients with brain disease.

There are several considerations when planning brain CT or MRI. Imaging requires general anesthesia, and animals with brain disease can be at risk of developing increased intracranial pressure. Anesthetic personnel must be familiar with anesthetizing and monitoring veterinary patients with brain disease, and be prepared to deal with any complications. Most important are maintaining adequate blood pressure and oxygenation and avoiding hypercapnia during anesthesia and recovery. The imaging staff should be familiar with veterinary anatomy to properly position the patient and obtain diagnostic quality images. The lesion must be accurately localized, based on the history and examination, so that the appropriate region is imaged. Scanning multiple regions of the spine and the brain in an attempt to chance on a clinically significant lesion increases cost for the client and subjects the patient to increased anesthetic time. An appropriate list of differential diagnoses is important, especially with MRI, for which specific imaging sequences and planes are best tailored to detect the suspected diseases. Based on the clinical features and imaging results, analysis of CSF is often indicated in patients with brain disease. The best time to collect CSF is while the patient is still anesthetized for imaging. Before imaging is undertaken, there must be close communication between the attending veterinarian and radiologist. Any potential treatment should be anticipated, and, if necessary, the neurosurgeon, neurologist, or radiation oncologist is consulted early on, so that the necessary images are obtained. Otherwise, the patient may be subjected to a second imaging procedure and the client is faced with additional expense.

Infectious and inflammatory diseases are common causes of brain disease. Analysis of CSF is usually crucial in the diagnosis of these conditions. Indications for CSF collection are suspected encephalitis or meningitis, imaging results suggestive of inflammatory disease, and patients with brain disease in which other diagnostic tests are normal or inconclusive. In patients with brain disease, CSF is usually collected from the cisterna magna. The primary contraindication for CSF collection is caudal cerebellar herniation with obliteration of the cisterna magna. Patients with increased intracranial pressure or a substantial mass effect on brain imaging may be at risk of developing dangerous shifts in brain tissue if CSF is removed from the spinal subarachnoid space. Ideally, these conditions should be ruled out with CT or MRI before CSF is collected.

Usually 1 to 2 mL of CSF is adequate for routine analysis, which includes nucleated cell count, protein quantification, and cytology. A portion of fluid is saved for further analysis, such as infectious disease testing and culture, if indicated by initial analysis. Cell count and cytology preparations are performed as soon as possible. If a delay of more than 8 hours is anticipated, hetastarch (1:1, volume basis) or serum (20%, volume basis) is added to the CSF, which will preserve the sample for at least 48 hours.[9]

SUMMARY

If the clinical process outlined in this article is adhered to, it is usually possible to define where the lesion is, and what the lesion is. An accurate diagnosis enables the veterinarian to recommend the proper treatment, and is helpful in predicting prognosis.

However, even after the most diligent assessment, the diagnosis may remain elusive. In such cases, several general rules may help:

1. Avoid premature closure of diagnosis. Often this is the result of early fixation on some item in the history or examination, which closes the mind to alternative diagnoses.
2. Realize that a common disease presenting with atypical features is more likely than a rare disease with classic features.
3. If several of the main features of a disease are lacking, an alternative diagnosis should always be entertained.
4. Do not order ancillary diagnostic tests without a clear idea of how the expected findings will influence management of the patient.[10]
5. Early in the course of brain disease, deficits may be subtle and nonspecific. As the disease progresses, the signs often become more obvious and specific, clarifying the diagnosis. Often the most useful test in neurology is a second history and examination.

ACKNOWLEDGMENTS

The author thanks Dr Curtis Probst for careful review of this article.

REFERENCES

1. Thomas WB, Dewey CW. Performing the neurologic examination. In: Dewey CW, editor. A practical guide to canine and feline neurology. 2nd edition. Ames (IA): Wiley-Blackwell; 2009. p. 53–74.
2. Bagley RS. Clinical examination of the animal with suspected neurologic disease. In: Fundamentals of veterinary clinical neurology. Ames (IA): Blackwell; 2005. p. 57–107.
3. Lorenz MD, Kornegay JN. Neurologic history and examination. In: Handbook of veterinary neurology. St. Louis (MO): Saunders; 2004. p. 3–44.
4. Bailey CS, Kitchell RL. Cutaneous sensory testing in the dog. J Vet Intern Med 1987;1:128–35.
5. Tipold A. Diagnosis of inflammatory and infectious diseases of the central nervous system in dogs: a retrospective study. J Vet Intern Med 1995;9:304–14.
6. Ramsey IK, Chandler KE, Franklin RJM. A movement disorder in boxer pups. Vet Rec 1999;144:179–80.
7. Penderis J, Franklin RJM. Dyskinesia in an adult bichon frise. J Small Anim Pract 2001;42:24–5.
8. Kube SA, Vernau KM, LeCouteur RA. Dyskinesia associated with oral phenobarbital administration in a dog. J Vet Intern Med 2006;20:1238–40.
9. Fry MM, Vernau W, Kass PH, et al. Effects of time, initial composition, and stabilizing agents on the results of canine cerebrospinal fluid analysis. Vet Clin Pathol 2006;35.72–7.
10. Adams RD, Brown RH. Approach to the patient with neurologic disase. In: Principles of neurology. 8th edition. New York: McGraw Hill; 2009. p. 3–10.

MRI of Brain Disease in Veterinary Patients Part 1: Basic Principles and Congenital Brain Disorders

Silke Hecht, Dr Med Vet*, William H. Adams, DVM

KEYWORDS

- Magnetic resonance imaging • Brain • Dog • Cat
- Basic principles • Congenital disorders

Magnetic resonance imaging (MRI) is the imaging modality of choice in the diagnosis of brain diseases in human patients and is increasingly available in veterinary practice.[1,2] Advantages of MRI over computed tomography (CT) include improved contrast resolution, capabilities in multiplanar image acquisition, availability of specialized sequences, and use of nonionizing radiation. Disadvantages include longer acquisition time and less spatial resolution compared with CT. Although CT might be preferred to MRI in cases of acute head trauma where evaluation of small bony structures and minimization of anesthesia time are crucial, MRI is the superior imaging modality in the evaluation of most intracranial disorders.

BASIC MRI PRINCIPLES

In-depth review of MR physics is beyond the scope of this article. A short overview of basic principles is provided as a basis for understanding pulse sequences and appearance of pathologic changes on MR images. Diagnostic MRI images hydrogen protons, which are ubiquitous in biologic tissues.[3,4] As most pathologic processes result in the alteration of content, distribution, and ambient environment of hydrogen protons of tissues, MRI is an appropriate and sensitive modality for imaging of disease. When a patient is placed in an MR scanner, the hydrogen protons align along the main magnetic field. An excitation radiofrequency pulse is applied, which changes

Department of Small Animal Clinical Sciences, University of Tennessee College of Veterinary Medicine, 2407 River Drive, Knoxville, TN 37996, USA
* Corresponding author.
E-mail address: shecht@utk.edu (S. Hecht).

Vet Clin Small Anim 40 (2010) 21–38
doi:10.1016/j.cvsm.2009.09.005
0195-5616/09/$ – see front matter © 2010 Elsevier Inc. All rights reserved.

the energy state of the protons and results in their misalignment with the main magnetic field. As the protons return to their original energy level and realign with the main magnetic field, radiofrequency energy is emitted, creating a signal that is detected by a receiver coil. From its highest initial intensity immediately following excitation, the signal fades because of 2 simultaneous processes: The hydrogen protons align again with the main magnetic field (spin-lattice relaxation; T1 relaxation), and protons interfere with each other resulting in loss of transverse magnetization (spin-spin relaxation; T2 relaxation).[5,6] Differences in relaxation times of different tissues create differences in signal intensity emitted by tissues, resulting in tissue contrast. In general terms, water (pure fluid) has long relaxation times, various soft tissues have intermediate relaxation times, and fat has short relaxation times. Other contrast parameters intrinsic to individual tissues are the proton density, flow, and apparent diffusion coefficient (ADC).[3,4]

MRI SEQUENCES

MRI sequences are designed to acquire information by exploiting differences in behavior of hydrogen protons in varied tissues in changing magnetic fields.[4] MRI technology is constantly evolving, and more and varied sequences are becoming available. Commonly used MRI sequences for brain imaging include T1-weighting (T1-W, pre- and postcontrast), T2-weighting (T2-W), fluid attenuated inversion recovery (FLAIR), and T2*-weighting (T2*-W). Proton density weighting (PD-W), diffusion-weighted imaging (DWI), perfusion-weighted imaging (PWI), fat suppression techniques (short tau inversion recovery [STIR] and chemical fat suppression [fat saturation (FatSat)]), and ultrafast spin echo (SE) sequences. Magnetic resonance angiography (MRA), high-resolution sequences, and dynamic studies are less commonly performed but may be considered for certain indications. At the time of writing, functional MRI, diffusion tensor tractography, magnetization transfer imaging, and MR spectroscopy are not routinely performed in veterinary patients and are discussed elsewhere.[3,4,7,8]

T1-W

On T1-W images, contrast between tissues depends predominantly on differences in T1 relaxation times. Fat has short T1 relaxation time and is hyperintense, whereas fluid has long T1 relaxation time and appears hypointense. Soft tissues have somewhat variable intermediate T1 relaxation times and have medium intensity. After uptake of administered paramagnetic contrast agents, physiologically, contrast-enhancing tissues (eg, pituitary gland) and contrast-enhancing pathologic lesions (eg, certain brain tumors) are hyperintense (**Fig. 1**).[3,4]

T2-W

On T2-W images, contrast between tissues depends predominantly on differences in T2 relaxation times. Fluid and tissues with increased fluid content ("juicy tissues") appear strongly hyperintense.[9] Intensity of fat is variable. A T2-W image can be considered a "pathology" scan, because abnormal fluid collections and tissues with abnormal increased fluid content (edema, inflammation, neoplasia, and so forth) will appear hyperintense (**Fig. 2**).[3,4,10]

FLAIR

FLAIR images are useful in conjunction with T2-W images in evaluating and characterizing T2 hyperintense lesions. Using FLAIR, pure fluid (cerebrospinal fluid [CSF] and

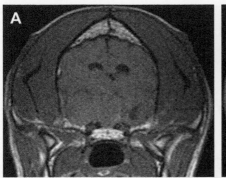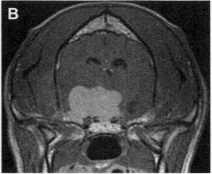

Fig. 1. Transverse T1-W images of a 9-year-old golden retriever pre- (A) and postadministration (B) of contrast medium. Fat associated with the subcutaneous tissues and bone marrow is hyperintense, and fluid (cerebrospinal fluid [CSF] within ventricles) is hypointense. A large intracranial mass (meningioma) is present, which is isointense to brain parenchyma on precontrast image and hyperintense on postcontrast image. Note mass effect (midline shift and compression of right lateral ventricle) on precontrast image.

fluid in cystic lesions) is suppressed and becomes hypointense, whereas solid lesions remain hyperintense, facilitating differentiation (**Fig. 3**). Additionally, this sequence increases conspicuity of small lesions bordering a fluid-filled ventricle or subarachnoid space (**Fig. 4**).[2,11,12] Without modification of acquisition parameters, FLAIR is unable to suppress the signal from fluids containing high protein, cell components, or blood by-products, a potential pitfall when interpreting images.[9,13] FLAIR images were initially exclusively acquired before contrast administration. However, postcontrast FLAIR images are very sensitive in the detection of contrast-enhancing lesions and may be used as an alternative to postcontrast T1-W imaging.[14]

T2*-W

A T2*-W sequence is very susceptible to external magnetic field inhomogeneities. Gas interfaces, soft tissue mineralization, fibrous tissue, and certain blood degradation products (eg, methemoglobin) cause magnetic field inhomogeneities, which appear

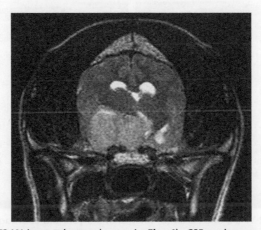

Fig. 2. Transverse T2-W image (same dog as in **Fig. 1**). CSF and mass are hyperintense to brain parenchyma.

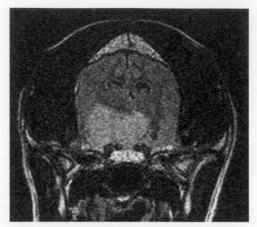

Fig. 3. Transverse FLAIR image (same dog as **Figs. 1** and **2**). The mass remains hyperintense, whereas CSF is attenuated, now appearing as a signal void.

as a signal void (susceptibility artifact) on T2*-W images.[15] T2*-W is most commonly used to identify intracranial hemorrhage and differentiate it from other intracranial lesions (**Fig. 5**).[16] Additional indications include identification of intracranial mineralization (eg, in meningiomas) or abnormal gas pockets (eg, in brain abscesses).

PD-W

PD-W images are acquired by minimizing T1 and T2 relaxation effects on image contrast. Although this sequence is used extensively in musculoskeletal MRI, it only plays a minor role in brain imaging.[2]

DWI and PWI

DWI and PWI are important sequences in imaging of brain tumors[17] and especially, in imaging of cerebral ischemia.[18] DWI is able to demonstrate "Brownian motion" (ie, random movement) of water molecules in brain tissue. As diffusion in biologic

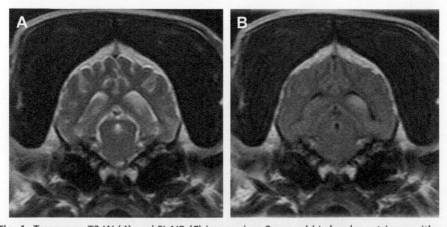

Fig. 4. Transverse T2-W (*A*) and FLAIR (*B*) images in a 9-year-old Labrador retriever with an ischemic infarct as a sequel to intravascular lymphoma. The T2-hyperintense area ventral to the left lateral ventricle is more conspicuous on FLAIR than on T2-W image.

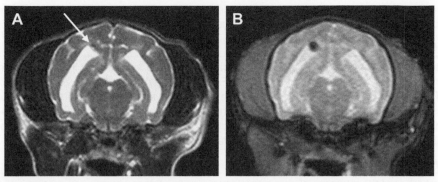

Fig. 5. Transverse T2-W (*A*) and T2*-W (*B*) images in a 13-year-old Yorkshire terrier with presumptive small hemorrhagic infarcts secondary to chronic renal disease and hypertension. On T2-W image, there is a subtle hypointensity associated with the right occipital lobe immediately dorsal to the right lateral ventricle (*arrow*). The lesion is more conspicuous on T2*-W image because of increased sensitivity of this sequence to susceptibility artifacts created by the presence of hemoglobin degradation products.

tissues is not truly random because of the presence of physiologic boundaries (cell membranes and so forth) it is referred to as "apparent diffusion," disturbance of which will appear as abnormal signal intensity on DWI.[19] In acute cerebral ischemia, restricted diffusion occurs secondary to failure of the cell membrane ion pump and subsequent cytotoxic edema. An acute stroke is characterized by marked hyperintensity on a DWI and hypointensity on a synthesized ADC map derived from 2 or more DWI (**Fig. 6**). PWI allows estimation of blood volume passing through the capillary bed per unit of time. This is most commonly accomplished by tracing the passage of a bolus of contrast agent through the cerebral vasculature.[19] Perfusion imaging is often used in combination with DWI in patients with acute ischemic stroke, where the difference between diffusion and perfusion abnormalities provides a measure of the ischemic penumbra (area of reversible ischemia that can be salvaged if blood flow is re-established promptly).

STIR and FatSat

Both techniques result in suppression of signal from fat, which makes them highly valuable in orthopedic and spinal imaging.[4,20] They are not commonly used in brain

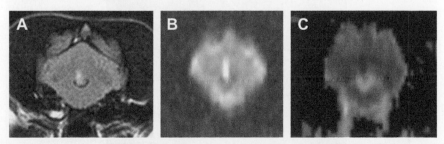

Fig. 6. Transverse FLAIR image (*A*), DWI (*B*), and ADC map (*C*) of a 5-year-old Shi Tzu with a presumptive ischemic infarct. There is a small wedge-shaped hyperintensity within the cerebellum dorsal to the fourth ventricle on FLAIR image, which remains hyperintense on DWI and appears hypointense on the ADC map indicating restricted diffusion. Hyperintense material in the dependent part of the right tympanic bulla is consistent with otitis media (*Courtesy of* Dr Andrea Matthews, University of Tennessee, Knoxville, TN).

imaging but may be considered in select cases, for example, to differentiate a contrast-enhancing lesion from normal tissue, such as bone marrow fat.

Ultrafast SE Techniques

These sequences are heavily T2-W and can be used to image noncirculating liquid structures (eg, pancreatobiliary tract, CSF-filled spaces) (**Fig. 7**).[21,22] "Quick-brain" MR imaging was initially introduced as an alternative technique to CT scanning for assessing children with hydrocephalus. Other indications in humans include macrocephaly, Chiari malformation, intracranial cysts, screening before lumbar puncture, screening for congenital anomalies, and trauma.[23]

MRA

Evaluation of the intracranial circulation in humans provides valuable information in the diagnosis and prognosis of various abnormalities, such as aneurysms, arterial and venous steno-occlusive diseases, inflammatory arterial diseases, and congenital vascular abnormalities.[24] Conventional MRA is usually performed by demonstrating flow-related enhancement (time-of-flight MRA) or demonstrating phase shifts of moving spins (phase shift MRA). Contrast-enhanced MRA is considered superior to conventional MRA.[25] Although intracranial vascular abnormalities are infrequently reported in the veterinary literature, MRA might be considered as a quick and low-risk procedure to evaluate intracranial vessels.[15,26]

High-resolution Sequences

Acquisition of high-resolution images can be helpful in select cases, for example, when detailed evaluation of the inner ear[27] or pituitary gland[28] is required (**Fig. 8**). Specific 3-dimensional (3D) sequences allow acquisition of slices less than 1 mm thick, and they have the added advantage of providing a dataset for 2D and 3D reconstructions without needing to acquire additional imaging planes.

Dynamic Studies

In human medicine, dynamic MRI studies of the brain are performed for assessment of cerebral perfusion[19] and evaluation of brain tumors.[29] A protocol for dynamic MRI of

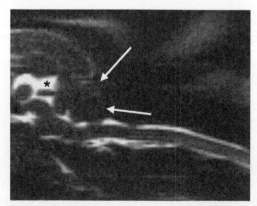

Fig. 7. Sagittal ultrafast heavily T2-W SE image of the caudal head/cranial cervical spine in a Cavalier King Charles Spaniel with mild Chiari-like malformation. There is attenuation of the subarachnoid space caudal to the cerebellum (*arrows*), indicating crowding of the caudal cranial fossa. Mild ventriculomegaly and mild dilation of the quadrigeminal cistern (*) are also noted.

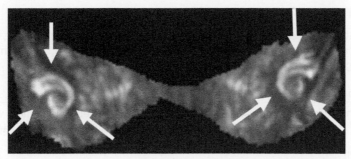

Fig. 8. High resolution 3-dimensional image of the inner ear (*arrows*) in a normal 11-year-old Jack Russell terrier.

the pituitary gland in dogs has been described,[30] which may aid in the diagnosis in pituitary microadenomas.

CONTRAST MEDIA IN MRI

MRI contrast agents most commonly used in veterinary medicine are gadolinium-based.[31] Contrast medium is administered at a dose of 0.1 mmol/kg, which may be increased to improve detection of poorly enhancing lesions. Enhancement is seen if a lesion is vascularized and has disrupted the blood-brain barrier. Gadolinium-based contrast media mostly affect T1 relaxation and therefore enhancing lesions appear hyperintense on T1-W images. Certain normal intracranial structures outside of the blood brain barrier, such as the pituitary gland, choroid plexus, and blood vessels, show physiologic contrast uptake. Although nephrogenic systemic fibrosis has been reported as a serious complication after administration of gadolinium-based contrast agents in humans,[32] adverse systemic effects have not been described in cats[33] or dogs.[34]

APPROACH TO THE MR EXAMINATION OF THE BRAIN

Many disorders of the brain can result in similar MR findings, and some intracranial abnormalities can be detected as incidental findings unrelated to a patient's clinical presentation. Therefore, familiarity with signalment (species, breed, sex, and age) and pertinent history (clinical signs, time of onset of clinical signs, course of disease, and concurrent or previous diseases) are crucial when evaluating brain MRI scans. Intracranial lesions may be extra-axial (ie, originating outside actual brain parenchyma) or intra-axial (originating from brain parenchyma).[16,35,36] Differential diagnoses for extra-axial lesions include certain neoplastic (eg, meningioma, nasal tumor, and so forth), inflammatory (eg, meningitis), and traumatic lesions (eg, epidural/subdural hematoma). Differential diagnoses for solitary intra-axial lesions include neoplasia, hematoma, cyst, abscess/granuloma, and infarct. Although inflammatory brain diseases usually manifest as multifocal lesions, solitary masses may be encountered on occasion. Masses in specific locations may allow a presumptive diagnosis of certain tumor types (eg, pituitary tumors, nerve sheath tumors, medulloblastoma, and so forth). Differential diagnoses for multifocal brain lesions include metabolic/toxic brain disease, inflammatory brain disease, infarcts, and certain intracranial neoplasms (lymphoma, disseminated histiocytic sarcoma, metastases, and occasionally, meningiomas).

ASSOCIATED FINDINGS IN INTRACRANIAL DISEASE

Various pathologic sequelae can be associated with various brain diseases, including hydrocephalus, vasogenic edema, mass effect, brain herniation, and hemorrhage. Hemorrhage will be covered in the second companion article.

Hydrocephalus

Hydrocephalus is defined as abnormal accumulation of cerebrospinal fluid within the cranium.[37] It is a multifactorial disorder that can be classified in various ways:

1. Location:
   - Ventricular system (internal hydrocephalus) versus subarachnoid space (external hydrocephalus)
2. Etiology:
   - Congenital versus acquired
   - Obstructive versus nonobstructive
     - ○ Obstructive hydrocephalus: blockage of CSF flow, for example, secondary to an intracranial space-occupying lesion or congenital stenosis of mesencephalic aqueduct or lateral apertures
     - ○ Compensatory hydrocephalus: decreased volume of brain parenchyma, for example, following trauma or infarction (Hydrocephalus ex vacuo)
     - ○ Decreased resorption (secondary to inflammatory processes or due to under-development of arachnoid villi) or increased production (seen in choroid plexus tumors) of CSF (very rare)
3. Morphology:
   - Communicating (communication between the ventricular system and subarachnoid space) versus noncommunicating (no communication between the ventricular system and subarachnoid space)
4. Pressure:
   - Hypertensive (increased pressure within dilated CSF-filled space, for example, secondary to obstruction) versus normotensive (eg, hydrocephalus ex vacuo)

MRI findings in hydrocephalus include dilation of one or more ventricles or dilation of the subarachnoid space.[36,38] In most cases, abnormal CSF accumulation appears hyperintense on T2-W images, hypointense on T1-W images, and attenuated on FLAIR. If CSF contains abnormal cells or protein (eg, in cases of inflammation or intraventricular hemorrhage), altered signal intensity may be observed. Hypertensive hydrocephalus may be associated with periventricular edema characterized by periventricular T2 hyperintensity,[39] which is most obvious on FLAIR images (**Fig. 9**).[40] Depending on cause, potential concurrent findings in cases of hydrocephalus include other congenital anomalies, an intracranial mass, and trauma. Imaging diagnoses of pathologic hydrocephalus can be challenging. In one study describing ultrasound evaluation of canine lateral ventricles, normal lateral ventricular height was reported to be 0% to 14% of dorsoventral height of the cerebral hemisphere, moderate ventricular enlargement was defined as 15% to 25% of ventricular height to the cerebral hemisphere, and more than 25% was considered consistent with severe ventricular enlargement.[41] However, ventriculomegaly and ventricular asymmetry are common findings in asymptomatic animals and may or may not represent a clinically significant change.[42–46] Progressive dilation of ventricles and subarachnoid space are also anticipated findings with increasing age.[47,48] Therefore, imaging diagnosis, especially of mild ventricular or subarachnoid space dilation, should be judged in light of clinical presentation.

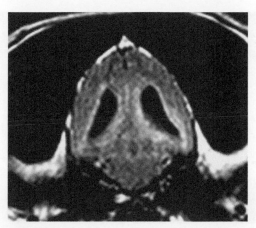

Fig. 9. Transverse FLAIR image of a dog with obstructive hydrocephalus demonstrating periventricular T2 hyperintensity (edema).

Vasogenic Edema

Vasogenic brain edema may be seen concurrently with several intracranial diseases. Under normal circumstances, exchange of substances between the blood and the brain is limited by the blood-brain barrier. Damage to brain capillaries results in leakage of fluid into the extracellular space (vasogenic edema). The edema migrates along the white matter fiber tracts and may create a mass effect. Vasogenic edema appears hyperintense on T2-W MR images and hypointense on T1-W images, and it often has the same signal intensity as the lesion causing the edema (**Fig. 10**A). After contrast medium administration, gadolinium leaks out of damaged capillaries, resulting in increased signal intensity of the lesion responsible for the edema, whereas the edema remains hypointense on postcontrast T1-W images (**Fig. 10**B).[2,9]

Mass Effect

Space-occupying lesions within the cranial vault (eg, tumor, abscess/granuloma, edema, hydrocephalus) are commonly associated with a mass effect, which is indicated by displacement of the falx cerebri or compression of the ventricular system.[49]

Brain Herniation

Increase in intracranial pressure (eg, due to an intracranial mass) can lead to compression and displacement of brain parenchyma.[50–52] Foramen magnum herniation (herniation of the caudal portion of the cerebellum into and through the foramen magnum) and caudal transtentorial herniation (displacement of portions of the cerebral cortex ventral to the tentorium cerebelli) are most common and are best evaluated on sagittal images (**Fig. 11**).

Seizures and Cerebral Necrosis

The relationship between seizures and brain injury remains diagnostically challenging.[37] In human patients, it has been shown that severe seizure activity causes reversible changes in certain areas of the brain, such as the neocortex, hippocampus, and amygdala.[53,54] Brain parenchymal changes, including edema, neovascularization, reactive astrocytosis, and acute neuronal necrosis, have been reported in dogs with

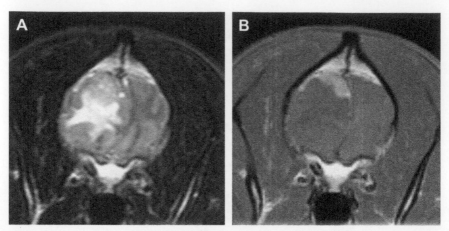

Fig. 10. Vasogenic edema in a dog with an intracranial mass, presumptive meningioma. On T2-W image (*A*) there is extensive hyperintensity associated with the white-matter tracts of the right cerebral hemisphere. On T1-W postcontrast image (*B*) there is homogenous enhancement of a plaque-like mass extending ventral to the right frontal bone and coursing ventrally with the falx cerebri. Edematous brain parenchyma appears hypointense on this image, and mass effect is indicated by leftward displacement of the falx.

seizures.[55] These lesions appeared as unilateral or bilateral T2 hyperintense and T1 hypointense foci, with variable contrast enhancement associated with piriform or temporal lobes (**Fig. 12**). Changes resolved on recheck examination, indicating that they most probably represented sequelae to seizures rather than their underlying cause. Cerebral cortical necrosis (polioencephalomalacia) appearing as increased T1 and T2 signal intensity of the gray matter of temporal and parietal lobes with mild contrast enhancement has been reported in a dog with seizures.[56] Signal characteristics were attributed to large numbers of fat-containing macrophages found within these areas on histopathologic examination. Necrosis of hippocampus and piriform lobes in cats with seizures has been described as bilaterally symmetric T2 hyperintensity of hippocampus and piriform lobes with variable contrast enhancement.[57,58] In these studies, structural brain damage was thought to be the underlying cause of seizures. In some cases, it may not be possible to determine whether brain changes

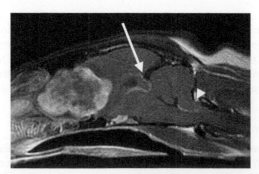

Fig. 11. Sagittal T1-W post contrast image of the brain in an 8-year-old cat with a large intracranial mass and secondary foramen magnum (*arrowhead*) and subtentorial (*arrow*) brain herniation.

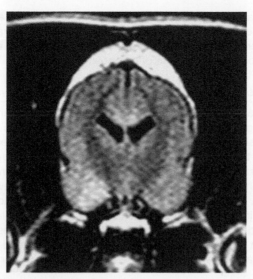

Fig. 12. Transverse FLAIR image of a 9-year-old boxer presented with seizures. There are asymmetric T2 hyperintense areas associated with the piriform lobes and hippocampus bilaterally.

found on MRI or histopathology represent the underlying cause or the result of seizures.[37,56]

CONGENITAL BRAIN DISORDERS
Forebrain (Telencephalon and Diencephalon)

Imaging findings in congenital abnormalities of the cerebrum are infrequently reported in the veterinary literature. Congenital hydrocephalus is most commonly seen in toy and brachycephalic breed dogs and appears as dilation of the ventricular system of variable severity.[59] In hydranencephaly, there is near complete destruction or lack of development of the neocortex.[37] MRI findings have been described in 2 kittens with hydranencephaly attributed to intrauterine parvovirus infection.[60] Affected animals showed reduction of size of one or both cerebral cortices to a thin mantle surrounding a large, centrally located cavity. Porencephaly appears as cystic cavities in the cerebrum due to cell destruction or failure of development.[37] These cavities show signal typical of CSF on MRI and may communicate with ventricles or the subarachnoid space.[40] Lissencephaly is a brain malformation characterized by a paucity of hypoplastic gyri and thickening of the cerebral cortex. MRI findings in 2 Lhasa Apso dogs with lissencephaly included a smooth cerebral surface and a thick neocortex with absence of the corona radiata.[61] Agenesis of the corpus callosum has been reported to result in abnormal appearance of the cingulate gyrus.[40] Holoprosencephaly is characterized by an absence or reduction in size of midline prosencephalic structures (corpus callosum, septum pellucidum, septal nuclei, fornix, and optic nerves), incomplete separation of normally paired forebrain structures (lateral ventricles, cingulate gyri, and caudate nuclei), and hydrocephalus.[62] Protrusion of meninges and meninges along with brain tissue through a calvarial defect are termed meningocele and meningoencephalocele, respectively.[37] MR diagnoses of a frontoethmoidal meningoencephalocele in a German shepherd dog[63] and an ethmoidal encephalocele in a mixed-breed dog[64] have been reported. Rathke cleft cysts are pituitary cysts containing mucoid or, less commonly, serous fluid and cellular debris, and they appear as cystic lesions in the middle cranial fossa, which are hypointense on T1-W images, hyperintense on T2-W images, may show mild ring enhancement, and may not suppress on FLAIR because of composition of fluid.[40,65]

Midbrain and Hindbrain (Mesencephalon, Metencephalon, Myelencephalon)

Intracranial intra-arachnoid cysts are considered developmental anomalies that arise from splitting/duplication of the arachnoidea in early embryonic development and occur in close association with an intracranial arachnoid cistern. Quadrigeminal cistern cysts dorsal to the quadrigeminal plate are most common, but cerebellomedullary cistern cysts have also been reported.[66,67] Intracranial intra-arachnoid cysts contain fluid isointense to CSF, with attenuation on FLAIR and no evidence of contrast enhancement (**Fig. 13**). Hemorrhage into intracranial intra-arachnoid cysts may change the signal intensity.[68] Quadrigeminal cysts are of variable significance and are frequently incidental.[69] In one study, occipital lobe compression greater than 14% by the cyst on median-sagittal image was always associated with clinical signs, whereas no association was found between degree of cerebellar compression and clinical signs.[66]

Chiari malformations are a group of structural defects involving brainstem, cerebellum, upper spinal cord, and surrounding bony structures in humans.[70] Secondary formation of a cystic cavity within the cervical spinal cord parenchyma or dilation of the central canal (syringohydromyelia) are common. A disorder similar to Chiari type I malformation in humans termed "Chiari-like malformation and syringomyelia" has been reported in dogs.[71–73] Cavalier King Charles spaniels are most commonly affected, but the disease is seen in various breeds and can be found in symptomatic and asymptomatic animals.[74] The condition is characterized by crowding of the caudal fossa, resulting in attenuation of the subarachnoid space surrounding the cerebellum, compression and, in severe cases, herniation of the cerebellum into or through the foramen magnum, best demonstrated on T2-W median-sagittal image. Additional findings include a focal bending of the cranial aspect of the spinal cord, hydrocephalus and syringohydromyelia (**Fig. 14**).[75,76]

Cerebellar hypoplasia can occur as a primary developmental defect or secondary to in utero or perinatal viral infection, most commonly parvovirus.[37,77] MRI diagnosis is

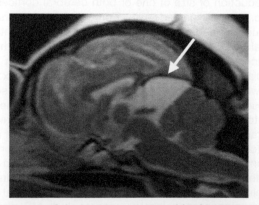

Fig. 13. Sagittal T2-W image of the brain in a 10-year-old Pekingese presented with cervical intervertebral disk extrusion, demonstrating an incidental quadrigeminal cistern cyst rostral to the cerebellum (*arrow*).

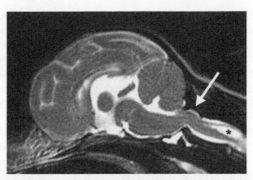

Fig. 14. Sagittal T2-W image of a Cavalier King Charles spaniel with Chiari-like malformation and syringomyelia. There is crowding of the caudal fossa resulting in attenuation of the subarachnoid space and compression of the cerebellum, dorsal angulation of the spinal cord at the level of the foramen magnum and odontoid process of C2 (*arrow*), mild hydrocephalus, and syringohydromyelia (*).

best made on sagittal T2-W image. The cerebellum may appear small, with increased CSF signal noted around and extending into the folia.[40] Subtotal agenesis of the cerebellum in a Shi Tzu was characterized by absence of most of the cerebellum with normal size of the caudal fossa.[78] Isolated hypoplasia of the cerebellar vermis has been reported in a miniature Schnauzer.[79] In 2 kittens, MR findings of cerebellar cyst and the small size of the cerebellum were attributed to intrauterine parvovirus infection.[60] Congenital cerebellar abnormalities may not always be apparent on MRI examination. No abnormalities were detected in Coton de Tulear dogs with neonatal cerebellar ataxia.[80] Differentiation of true cerebellar hypoplasia from degenerative disease (cerebellar atrophy, abiotrophy, and degeneration) is not possible solely based on imaging findings.

The Dandy-Walker malformation complex in human patients refers to a group of congenital central nervous system anomalies that primarily involve the cerebellum and adjacent tissues.[81] The primary abnormality is partial or complete absence of

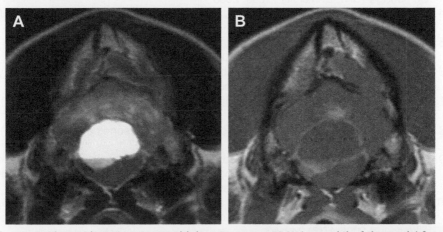

Fig. 15. Epidermoid cyst in a 3-year-old dog. Transverse T2-W image (*A*) of the caudal fossa shows a heterogeneous mass consisting of a cystic component dorsally and solid component ventrally, with ring and solid component enhancement present on T1-W image following contrast medium administration (*B*).

the cerebellar vermis and cystic dilation of the fourth ventricle. Additional abnormalities, such as hydrocephalus, stenosis of the mesencephalic aqueduct, and absence of the corpus callosum, may be present.[37] MRI findings in a golden retriever with Dandy-Walker malformation included generalized ventricular enlargement, extension of the cystic fourth ventricle into the supratentorial space with displacement of the occipital lobes, absence of cerebellar vermis, reduced size of the cerebellar hemispheres, widening and irregular gyrification of cerebral sulci, and absence of the corpus callosum.[82]

A case of cerebellar ependymal cyst has been reported in a Staffordshire terrier.[83] On MRI, the area of the cerebellum was almost completely replaced by a fluid collection independent of the fourth ventricle and isointense to CSF.

Intracranial epidermoid and dermoid cysts are benign space-occupying lesions that originate from remnants of ectodermal tissue because of defects of neural tube closure.[37] They are often located in the cerebellopontine angle or the fourth ventricle. Signal intensity is variable and dependent on cyst content. Cysts with a high lipid content appear hyperintense on T1-W and T2-W images,[84] whereas cysts with lower lipid content appear hypointense on T1-W images and hyperintense on T2-W images.[85,86] Dermoid cysts containing adnexa (eg, hair) may show suspended low intensity foci in all sequences.[84] Cysts often contain protein and keratin and therefore, do not attenuate on FLAIR.[86] They usually do not show contrast enhancement, although ring enhancement may occasionally be noted (**Fig. 15**).

REFERENCES

1. Thomson CE, Kornegay JN, Burn RA, et al. Magnetic resonance imaging - a general overview of principles and examples in veterinary neurodiagnosis. Vet Radiol Ultrasound 1993;34(1):2–17.
2. Tidwell AS, Jones JC. Advanced imaging concepts: a pictorial glossary of CT and MRI technology. Clin Tech Small Anim Pract 1999;14(2):65–111.
3. McRobbie DW, Moore EA, Graves MJ, et al. MRI - from picture to Proton. Cambridge (UK): University Press; 2003.
4. Westbrook C, Kaut Roth C, Talbot J. MRI in practice. Oxford (UK): Blackwell Publishing Ltd; 2005.
5. Pooley RA. AAPM/RSNA physics tutorial for residents: fundamental physics of MR imaging. Radiographics 2005;25(4):1087–99.
6. Faulkner W. Rad tech's guide to MRI: basic physics, instrumentation, and quality control. Malden (MA): Blackwell Science, Inc.; 2002.
7. Mikulis DJ, Roberts TP. Neuro MR: protocols. J Magn Reson Imaging 2007;26(4): 838–47.
8. Roberts TP, Mikulis D. Neuro MR: principles. J Magn Reson Imaging 2007;26(4): 823–37.
9. Tidwell AS. Principles of computed tomography and magnetic resonance imaging. In: Thrall DE, editor. Textbook of veterinary diagnostic radiology. 5th edition. St. Louis (MO): Saunders Elsevier; 2007. p. 50–77.
10. Sage JE, Samii VF, Abramson CJ, et al. Comparison of conventional spin-echo and fast spin-echo magnetic resonance imaging in the canine brain. Vet Radiol Ultrasound 2006;47(3):249–53.
11. Benigni L, Lamb CR. Comparison of fluid-attenuated inversion recovery and T2-weighted magnetic resonance images in dogs and cats with suspected brain disease. Vet Radiol Ultrasound 2005;46(4):287–92.

12. Cherubini GB, Platt SR, Howson S, et al. Comparison of magnetic resonance imaging sequences in dogs with multi-focal intracranial disease. J Small Anim Pract 2008;49(12):634–40.
13. Essig M, Bock M. Contrast optimization of fluid-attenuated inversion-recovery (FLAIR) MR imaging in patients with high CSF blood or protein content. Magn Reson Med 2000;43(5):764–7.
14. Falzone C, Rossi F, Calistri M, et al. Contrast-enhanced fluid-attenuated inversion recovery vs. contrast-enhanced spin echo T1-weighted brain imaging. Vet Radiol Ultrasound 2008;49(4):333–8.
15. Wessmann A, Chandler K, Garosi L. Ischaemic and haemorrhagic stroke in the dog. Vet J 2009;180(3):290–303.
16. Robertson ID. Magnetic resonance imaging features of brain disease in small animals. In: Thrall DE, editor. Textbook of veterinary diagnostic radiology. 5th edition. St. Louis (MO): Saunders Elsevier; 2007. p. 142–59.
17. Pomper MG, Port JD. New techniques in MR imaging of brain tumors. Magn Reson Imaging Clin N Am 2000;8(4):691–713.
18. Roberts TP, Rowley HA. Diffusion weighted magnetic resonance imaging in stroke. Eur J Radiol 2003;45(3):185–94.
19. Crawley AP, Poublanc J, Ferrari P, et al. Basics of diffusion and perfusion MRI. Appl Radiol 2003;32(4):13–23.
20. Scarabino T, Giannatempo GM, Popolizio T, et al. [Fast spin echo imaging of vertebral metastasis: comparison of fat suppression techniques (FSE-CHESS, STIR-FSE)]. Radiol Med 1996;92(3):180–5 [in Italian].
21. Pease A, Sullivan S, Olby N, et al. Value of a single-shot turbo spin-echo pulse sequence for assessing the architecture of the subarachnoid space and the constitutive nature of cerebrospinal fluid. Vet Radiol Ultrasound 2006;47(3):254–9.
22. Tang Y, Yamashita Y, Takahashi M. Ultrafast T2-weighted imaging of the abdomen and pelvis: use of single shot fast spin-echo imaging. J Magn Reson Imaging 1998;8(2):384–90.
23. Missios S, Quebada PB, Forero JA, et al. Quick-brain magnetic resonance imaging for nonhydrocephalus indications. J Neurosurg Pediatr 2008;2(6): 438–44.
24. Ozsarlak O, Van Goethem JW, Maes M, et al. MR angiography of the intracranial vessels: technical aspects and clinical applications. Neuroradiology 2004;46(12): 955–72.
25. Anzalone N. Contrast-enhanced MRA of intracranial vessels. Eur Radiol 2005; 15(Suppl 5):E3–10.
26. Sager M, Assheuer J, Trummler H, et al. Contrast-enhanced magnetic resonance angiography (CE-MRA) of intra- and extra-cranial vessels in dogs. Vet J 2009; 179(1):92–100.
27. Garosi LS, Dennis R, Penderis J, et al. Results of magnetic resonance imaging in dogs with vestibular disorders: 85 cases (1996–1999). J Am Vet Med Assoc 2001;218(3):385–91.
28. van der Vlugt-Meijer RH, Meij BP, Voorhout G. Thin-slice three-dimensional gradient-echo magnetic resonance imaging of the pituitary gland in healthy dogs. Am J Vet Res 2006;67(11):1865–72.
29. Senturk S, Oguz KK, Cila A. Dynamic contrast-enhanced susceptibility-weighted perfusion imaging of intracranial tumors: a study using a 3T MR scanner. Diagn Interv Radiol 2009;15(1):3–12.
30. Graham JP, Roberts GD, Newell SM. Dynamic magnetic resonance imaging of the normal canine pituitary gland. Vet Radiol Ultrasound 2000;41(1):35–40.

31. Kuriashkin IV, Losonsky JM. Contrast enhancement in magnetic resonance imaging using intravenous paramagnetic contrast media: a review. Vet Radiol Ultrasound 2000;41(1):4–7.
32. Bhave G, Lewis JB, Chang SS. Association of gadolinium based magnetic resonance imaging contrast agents and nephrogenic systemic fibrosis. J Urol 2008; 180(3):830–5.
33. Pollard RE, Puchalski SM, Pascoe PJ. Hemodynamic and serum biochemical alterations associated with intravenous administration of three types of contrast media in anesthetized cats. Am J Vet Res 2008;69(10):1274–8.
34. Pollard RE, Puchalski SM, Pascoe PJ. Hemodynamic and serum biochemical alterations associated with intravenous administration of three types of contrast media in anesthetized dogs. Am J Vet Res 2008;69(10):1268–73.
35. Kraft SL, Gavin PR. Intracranial neoplasia. Clin Tech Small Anim Pract 1999;14(2): 112–23.
36. Thomas WB. Nonneoplastic disorders of the brain. Clin Tech Small Anim Pract 1999;14(3):125–47.
37. Summers BA, Cummings JF, de Lahunta A. Veterinary neuropathology. St. Louis (MO): Mosby; 1995.
38. Dewey CW, Coates JR, Ducote JM, et al. External hydrocephalus in two cats. J Am Anim Hosp Assoc 2003;39(6):567–72.
39. Drake JM, Potts DG, Lemaire C. Magnetic resonance imaging of silastic-induced canine hydrocephalus. Surg Neurol 1989;31(1):28–40.
40. Matiasek LA. Malformations of the brain and neurocranium - magnetic resonance imaging features. Newmarket: European Association of Veterinary Diagnostic Imaging (EAVDI). EAVDI Yearbook 2008. p. 1–30.
41. Spaulding KA, Sharp NJH. Ultrasonographic imaging of the lateral cerebral ventricles in the dog. Vet Radiol 1990;31(2):59–64.
42. De Haan C, Kraft SL, Gavin PR, et al. Normal variation in size of the lateral ventricles of the labrador retriever dog as assessed by magnetic resonance imaging. Vet Radiol Ultrasound 1994;35(2):83–6.
43. Kii S, Uzuka Y, Taura Y, et al. Magnetic resonance imaging of the lateral ventricles in beagle-type dogs. Vet Radiol Ultrasound 1997;38(6):430–3.
44. Vite CH, Insko EK, Schotland HM, et al. Quantification of cerebral ventricular volume in English bulldogs. Vet Radiol Ultrasound 1997;38(6):437–43.
45. Vullo T, Korenman E, Manzo RP, et al. Diagnosis of cerebral ventriculomegaly in normal adult beagles using quantitative MRI. Vet Radiol Ultrasound 1997;38(4): 277–81.
46. Esteve-Ratsch B, Kneissl S, Gabler C. Comparative evaluation of the ventricles in the Yorkshire Terrier and the German Shepherd dog using low-field MRI. Vet Radiol Ultrasound 2001;42(5):410–3.
47. Hasegawa D, Yayoshi N, Fujita Y, et al. Measurement of interthalamic adhesion thickness as a criteria for brain atrophy in dogs with and without cognitive dysfunction (dementia). Vet Radiol Ultrasound 2005;46(6):452–7.
48. Kimotsuki T, Nagaoka T, Yasuda M, et al. Changes of magnetic resonance imaging on the brain in beagle dogs with aging. J Vet Med Sci 2005;67(10):961–7.
49. Thomas WB, Wheeler SJ, Kramer R, et al. Magnetic resonance imaging features of primary brain tumors in dogs. Vet Radiol Ultrasound 1996;37(1):20–7.
50. Kornegay JN, Oliver JE Jr, Gorgacz EJ. Clinicopathologic features of brain herniation in animals. J Am Vet Med Assoc 1983;182(10):1111–6.
51. Bagley RS. Pathophysiologic sequelae of intracranial disease. Vet Clin North Am Small Anim Pract 1996;26(4):711–33.

52. Walmsley GL, Herrtage ME, Dennis R, et al. The relationship between clinical signs and brain herniation associated with rostrotentorial mass lesions in the dog. Vet J 2006;172(2):258–64.
53. Aykut-Bingol C, Tekin S, Ince D, et al. Reversible MRI lesions after seizures. Seizure 1997;6(3):237–9.
54. Chan S, Chin SS, Kartha K, et al. Reversible signal abnormalities in the hippo-campus and neocortex after prolonged seizures. AJNR Am J Neuroradiol 1996; 17(9):1725–31.
55. Mellema LM, Koblik PD, Kortz GD, et al. Reversible magnetic resonance imaging abnormalities in dogs following seizures. Vet Radiol Ultrasound 1999;40(6): 588–95.
56. Mariani CL, Platt SR, Newell SM, et al. Magnetic resonance imaging of cerebral cortical necrosis (polioencephalomalacia) in a dog. Vet Radiol Ultrasound 2001;42(6):524–31.
57. Fatzer R, Gandini G, Jaggy A, et al. Necrosis of hippocampus and piriform lobe in 38 domestic cats with seizures: a retrospective study on clinical and pathologic findings. J Vet Intern Med 2000;14(1):100–4.
58. Schmied O, Scharf G, Hilbe M, et al. Magnetic resonance imaging of feline hippo-campal necrosis. Vet Radiol Ultrasound 2008;49(4):343–9.
59. Dewey CW. Encephalopathies: disorders of the brain. In: Dewey CW, editor. A practical guide to canine and feline neurology. Ames (IA): Iowa State Press; 2003. p. 99–178.
60. Sharp NJ, Davis BJ, Guy JS, et al. Hydranencephaly and cerebellar hypoplasia in two kittens attributed to intrauterine parvovirus infection. J Comp Pathol 1999; 121(1):39–53.
61. Saito M, Sharp NJ, Kortz GD, et al. Magnetic resonance imaging features of lissencephaly in 2 Lhasa Apsos. Vet Radiol Ultrasound 2002;43(4):331–7.
62. Sullivan SA, Harmon BG, Purinton PT, et al. Lobar holoprosencephaly in a Minia-ture Schnauzer with hypodipsic hypernatremia. J Am Vet Med Assoc 2003; 223(12):1783–7.
63. Kärkkäinen M. Low- and high-field strength magnetic resonance imaging to eval-uate the brain in one normal dog and two dogs with central nervous system disease. Vet Radiol Ultrasound 1995;36(6):528–32.
64. Jeffery N. Ethmoidal encephalocoele associated with seizures in a puppy. J Small Anim Pract 2005;46(2):89–92.
65. Hasegawa D, Uchida K, Kobayashi T, et al. Imaging diagnosis - Rathke's cleft cyst. Vet Radiol Ultrasound 2009;50(3):298–300.
66. Matiasek LA, Platt SR, Shaw S, et al. Clinical and magnetic resonance imaging char-acteristics of quadrigeminal cysts in dogs. J Vet Intern Med 2007;21(5):1021–6.
67. Vernau KM, Kortz GD, Koblik PD, et al. Magnetic resonance imaging and computed tomography characteristics of intracranial intra-arachnoid cysts in 6 dogs. Vet Radiol Ultrasound 1997;38(3):171–6.
68. Vernau KM, LeCouteur RA, Sturges BK, et al. Intracranial intra-arachnoid cyst with intracystic hemorrhage in two dogs. Vet Radiol Ultrasound 2002;43(5): 449–54.
69. Duque C, Parent J, Brisson B, et al. Intracranial arachnoid cysts: are they clinically significant? J Vet Intern Med 2005;19(5):772–4.
70. Tubbs RS, Shoja MM, Ardalan MR, et al. Hindbrain herniation: a review of embryological theories. Ital J Anat Embryol 2008;113(1):37–46.
71. Cappello R, Rusbridge C. Report from the Chiari-like malformation and syringo-myelia working group round table. Vet Surg 2007;36(5):509–12.

72. Rusbridge C, Greitz D, Iskandar BJ. Syringomyelia: current concepts in pathogenesis, diagnosis, and treatment. J Vet Intern Med 2006;20(3):469–79.
73. Rusbridge C, Knowler SP. Inheritance of occipital bone hypoplasia (Chiari type I malformation) in Cavalier King Charles spaniels. J Vet Intern Med 2004;18(5): 673–8.
74. Couturier J, Rault D, Cauzinille L. Chiari-like malformation and syringomyelia in normal cavalier King Charles spaniels: a multiple diagnostic imaging approach. J Small Anim Pract 2008;49(9):438–43.
75. Lu D, Lamb CR, Pfeiffer DU, et al. Neurological signs and results of magnetic resonance imaging in 40 cavalier King Charles spaniels with Chiari type 1-like malformations. Vet Rec 2003;153(9):260–3.
76. Kitagawa M, Kanayama K, Sakai T. Quadrigeminal cisterna arachnoid cyst diagnosed by MRI in five dogs. Aust Vet J 2003;81(6):340–3.
77. Schatzberg SJ, Haley NJ, Barr SC, et al. Polymerase chain reaction (PCR) amplification of parvoviral DNA from the brains of dogs and cats with cerebellar hypoplasia. J Vet Intern Med 2003;17(4):538–44.
78. Kitagawa M, Kanayama K, Sakai T. Subtotal agenesis of the cerebellum in a dog. Aust Vet J 2005;83(11):680–1.
79. Choi H, Kang S, Jeong S, et al. Imaging diagnosis-cerebellar vermis hypoplasia in a miniature schnauzer. Vet Radiol Ultrasound 2007;48(2):129–31.
80. Coates JR, O'Brien DP, Kline KL, et al. Neonatal cerebellar ataxia in Coton de Tulear dogs. J Vet Intern Med 2002;16(6):680–9.
81. Patel S, Barkovich AJ. Analysis and classification of cerebellar malformations. Am J Neuroradiol 2002;23(7):1074–87.
82. Schmidt MJ, Jawinski S, Wigger A, et al. Imaging diagnosis-Dandy walker malformation. Vet Radiol Ultrasound 2008;49(3):264–6.
83. Wyss-Fluehmann G, Konar M, Jaggy A, et al. Cerebellar ependymal cyst in a dog. Vet Pathol 2008;45(6):910–3.
84. Targett MP, McInnes E, Dennis R. Magnetic resonance imaging of a medullary dermoid cyst with secondary hydrocephalus in a dog. Vet Radiol Ultrasound 1999;40(1):23–6.
85. Platt SR, Graham J, Chrisman CL, et al. Canine intracranial epidermoid cyst. Vet Radiol Ultrasound 1999;40(5):454–8.
86. Steinberg T, Matiasek K, Bruhschwein A, et al. Imaging diagnosis–intracranial epidermoid cyst in a Doberman Pinscher. Vet Radiol Ultrasound 2007;48(3): 250–3.

MRI of Brain Disease in Veterinary Patients Part 2: Acquired Brain Disorders

Silke Hecht, Dr Med Vet*, William H. Adams, DVM

KEYWORDS

- Magnetic resonance imaging • Cat • Dog • Neoplasia
- Inflammation • Infarct

INFLAMMATORY BRAIN DISEASES

Inflammatory brain diseases can affect brain parenchyma (encephalitis), meninges (meningitis), or both (meningoencephalitis).[1] Depending on the underlying causes, involvement of the spinal cord (myelitis/meningomyelitis) may occur. Encephalitis may cause no detectable abnormalities on magnetic resonance imaging (MRI), or may manifest as multifocal (rather than focal or diffuse) lesions associated with brain parenchyma that typically appear hyperintense on T2-weighted (T2-W) images, and hypointense on T1-weighted (T1-W) images.[2–4] Fluid attenuated inversion recovery (FLAIR) has higher sensitivity than conventional spin-echo sequences in detecting subtle brain lesions in dogs with clinical signs of multifocal brain disease, and its use is encouraged in all of these cases.[5] Meningitis may not be detected with MRI, or may appear as meningeal enhancement following administration of contrast medium.[2–4,6]

Infectious Inflammatory Brain Diseases

Canine distemper virus (CDV) and feline infectious peritonitis virus (FIPV) are the most common causes of viral encephalitis in dogs and cats, respectively. In acute CDV infection, T2 hyperintense lesions, and loss of contrast between gray and white matter on T2-W images, may be found in cerebellum or brainstem, corresponding to areas of demyelination.[7] T2 hyperintense areas are occasionally seen in the temporal lobes, which may be related to infection or postictal edema. MRI findings in chronic distemper meningoencephalitis include essentially bilaterally symmetric T2 hyperintensity of the cortical gray/white matter junction of the parietal and frontal lobes, T2

Department of Small Animal Clinical Sciences, University of Tennessee College of Veterinary Medicine, 2407 River Drive, Knoxville, TN 37996, USA
* Corresponding author.
E-mail address: shecht@utk.edu (S. Hecht).

Vet Clin Small Anim 40 (2010) 39–63
doi:10.1016/j.cvsm.2009.09.006
0195-5616/09/$ – see front matter © 2010 Elsevier Inc. All rights reserved.

hyperintensity of the arbor vitae of the cerebellum with partial loss of cerebellar cortical gray/white matter demarcation, subtle focal T2 hyperintensity of the pons, and meningeal contrast enhancement.[8] In feline infectious peritonitis (FIP), MRI may show T2 hyperintensity and contrast enhancement of ventricular lining, choroid plexus and meninges compatible with ependymitis, choroiditis, and meningitis (**Fig. 1**).[1,4,9] Concurrent hydrocephalus is common, and herniation of the cerebellum secondary to increased intracranial pressure is possible.[4]

Mechanisms of bacterial infection of the central nervous system (CNS) in cats and dogs include hematogenous spread, contiguous infection from adjacent structures (inner ears, cribriform plate, sinuses, eyes, and vertebrae), direct inoculation (trauma, bite wound, and surgery), and migration of foreign bodies or aberrant parasites. In addition to meningitis (**Fig. 2**) and meningoencephalomyelitis, CNS infection may result in focal parenchymal abscesses or empyema in subdural or epidural locations.[10] MRI features of intracranial infection secondary to plant foreign-body migration,[11] due to hematogenous spread from a mediastinal abscess,[12] secondary to bacterial endocarditis,[13] secondary to local extension from a retrobulbar abscess,[14] and as complication of otitis media or interna,[15] have been described. Intracranial abscesses are typically hypointense on T1-W and hyperintense on T2-W images, with strong peripheral contrast enhancement and associated brain edema. Concurrent meningitis appearing as meningeal enhancement is common. Presumed rupture of an abscess into the ventricular system in a dog resulted in failure of cerebrospinal fluid (CSF) to suppress on FLAIR.[16]

Fungal infections have been reported to affect the CNS, with varied MRI findings.[17] Imaging findings in cats with CNS cryptococcosis include solitary or multifocal mass lesions that are typically hyperintense on T2-W images and show variable degrees of contrast enhancement. Diffuse and patchy meningeal, ependymal, and choroid plexus enhancement are also possible.[17–19] In dogs with cryptococcosis, T1 hypointense and T2 hyperintense lesions with multifocal (ring) enhancement and meningeal enhancement have been reported.[17,20,21] Extension of a cryptococcal fungal granuloma through the cribriform plate was observed in 1 dog.[17] *Cladophialophora bantiana* meningoencephalitis appeared as an irregularly shaped area of increased T2 signal intensity and

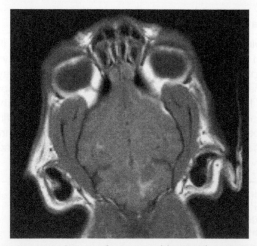

Fig. 1. Dorsal T1-W postcontrast image of a 2-year-old cat with presumptive diagnosis of FIP. There is contrast enhancement associated with meninges and ventricular lining, consistent with meningitis and ependymitis.

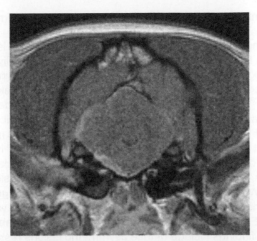

Fig. 2. Meningitis in a 5-year-old pug secondary to otitis media. On transverse T1-W post-contrast image, extensive enhancement and thickening of the meninges of the right cerebellum and brainstem are noted, along with enhancement of the external ear canal. Low-signal material within the right tympanic bulla does not show evidence of contrast enhancement consistent with exudate.

mass effect in the cerebral white matter of the parietal and temporal lobes of a dog, with nonuniform contrast enhancement of mass and meninges observed on postcontrast images.[22] The same organism in a cat appeared as a large uniformly contrast-enhancing mass involving the cerebellum and pons.[23] MRI findings in a cat with histoplasmosis included a single high-signal T2/low-signal T1 uniformly contrast-enhancing intra-axial mass of the frontal lobe with severe concurrent edema.[23]

Parasitic meningoencephalitis in dogs and cats is caused by aberrant migration of parasites such as *Dirofilaria*, *Baylisascaris*, *Cuterebra*, *Taenia*, *Ancylostoma*, *Toxascaris* and *Angiostronglylus*.[24] MRI features include focal or multifocal parenchymal lesions of variable signal intensity, and peripheral parenchymal or meningeal contrast enhancement.[21,25–27] Intraparenchymal hemorrhage is a common feature in parasite migration, and T2*-W images are useful in establishing a presumptive diagnosis.

Protozoal meningoencephalitis may be caused by *Toxoplasma* and *Neospora* infection in dogs and *Toxoplasma* infection in cats.[24] MRI in a dog with neosporosis demonstrated T2 hyperintensity of the vermis and cerebellar hemispheres with subtle contrast enhancement.[21] CNS toxoplasmosis in cats appeared as multifocal, indistinct, contrast-enhancing parenchymal lesions which were iso- to hypointense on T1-W images, hyperintense on T2-W images, and were associated with edema.[4]

Noninfectious Inflammatory Brain Diseases

Several inflammatory conditions unrelated to infectious agents have been identified in several different canine breeds.[28]

Granulomatous meningoencephalitis (GME) is an inflammatory CNS disorder of uncertain cause that can affect any breed but most often occurs in young to middle-aged toy-breed dogs.[29] The disease can affect the brain or spinal cord. On MRI, GME lesions can be focal or multifocal, and commonly affect the brain stem. Although the disease has a predilection for white matter, it is not associated with distinct topography.[28] Lesions are typically hyperintense on T2-W and FLAIR images, iso- to hypointense on T1-W images, and variably contrast-enhancing, ranging from none to intense contrast uptake (**Fig. 3**).[30–32] Meningeal enhancement may[6] or may not[30] be observed.

Necrotizing meningoencephalitis (NME) is of uncertain cause and is characterized by cavitary necrosis in the neuroparenchyma. The disease was initially described in the pug breed ("pug dog encephalitis"),[33] but similar disorders have since been reported in other small breeds, including the Maltese,[34] Chihuahua,[35] Pekingese,[36] French bulldog,[37] Shi Tzu,[28] and Lhasa apso.[28] A distinct form of NME, described mainly in Yorkshire terriers, has been termed necrotizing leukoencephalitis (NLE).[28] Descriptions of imaging findings in this group of inflammatory brain disorders are not available for all breeds affected, but there seem to be breed-specific differences.[38] In almost all cases of NLE reported in Yorkshire terriers, lesions were found to be associated with the cerebrum and brainstem. On magnetic resonance (MR) images, these lesions appear iso- to hypointense on T1-W images, hyperintense on T2-W and FLAIR images, and show variable contrast enhancement.[28,39–42] Concurrent hydrocephalus of variable severity is possible. Unlike NLE, NME in pugs usually does not involve the cerebellum, brainstem, or spinal cord. MRI findings include diffuse asymmetric lesions restricted to the forebrain, affecting both cerebral hemispheres.[28,38,43] Lesions are nonuniformly hyperintense on T2-W, isointense to hypointense on T1-W images, and affect gray and white matter, resulting in loss of gray/white matter distinction (**Fig. 4**). Additional MRI findings include variable degrees of contrast enhancement of brain and meninges, asymmetry of lateral ventricles, brain herniation, and T2/FLAIR hyperintensity associated with hippocampus and piriform lobes. MRI of the brain in 2 Chihuahuas with NME demonstrated multifocal loss of cortical gray/white matter demarcation with hypointensity on T1-W, hyperintensity on T2-W/FLAIR images, and slight contrast enhancement.[35] In 1 dog there was involvement of the medulla, and asymmetric hydrocephalus was noted in the second animal. A French bulldog had asymmetry of both lateral ventricles, cerebrum, midbrain, and several distinct T2 hyperintense white matter foci of the forebrain and the brain stem, with variable contrast enhancement.[37]

Other Inflammatory Intracranial Diseases

Idiopathic eosinophilic meningitis/meningoencephalitis in dogs may not show abnormalities on MRI, or may have variable findings including patchy regions of T2

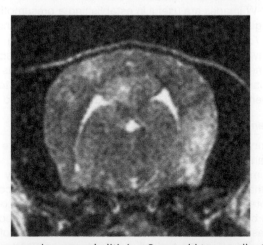

Fig. 3. Granulomatous meningoencephalitis in a 2-year-old toy poodle. On transverse T2-W image, multifocal hyperintense lesions are associated with both cerebral hemispheres.

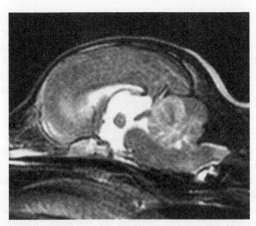

Fig. 4. NME in an 8-year-old Maltese. Sagittal T2-W image demonstrates multiple poorly circumscribed hyperintense lesions within the cerebrum, cerebellum, brainstem, and spinal cord.

hyperintensity and contrast enhancement in the cerebral cortex, solitary or multiple masses, meningeal enhancement, and enlargement and contrast enhancement of cranial nerves.[21] A case of lymphocytic meningoencephalitis in a cat was characterized by focal T1 isointense and T2 hyperintense contrast-enhancing lesions.[4] No intracranial abnormalities were detected on MRI in a cat with histiocytic encephalitis.[4] Trigeminal neuritis in dogs is characterized by diffuse enlargement of the nerve without a mass lesion. Affected nerves are isointense to brain parenchyma on T1-W and PD-W images, isointense or hyperintense on T2-W images, and show contrast enhancement.[44]

CEREBROVASCULAR DISEASE

The term "cerebrovascular diseases" refers to all disorders in which there is an area of brain transiently or permanently affected by ischemia or bleeding, or in which 1 or more blood vessels of the brain are primarily impaired by a pathologic process.[45]

Intracranial Aneurysms and Cerebrovascular Malformations

An aneurysm is an abnormal focal enlargement of an artery of variable cause.[46] Patent aneurysms appear as signal void on T1-W and T2-W images, representing fast flowing blood. Small aneurysms, and aneurysms with turbulent flow, are unreliably shown on conventional MRI, and are better demonstrated by magnetic resonance angiography (MRA).[46,47] A case of a presumed aneurysm, most likely the result of traumatic arteriovenous fistulization, has been described in a dog.[48] On computerized tomography (CT) images, an expansile enhancing mass was present along the intracranial cavernous sinus and extended through the orbital fissure into the retrobulbar space. With MRI, the structure appeared as a signal void due to the presence of rapidly flowing blood. The vascular origin of the lesion was confirmed with MRA.

Cerebrovascular malformations are congenital anomalies of brain vasculature.[49] Different types include arteriovenous malformations (clusters of abnormal arteries and veins with direct arterial-to-venous shunts), venous malformations (anomalous veins separated by normal neural parenchyma), cavernous malformations (masses of contiguous sinusoidal vessels with no intervening parenchyma), and telangiectasias (masses of small capillary-type vessels separated by normal parenchyma). Animals with cerebrovascular abnormalities usually present with intracranial hemorrhage, and imaging findings are consistent with hemorrhagic stroke (see later).[1,39] Identification of associated large vessels suggests vascular malformation as the underlying cause of spontaneous intracranial hemorrhage. However, compression or obliteration of vessels by hematoma, extremely slow flow, and thrombosis may obscure the abnormal vessels, and specialized techniques (catheter angiography, repeat MRI or MRA) may be needed to achieve a diagnosis.[46]

Stroke (Cerebrovascular Accident, Infarct)

A stroke is a suddenly developing focal neurologic deficit resulting from an intracranial vascular event.[50] In ischemic stroke, blood flow to an area of tissue is compromised due to intracranial arterial or venous obstruction. Hemorrhagic stroke results from rupture of intracranial blood vessels.

Ischemic strokes can be categorized according to anatomic site, size, age, type (pallid or hemorrhagic), pathology (arterial vs venous), mechanism (thrombotic, embolic, hemodynamic), and etiology.[45] Causes of ischemic stroke in dogs include atherosclerosis associated with primary hypothyroidism,[51] hypertension and diabetes,[52] embolic metastatic tumor cells,[51] chronic renal disease,[51–53] hyperadrenocorticism,[51,53] intravascular lymphoma,[54,55] septic thromboemboli,[56] fibrocartilaginous embolism,[57] migrating parasite or parasitic emboli (Dirofilaria immitis),[58] and a hypercoagulable state associated with hyperadrenocorticism, protein losing nephropathy (PLN), or neoplasia.[53] In approximately 50% of dogs with ischemic stroke, no underlying medical condition is identified.[53] Territorial infarcts occur when one of the main arteries supplying the brain is occluded. Lacunar infarcts are defined as subcortical infarcts limited to the vascular territory of an intraparenchymal superficial or deep perforating artery.[59] Small-breed dogs are more likely to have territorial cerebellar infarcts, and large-breed dogs are more likely to have lacunar thalamic or midbrain infarcts.[53] Cavalier King Charles spaniels and greyhounds may be predisposed for infarcts.[53,60] Watershed infarcts, defined as infarcts in the boundary zone between large artery territories,[59] do not seem to be common in veterinary patients.[53] Diffusion weighted imaging (DWI) is sensitive to alterations in brain parenchyma following stroke, and is capable of demonstrating abnormalities within minutes of an event.[61] Restricted diffusion (impairment of normal Brownian motion) occurs secondary to failure of the cell membrane ion pump and subsequent cytotoxic edema. This appears as marked hyperintensity on DWI, and hypointensity on a synthesized apparent diffusion coefficient (ADC) map derived from 2 or more DWI.[62] On conventional MRI sequences, changes will be apparent within 12 to 24 hours of onset. Although MRI findings in ischemic stroke may be similar to changes seen with other brain parenchymal diseases, certain distinguishing characteristics exist (**Fig. 5**).[52,53,60,63–65] An ischemic infarct appears as a homogeneous T2 hyperintense area with sharp demarcation between affected and nonaffected parenchyma, and minimal to no mass effect. Lesions are typically confined to gray matter, but may involve white matter in severe cases.[65] Faint diffuse or peripheral contrast enhancement may be noted and has been reported in patients imaged between 1 and 45 days postonset of neurologic signs.[60] Reperfusion injury of an ischemic infarct can occur, resulting in hemorrhagic infarction.[59]

Hemorrhagic stroke can be classified according to anatomic site (intraparenchymal, epidural, subdural, subarachnoid, and intraventricular), size, age, and cause (eg, intracranial neoplasia,[66] von Willebrand factor deficiency[67] and other coagulopathies, parasite migration,[25,27] cerebral vascular malformation,[39] idiopathic). The appearance of hemorrhage on MRI changes over time, allowing staging of a hematoma using conventional MRI sequences (**Table 1**).[68,69] However, there is considerable variability

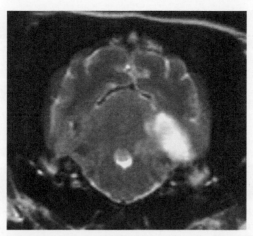

Fig. 5. Transverse T2-W image of the caudal fossa in a dog, demonstrating a wedge-shaped hyperintensity associated with the left cerebellar hemisphere consistent with an ischemic infarct.

in the appearance of hemorrhage on MRI. Hemorrhage in areas with high ambient oxygen (ventricles; epidural, subdural, and subarachnoid space) "ages" more slowly than parenchymal or neoplastic hematomas, with a resultant change in time course of degradation.[68] Deoxyhemoglobin, intracellular methemoglobin, hemosiderin, and ferritin have high magnetic susceptibility and are depicted with high sensitivity on T2*-W images (**Fig. 6**A).[70] Intraparenchymal hemorrhage appears as mass lesion(s) of variable size and intensity,[71] and (sub)acute parenchymal hemorrhage is often associated with brain edema. In the acute stage, there is no contrast enhancement of the hematoma. However, with time, neovascularization in the surrounding brain tissue develops, resulting in ring enhancement of the lesion.[69] Identification of underlying cause of intraparenchymal hemorrhage can be challenging. The signal of hematomas secondary to neoplasms is more heterogeneous and complex than in spontaneous hematomas because of the presence of hemorrhagic components of varied age and, therefore, hemoglobin state, presence of nonhemorrhagic areas,

Table 1
Change of appearance of intracranial hemorrhage over time

Stage	Time Frame	Hemoglobin State	Intensity (T1-W)	Intensity (T2-W)
Hyperacute	<12–24 h	Intracellular oxyhemoglobin	Isointense or hypointense	Hyperintense
Acute	1–3 d	Intracellular deoxyhemoglobin	Isointense or hypointense	Hypointense
Early subacute	>3 d	Intracellular methemoglobin	Hyperintense	Hypointense
Late subacute	>7 d	Extracellular methemoglobin	Hyperintense	Hyperintense
Chronic	>14 d	Hemosiderin and ferritin	Hypointense	Hypointense

Data from Bradley Jr WG. MR appearance of hemorrhage in the brain. Radiology 1993;189(1):15–26 and Parizel PM, Makkat S, Van Miert E, et al. Intracranial hemorrhage: principles of CT and MRI interpretation. Eur Radiol 2001;11(9):1770–83.

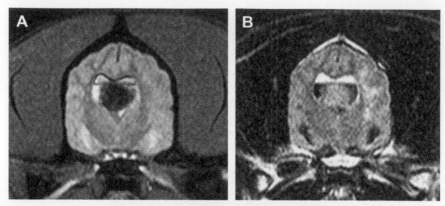

Fig. 6. Acute hemorrhagic stroke of undetermined cause in an 8-year-old boxer. The dog was positioned in dorsal recumbency for the examination. On T2*-W image (*A*) a large interventricular susceptibility artifact, consistent with hemorrhage, is noted. On FLAIR image (*B*) a fluid-fluid level between hypointense CSF and hyperintense CSF/blood mixture in the dependent part of the ventricles is noted.

and, in some instances, presence of necrotic-cystic components.[72] Epidural hemorrhage assumes a focal biconvex configuration that may cross dural folds, such as falx and tentorium, but not sutures, whereas subdural hemorrhage appears as a peripheral crescent-shaped collection of blood that may cross suture lines but is limited by the falx cerebri and tentorium cerebelli.[1,68,69] Subarachnoid and intraventricular hemorrhages result in admixture of blood and CSF. If massive bleeding has occurred, separation of intraventricular fluid into hemorrhagic and nonhemorrhagic strata may be observed (**Fig. 6**B). Subarachnoid or intraventricular thrombus may be present.[68]

Other Vascular Disorders

Feline ischemic encephalopathy (FIE) is a syndrome of cerebral infarction affecting adult cats, which is attributed to aberrant *Cuterebra* spp larval migration in the brain and toxin release by the parasites.[50,73] MRI findings in chronic FIE include asymmetry of the cerebral hemispheres and bilateral symmetric enlargement of the subarachnoid space over the temporal lobes in areas supplied by the middle cerebral artery.[74] MRI-detectable histopathologic lesions include parasitic tracks, superficial laminar cerebrocortical necrosis, cerebral infarction, subependymal rarefaction and astrogliosis, and subpial astrogliosis.[73]

In global brain ischemia (GBI) the entire brain is affected by a transient period of complete ischemia, followed by reperfusion.[75] MRI findings include bilaterally symmetric increased T2/FLAIR signal intensity associated with gray matter and, to a lesser degree, with white matter of the occipital and parietal lobes and caudate nuclei/thalamus.[76,77] Bilaterally symmetric contrast enhancement in these areas may be observed.[77] In a report of a dog with GBI, repeat examination showed that lesions associated with gray matter decreased in extent and severity, and white matter changes resolved.[76]

METABOLIC, NUTRITIONAL, TOXIC, AND DEGENERATIVE ENCEPHALOPATHIES

Lysosomal storage diseases comprise a wide variety of inherited abnormalities that are characterized by the intracellular accumulation of 1 or more products of an interrupted degradative metabolic pathway.[24] Globoid cell leukodystrophy (Krabbe disease) is caused by mutations in the gene for galactocerebrosidase, and has been described in cairn terriers and west highland white terriers.[78] MRI findings include mild hydrocephalus, increased signal intensity in the corpus callosum on T1-W images, bilaterally symmetric increased signal intensity of the corpus callosum, centrum semiovale, internal capsule, corona radiata and cerebellar white matter on T2-W images, and symmetric enhancement of the corpus callosum, internal capsule, and corona radiata after administration of gadolinium.[79] Gangliosidoses are characterized by excessive neuronal accumulation of ganglioside. MRI findings have been reported in a golden retriever with G_{M2}-gangliosidoses and included mild cerebral atrophy and bilaterally symmetric T2 hyperintensity and T1 hypointensity to the caudate nucleus without evidence of contrast enhancement.[80] MRI examinations performed on 2 canine mutants with G_{M1} gangliosidosis (English springer spaniel and Portuguese water dog) demonstrated a relative increase in gray matter and an abnormal signal intensity of cerebral and cerebellar white matter on T2-W images.[81] Ceroid lipofuscinosis is characterized by the abnormal accumulation of lipoprotein pigment within cellular lysosomes. MRI findings include dilation of cerebral sulci and cerebellar fissures and ventriculomegaly.[82,83] In cats affected with α-mannosidosis, a decrease in ADC values of white and gray matter and an increase in T2 values of white matter have been reported, corresponding to neuronal swelling, abnormal myelin, and astrogliosis.[84,85] Mucopolysaccharidoses (MPS) are a group of diseases caused by different specific deficits of metabolism of glycosaminoglycan. No abnormalities were detected on MRI examination of the brain in schipperkes with MPS III.[86]

L-2-Hydroxyglutaric aciduria is an inborn error of metabolism that has been described in Staffordshire bull terriers.[87] MRI findings included bilaterally symmetric, diffuse regions of gray matter hyperintensity on T2-W images, and T1-W hypointensity most prominent in the thalamus, hypothalamus, dentate nucleus, basal ganglia, dorsal brainstem, cerebellar nuclei, and cerebellar gyri. These lesions did not exhibit a mass effect and did not show evidence of contrast enhancement.

Mitochondrial encephalopathies resembling subacute necrotizing encephalomyelopathy (Leigh syndrome) in humans have been described in Australian cattle dogs[88] and Alaskan Huskies,[89,90] and similar diseases have been suspected in English springer spaniels, Yorkshire terriers, and cats.[24] MRI findings in hereditary polioencephalomyelopathy in an Australian cattle dog included bilaterally symmetric abnormalities in areas corresponding to the interpositial nuclei in the cerebellum and the vestibular nuclei in the medulla, and in areas corresponding to the dorsal nuclei of the trapezoid body, pontine nuclei, caudal colliculi, and the dorsolateral reticular formation.[91] Lesions were isointense or hypointense on T1-W images, hyperintense on T2-W images, did not have a mass effect, and did not show evidence of contrast enhancement. MRI examination in an Alaskan husky with subacute necrotizing encephalopathy revealed bilateral cavitation extending from the thalamus to the medulla, with less-pronounced degenerative lesions in the caudate nucleus, putamen, and claustrum.[90]

Failure of the liver to remove toxic substances absorbed from the gastrointestinal tract may result in hepatic encephalopathy.[24] MRI findings in dogs and cats with congenital portosystemic shunt include brain atrophy, possibly unrelated to shunt, and bilaterally symmetric hyperintensity to the lentiform nuclei on T1-W images without contrast enhancement.[92]

Thiamine deficiency results in insufficient adenosine triphosphate (ATP) production in the brain, with subsequent neuronal dysfunction.[24] MRI findings in dogs include bilaterally symmetric multifocal T2, FLAIR, and postcontrast T1 hyperintensities in the red nuclei, caudal colliculi, vestibular nuclei of the brainstem, and the cerebellar nodulus,[93] or bilaterally symmetric T2 hyperintensities in caudate nuclei and rostral colliculi.[94] In cats, bilaterally symmetric T2, FLAIR, and T2* hyperintense nonenhancing lesions are observed associated with the lateral geniculate nuclei, caudal colliculi, periaqueductal gray matter, medial vestibular nuclei, cerebellar nodulus, and facial nuclei (**Fig. 7**),[95] with the caudal colliculi, medial vestibular nuclei, and facial nuclei also being hyperintense on T1-W images.

Myelinolysis is a brain disorder most commonly caused by rapid correction of hyponatremia in humans, but probably multifactorial.[96] Lesions were originally believed to be limited to the pons, but extrapontine locations including the thalamus, midbrain, cerebellum, basal nuclei, and cerebrocortical gray and white matter junctions have been reported. MRI findings in dogs include bilaterally symmetric T2/FLAIR hyperintense nonenhancing lesions within the thalamus,[97] caudate nuclei, and along the cerebrocortical gray-white matter junction.

A series of progressive neurologic diseases have been summarized under the term "spongy degeneration."[50] These conditions are primarily, but not exclusively, diseases of white matter, and may be hereditary. MRI findings in spongy degeneration of the CNS in a Labrador retriever included large, bilaterally symmetric T2 hyperintense and T1 hypointense nonenhancing lesions in the region of the deep cerebellar nuclei, and smaller lesions within the thalamus ventromedial to the lateral ventricles.[98]

Neuroaxonal dystrophy is a degenerative disease of the CNS characterized by degeneration of neurons and axons. MRI features in a papillon included cerebral and cerebellar atrophy.[99]

Cerebellar cortical abiotrophy refers to the degeneration of normal neuronal cell populations within the cerebellar cortex after birth, and has been reported in a variety of breeds.[50] Presumptive diagnosis is best made on sagittal T2-W images, in which the small size of the cerebellum is indicated by a marked increase in fluid separating the folia of the cerebellum (**Fig. 8**).[100–104] Differentiation of true abiotrophy from other causes of small cerebellar size (cerebellar atrophy, cerebellar hypoplasia) is not possible based on imaging findings.

TRAUMA

MRI findings in head trauma in dogs and cats are infrequently reported. Possible findings include fractures,[74,105] intracranial hemorrhage,[106,107] brain edema,[105] and

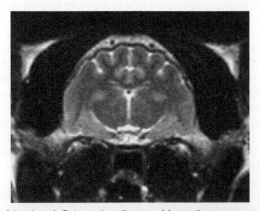

Fig. 7. Presumptive thiamine deficiency in a 7-year-old cat. On transverse T2-W image, there are bilaterally symmetric T2 hyperintense lesions associated with the thalamus, corresponding to the location of the lateral geniculate nuclei.

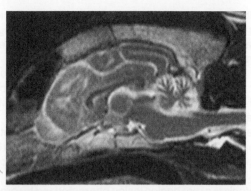

Fig. 8. Cerebellar abiotrophy in a 6-year-old Staffordshire terrier. Sagittal T2-W image demonstrates the small size of the cerebellum, indicated by increase in fluid separating the folia of the cerebellum.

parenchymal brain defects with compensatory CSF filling (hydrocephalus ex vacuo) (**Fig. 9**).[74] MRI appearance of traumatic intracranial hemorrhage corresponds to imaging features described earlier (see section on Stroke (Cerebrovascular Accident, Infarct)).

INTRACRANIAL NEOPLASTIC AND NONNEOPLASTIC MASS LESIONS

Numerous intracranial masses have been described in dogs and cats. They can be characterized by number, origin, location, size, margination, signal intensity, homogeneity, contrast enhancement, and concurrent imaging findings (eg, ventriculomegaly, changes associated with cranium or meninges, hemorrhage, mineralization, mass effect, edema, cystic or necrotic component).[66,108–112] Mass lesions can be subdivided based on location into intra-axial (arising from within the brain axis) and extra-axial.

Malformations, Hamartomas, Cysts, Borderline Tumors, and Tumorlike Lesions

A variety of conditions is included in this group,[50] and overlap exists with disorders described as congenital malformations and cerebrovascular disease. Cystic lesions

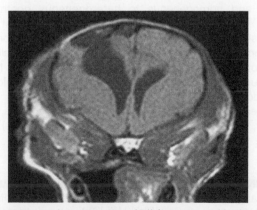

Fig. 9. Transverse T1-W image demonstrating skull fractures and hydrocephalus ex vacuo in an 8-year-old Pomeranian following presumed trauma.

of the brain (eg, arachnoid cysts, ependymal cysts, dermoid and epidermoid cysts) are discussed in the companion article elsewhere in this issue, and congenital disorders of intracranial vessels are discussed in the section on Intracranial Aneurysms and Cerebrovascular Malformations.

Hamartomas are masses formed by disorderly overgrowth of tissue elements normally present at that site.[50] MRI examination in a cat with cerebellar vascular hamartoma showed a heterogeneously T2 hyperintense mass lesion with heterogeneous contrast enhancement.[113]

Hemangiomas are borderline tumors with unclear distinction between hamartoma, malformation, and neoplasia.[50] MRI in a 13-month-old golden retriever with cerebral cavernous hemangioma revealed a large, contrast-enhancing, space-occupying cerebral mass.[114]

Meningioangiomatosis is a rare benign lesion characterized by proliferation of meningothelial cells surrounding small blood vessels.[50] MR examination in a 2-year-old Alaskan malamute showed a large T2 hyperintense mass associated with the cerebrum.[115]

Cholesterol granulomas due to progressive cholesterol accumulation in choroid plexuses are most commonly reported in horses.[50] MRI findings have been described in a cat.[116] An extensive, heterogeneous, space-occupying lesion was found in the area of the falx cerebri, extending from the olfactory bulbs to the tentorium cerebelli, with compression of both hemispheres and thalamus. The mass was mostly hyperintense on STIR, FLAIR, and T2-W images, and hypointense on T1-W images, with heterogeneous contrast enhancement. A peripheral hypointense rim was noted on all sequences, attributed to mineralization, hemorrhage, or cholesterol.

MR diagnosis of intracranial extension of a large nasal mucocele has been reported in a dog.[117] The mass was multilobulated and sharply marginated, hyperintense on T2-W and FLAIR images, isointense on T1-W images, with peripheral ring enhancement. Concurrent findings included mass effect and brain edema.

Meningeal Tumors

Meningiomas originate from the meningeal lining of the brain and are the most common brain tumors in dogs and cats.[110,118] They are typically single lesions, but multiple tumors may occasionally be found.[119] Meningiomas are typically in broad-based contact with underlying bone, have round/ovoid or plaquelike shape, are smoothly marginated, show expansile rather than infiltrative growth pattern, are hypointense to isointense on T1-W images, hyperintense on T2-W/FLAIR images, and show strong and homogeneous to heterogeneous contrast enhancement (**Fig. 10**).[66,108–110,118] Mineralization may be present, which is best demonstrated on T2*-W images. Possible concurrent findings include hyperostosis or pressure atrophy of adjacent bone, brain edema, and mass effect.[112,120] A "dural tail sign" (thickening and enhancement of the dura adjacent to an extra-axial mass) is frequently present and is strongly suggestive of meningioma.[121] Cystic meningiomas have been described and predominantly occur in the rostral cranial fossa.[122]

Other tumor types such as disseminated histiocytic sarcoma,[123] lymphoma,[110] granular cell tumor,[124] or metastases (meningeal carcinomatosis)[125] can affect the meninges and have variable appearance on MRI.

Glial Tumors

Glial tumors typically appear as single lesions. Astrocytomas are variable in appearance, with shapes ranging from an ovoid or amorphous mass to a diffuse infiltrate, with distinct to poorly defined margins.[66,108–110,112,126] Leptomeningeal involvement has been reported.[127] Lesions are hypointense to isointense on T1-W, and hyperintense

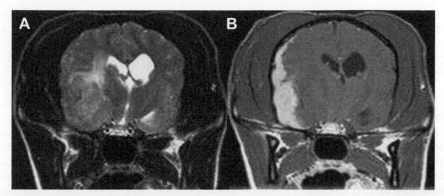

Fig. 10. Plaquelike meningioma in a dog. T2-W (*A*) and postcontrast T1-W (*B*) transverse images demonstrate a mass lesion extending along right temporal and parietal bone that is heterogeneously T2 hyperintense and shows strong homogeneous contrast enhancement. Edema is noted along the white-matter tracts. Deviation of the falx cerebri and compression of the right lateral ventricle are consistent with mass effect. Linear enhancement is noted at the periphery of the mass ("dural tail" sign).

on T2-W images, with contrast enhancement ranging from none to strong, with uniform, nonuniform, and ring-enhancing patterns. Concurrent brain edema is commonly seen.

MRI features of glioblastoma multiforme include heterogeneous increased T2 signal intensity with iso- to hypointense T1-W signal, sharp borders, necrosis, and peritumoral edema (**Fig. 11**).[128] Cyst formation is possible. Irregular margins and a pedunculated shape have been reported in 1 dog.[112] Ring enhancement is commonly seen.

Oligodendrogliomas appear as ovoid, indistinct, smooth to irregular masses, which are hypointense on T1-W and hyperintense on T2-W images, and are typically ring enhancing.[66,109,129,130] Concurrent edema is uncommon. Associated hemorrhage is common.[112]

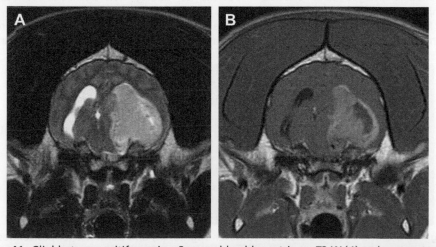

Fig. 11. Glioblastoma multiforme in a 2-year-old golden retriever. T2-W (*A*) and postcontrast T1-W (*B*) transverse images show a heterogeneously T2 hyperintense and inhomogeneously enhancing intra-axial mass with minimal mass effect and invasion of the left lateral ventricle.

Gliomatosis cerebri is a rare, tumorlike disease of glial cells, characterized by diffuse, widespread infiltration, with preservation of brain structures. MRI in a 9-year-old flat-coated retriever demonstrated ill-defined T2/FLAIR hyperintense non-contrast-enhancing areas associated with cerebral hemispheres, brainstem, and cerebellum.[131]

Ventricular Tumors

Choroid plexus tumors originate from the choroid plexus located within the ventricular system, and predominantly occur in the third and fourth ventricle. Choroid plexus papillomas (CPP) and choroid plexus carcinomas (CPC) are predominantly isointense to hyperintense on T1-W and T2-W images, typically with intense and homogeneous contrast enhancement (**Fig. 12**).[108,132] Signal heterogeneity can be observed secondary to cyst formation,[125] mineralization, hemorrhage, or necrosis. The most important feature in differentiating different tumor types is evidence of intraventricular or subarachnoid metastases detected in 35% of CPC but not in CPP.[132] Concurrent ventriculomegaly, perilesional, and periventricular edema are common.

Ependymal tumors (ependymomas) are derived from the lining epithelium of the ventricles and are uncommon in animals.[50] On MRI, ependymomas manifest as well-circumscribed smooth or lobulated tumors associated with the ventricular system. They are isointense on T1-W and hyperintense on T2-W images, show strong contrast enhancement, and are typically associated with hydrocephalus.[66,109,133]

Supraventricular location of meningiomas is common in cats, particularly involving the tela choroidea.[50] They are characterized by smooth margination, homogeneous contrast enhancement, and frequent hydrocephalus.

Primitive Neuroectodermal Tumors and Medulloblastomas

Primitive neuroectodermal tumors (PNETs) are a group of poorly differentiated neoplasms derived from primitive neuroectodermal cells.[50] MR findings in a dog with intracranial PNET include an ill-defined intra-axial mass, involving nasal sinus and frontal lobe, which was hypointense to isointense on T1-W images, hyperintense on T2-W images, and showed moderate to strong heterogeneous contrast enhancement.[112]

Medulloblastomas are malignant tumors occurring in young animals, which are almost exclusively located in the cerebellum.[50] On MRI, a medulloblastoma appears

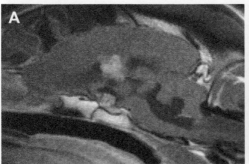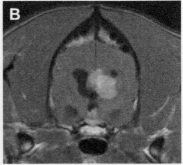

Fig. 12. CPC in a 4-year-old Labrador retriever. Sagittal (*A*) and transverse (*B*) postcontrast T1-W images show an irregularly marginated, strongly contrast-enhancing mass associated with the third ventricle and extending into the left lateral ventricle, with associated hydrocephalus. An additional smaller mass is observed associated with the third ventricle cranial and dorsal to the pituitary gland, which likely represents a metastasis.

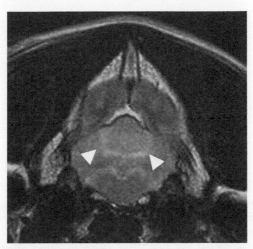

Fig. 13. Medulloblastoma in a 3-year-old mixed breed dog. Transverse FLAIR image shows indistinct T2 hyperintensity associated with the cerebellar vermis (*arrowheads*). No additional abnormalities were detected on other MR sequences.

as a heterogeneous cerebellar mass that is predominantly isointense to hypointense on T1-W images, hyperintense on T2-W images, and shows mild to strong contrast enhancement (**Fig. 13**).[134–136] Concurrent hemorrhage or cysts are possible.

Other CNS Tumors

MR findings have been reported in CNS lymphoma in dogs[112] and cats,[110] and disseminated histiocytic sarcoma in dogs.[112,123,137] Lesions can appear as ill- or well-defined, single or multifocal, intra-axial or extra-axial masses. These are typically isointense to hypointense on T1-W images and hyperintense on T2-W images, show moderate to strong contrast enhancement, and may be associated with edema and mass effect (**Fig. 14**). In cats with extra-axial lymphoma and dogs with extra-axial

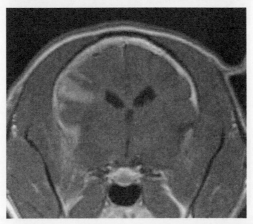

Fig. 14. Disseminated histiocytic sarcoma of the brain in an 11-year-old Norwich terrier. Transverse T1-W postcontrast image shows extensive meningeal and multifocal parenchymal enhancement of the right parietal and temporal lobes. (*Courtesy of* Dr Andrea Matthews, University of Tennessee, USA).

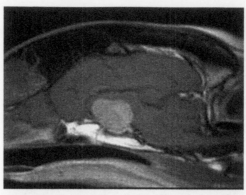

Fig. 15. Pituitary macroadenoma in a dog. Sagittal T1-W postcontrast image shows a smoothly marginated, homogeneously enhancing mass extending dorsally from the pituitary fossa.

histiocytic sarcoma, a "dural tail sign" has been reported after contrast medium administration,[110,123] mimicking a common finding in meningiomas.

Granular cell tumor is a descriptive term for a heterogeneous group of tumors. Intracranial granular cell tumors can be intra- or extra-axial, are typically hyperintense on T2-W images, and show strong contrast enhancement.[124,138,139] Concurrent finding include mass effect, transcalvarial extension, and meningeal enhancement.

CNS-associated Tumors

Pituitary tumors are characterized by their typical position in the pituitary fossa, which is best demonstrated on sagittal images (**Fig. 15**).[66,108,109,140] Pituitary microadenomas may not be readily apparent on conventional MR sequences,[141] and dynamic studies or specific thin-slice sections might be necessary to establish a diagnosis. Pituitary macroadenomas usually appear as well-circumscribed expansile T1 iso- to hypointense and T2/FLAIR hyperintense masses with strong contrast enhancement.

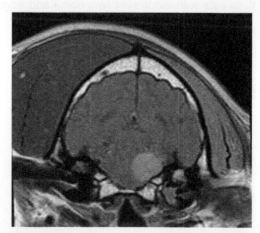

Fig. 16. Trigeminal nerve sheath tumor in a 6-year-old Labrador retriever. Transverse T1-W postcontrast image demonstrates a rounded, smoothly marginated, contrast-enhancing mass associated with the left brainstem. There is atrophy of the left temporalis and masseter muscles. A small amount of material isointense to soft tissue is present within the left tympanic bulla.

Pituitary hemorrhage may occur, resulting in susceptibility artifacts on gradient re-called echo (GRE) T2*-W images and alteration of signal intensity of the mass on pre- and postcontrast images. Pituitary carcinomas show more invasive growth than adenomas, and may invade adjacent basisphenoid bone and pharynx. They are typically inhomogeneous and show nonuniform contrast enhancement.

Craniopharyngiomas originate from remnants of the craniopharyngeal duct ectoderm, which are located above the sella turcica and, by expansion, compress the pituitary gland, optic chiasma, and hypothalamus.[50] MRI examination in 2 cats revealed large masses at the skull base, with extensive bone lysis and cerebral displacement.[142]

Trigeminal nerve sheath tumors are not uncommon in dogs.[50] MRI features include an extra-axial solitary or lobulated mass in the middle or caudal fossa which is typically isointense on T1-W images, isointense or hyperintense on T2-W images, and shows contrast enhancement (**Fig. 16**).[44,143] Atrophy of the temporalis and masseter muscles with increase in signal intensity of these muscles on T1-W images is typically present. Possible additional findings include distortion of the adjacent brain stem and enlarged skull foramina.

Nasal tumors (eg, adenocarcinoma, squamous cell carcinoma, chondrosarcoma, neuroesthesioblastoma) may invade the brain through the cribriform plate. Imaging findings include nasal masses of variable size, intensity, and contrast enhancement, with destruction of cribriform plate and intracranial extension of nasal mass. Cystic/necrotic areas associated with the tumor, and brain edema, are frequently present (**Fig. 17**).[110,144–147]

Tumors of the skull, such as multilobular osteochondrosarcoma or masses origi-nating from adjacent structures, may also extend into the cranial vault.[148]

Metastatic CNS Tumors

Many primary tumors, including hemangiosarcomas and carcinomas, have the poten-tial for wide dissemination, including spread to the CNS.[50,111] Metastases can appear

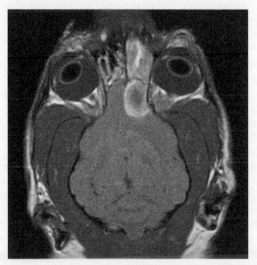

Fig. 17. Nasal squamous cell carcinoma in a 10-year-old miniature pinscher. Dorsal postcon-trast T1-W image shows a heterogeneously enhancing mass within the left nasal cavity, with turbinate destruction and invasion of the olfactory bulb through the cribriform plate.

as single or multiple lesions associated with brain parenchyma or meninges, often with associated brain edema. They are commonly rounded to ovoid, appear iso- to hypointense on T1-W images, and hyperintense on T2-W images.[66] Hemangiosarcoma metastases may be associated with hemorrhage. Strong and homogeneous or ring enhancement are commonly noted.

REFERENCES

1. Thomas WB. Nonneoplastic disorders of the brain. Clin Tech Small Anim Pract 1999;14(3):125–47.
2. Bohn AA, Wills TB, West CL, et al. Cerebrospinal fluid analysis and magnetic resonance imaging in the diagnosis of neurologic disease in dogs: a retrospective study. Vet Clin Pathol 2006;35(3):315–20.
3. Lamb CR, Croson PJ, Cappello R, et al. Magnetic resonance imaging findings in 25 dogs with inflammatory cerebrospinal fluid. Vet Radiol Ultrasound 2005;46(1):17–22.
4. Negrin A, Lamb CR, Cappello R, et al. Results of magnetic resonance imaging in 14 cats with meningoencephalitis. J Feline Med Surg 2007;9(2):109–16.
5. Cherubini GB, Platt SR, Howson S, et al. Comparison of magnetic resonance imaging sequences in dogs with multi-focal intracranial disease. J Small Anim Pract 2008;49(12):634–40.
6. Mellema LM, Samii VF, Vernau KM, et al. Meningeal enhancement on magnetic resonance imaging in 15 dogs and 3 cats. Vet Radiol Ultrasound 2002;43(1):10–5.
7. Bathen-Noethen A, Stein VM, Puff C, et al. Magnetic resonance imaging findings in acute canine distemper virus infection. J Small Anim Pract 2008;49(9):460–7.
8. Griffin JF, Young BD, Levine JM. Imaging diagnosis - canine chronic distemper meningoencephalitis. Vet Radiol Ultrasound 2009;50(2):182–4.
9. Foley JE, Lapointe JM, Koblik P, et al. Diagnostic features of clinical neurologic feline infectious peritonitis. J Vet Intern Med 1998;12(6):415–23.
10. Braund KG. Inflammatory diseases of the central nervous system. In: Braund KG, editor. Clinical neurology in small animals – localization, diagnosis and treatment. Ithaca (NY): International Veterinary Information Service; 2003. p. 1–45.
11. Mateo I, Lorenzo V, Munoz A, et al. Brainstem abscess due to plant foreign body in a dog. J Vet Intern Med 2007;21(3):535–8.
12. Smith PM, Haughland SP, Jeffery ND. Brain abscess in a dog immunosuppressed using cyclosporin. Vet J 2007;173(3):675–8.
13. Bach JF, Mahony OM, Tidwell AS, et al. Brain abscess and bacterial endocarditis in a Kerry Blue Terrier with a history of immune-mediated thrombocytopenia. J Vet Emerg Critl Care 2007;17(4):409–15.
14. Barrs VR, Nicoll RG, Churcher RK, et al. Intracranial empyema: literature review and two novel cases in cats. J Small Anim Pract 2007;48(8):449–54.
15. Sturges BK, Dickinson PJ, Kortz GD, et al. Clinical signs, magnetic resonance imaging features, and outcome after surgical and medical treatment of otogenic intracranial infection in 11 cats and 4 dogs. J Vet Intern Med 2006;20(3):648–56.
16. Seiler G, Cizinauskas S, Scheidegger J, et al. Low-field magnetic resonance imaging of a pyocephalus and a suspected brain abscess in a German Shepherd dog. Vet Radiol Ultrasound 2001;42(5):417–22.
17. Lavely J, Lipsitz D. Fungal infections of the central nervous system in the dog and cat. Clin Tech Small Anim Pract 2005;20(4):212–9.

18. Stevenson TL, Dickinson PJ, Sturges BK, et al. Magnetic resonance imaging of intracranial cryptococcosis in dogs and cats. Proceedings. Minneapolis (MN): ACVIM June 9–12, 2004.

19. Foster SF, Charles JA, Parker G, et al. Cerebral cryptococcal granuloma in a cat. J Feline Med Surg 2001;3(1):39–44.

20. O'Toole TE, Sato AF, Rozanski EA. Cryptococcosis of the central nervous system in a dog. J Am Vet Med Assoc 2003;222(12):1722–5.

21. Windsor RC, Sturges BK, Vernau KM, et al. Cerebrospinal fluid eosinophilia in dogs. J Vet Intern Med 2009;23(2):275–81.

22. Anor S, Sturges BK, Lafranco L, et al. Systemic phaeohyphomycosis (*Cladophialophora bantiana*) in a dog – clinical diagnosis with stereotactic computed tomographic-guided brain biopsy. J Vet Intern Med 2001;15(3):257–61.

23. Hecht S, Adams WH, Smith JR, et al. CT and MRI findings in intracranial fungal disease in dogs and cats. Proceedings 15th Congress of the International Veterinary Radiology Association. Buzios (Brazil): July 26–31, 2009.

24. Dewey CW. Encephalopathies: disorders of the brain. In: Dewey CW, editor. A practical guide to canine and feline neurology. Ames (IA): Iowa State Press; 2003. p. 99–178.

25. Garosi LS, Platt SR, McConnell JF, et al. Intracranial haemorrhage associated with *Angiostrongylus vasorum* infection in three dogs. J Small Anim Pract 2005;46(2):93–9.

26. Negrin A, Cherubini GB, Steeves E. *Angiostrongylus vasorum* causing meningitis and detection of parasite larvae in the cerebrospinal fluid of a pug dog. J Small Anim Pract 2008;49(9):468–71.

27. Wessmann A, Lu D, Lamb CR, et al. Brain and spinal cord haemorrhages associated with *Angiostrongylus vasorum* infection in four dogs. Vet Rec 2006; 158(25):858–63.

28. Higginbotham MJ, Kent M, Glass EN. Noninfectious inflammatory central nervous system diseases in dogs. Compend Contin Educ Vet 2007;29(8):488–97.

29. Braund KG. Granulomatous meningoencephalomyelitis. J Am Vet Med Assoc 1985;186(2):138–41.

30. Cherubini GB, Platt SR, Anderson TJ, et al. Characteristics of magnetic resonance images of granulomatous meningoencephalomyelitis in 11 dogs. Vet Rec 2006;159(4):110–5.

31. Kitagawa M, Kanayama K, Satoh T, et al. Cerebellar focal granulomatous meningoencephalitis in a dog: clinical findings and MR imaging. J Vet Med A Physiol Pathol Clin Med 2004;51(6):277–9.

32. Lobetti RG, Pearson J. Magnetic resonance imaging in the diagnosis of focal granulomatous meningoencephalitis in two dogs. Vet Radiol Ultrasound 1996; 37(6):424–7.

33. Cordy DR, Holliday TA. A necrotizing meningoencephalitis of pug dogs. Vet Pathol 1989;26(3):191–4.

34. Stalis IH, Chadwick B, Dayrell-Hart B, et al. Necrotizing meningoencephalitis of Maltese dogs. Vet Pathol 1995;32(3):230–5.

35. Higgins RJ, Dickinson PJ, Kube SA, et al. Necrotizing meningoencephalitis in five Chihuahua dogs. Vet Pathol 2008;45(3):336–46.

36. Cantile C, Chianini F, Arispici M, et al. Necrotizing meningoencephalitis associated with cortical hippocampal hamartia in a Pekingese dog. Vet Pathol 2001; 38(1):119–22.

37. Timmann D, Konar M, Howard J, et al. Necrotising encephalitis in a French bulldog. J Small Anim Pract 2007;48(6):339–42.

38. Flegel T, Henke D, Boettcher IC, et al. Magnetic resonance imaging findings in histologically confirmed Pug dog encephalitis. Vet Radiol Ultrasound 2008; 49(5):419–24.
39. Jull BA, Merryman JI, Thomas WB, et al. Necrotizing encephalitis in a Yorkshire terrier. J Am Vet Med Assoc 1997;211(8):1005–7.
40. Lotti D, Capucchio MT, Gaidolfi E, et al. Necrotizing encephalitis in a Yorkshire terrier: clinical, imaging, and pathologic findings. Vet Radiol Ultrasound 1999; 40(6):622–6.
41. Sawashima Y, Sawashima K, Taura Y, et al. Clinical and pathological findings of a Yorkshire terrier affected with necrotizing encephalitis. J Vet Med Sci 1996; 58(7):659–61.
42. von Praun F, Matiasek K, Grevel V, et al. Magnetic resonance imaging and pathologic findings associated with necrotizing encephalitis in two Yorkshire terriers. Vet Radiol Ultrasound 2006;47(3):260–4.
43. Kuwabara M, Tanaka S, Fujiwara K. Magnetic resonance imaging and histopathology of encephalitis in a Pug. J Vet Med Sci 1998;60(12):1353–5.
44. Schultz RM, Tucker RL, Gavin PR, et al. Magnetic resonance imaging of acquired trigeminal nerve disorders in six dogs. Vet Radiol Ultrasound 2007; 48(2):101–4.
45. National Institute of Neurological Disorders and Stroke. Special report from the National Institute of Neurological Disorders and Stroke. Classification of cerebrovascular diseases III. Stroke 1990;21(4):637–76.
46. Terbrugge KG, Rao KCVG. Intracranial aneurysms and vascular malformations. In: Lee SH, Rao KCVG, Zimmerman RA, editors. Cranial MRI and CT. 4th edition. New York: McGraw-Hill; 1999. p. 517–56.
47. Ozsarlak O, Van Goethem JW, Maes M, et al. MR angiography of the intracranial vessels: technical aspects and clinical applications. Neuroradiology 2004; 46(12):955–72.
48. Tidwell AS, Ross LA, Kleine LJ. Computed tomography and magnetic resonance imaging of cavernous sinus enlargement in a dog with unilateral exophthalmos. Vet Radiol Ultrasound 1997;38(5):363–70.
49. McCormick WF. Pathology of vascular malformations of the brain. In: Wilson CB, Stein BM, editors. Intracranial arteriovenous malformations of the brain. Baltimore (MD): Williams and Wilkins; 1984. p. 44–63.
50. Summers BA, Cummings JF, de Lahunta A. Veterinary neuropathology. St. Louis (MO): Mosby; 1995.
51. Joseph RJ, Greenlee PG, Carrillo JM, et al. Canine cerebrovascular disease. Findings in 17 cases. J Am Anim Hosp Assoc 1988;24:569–76.
52. Irwin JC, Dewey CW, Stefanacci JD. Suspected cerebellar infarcts in 4 dogs. J Vet Emerg Crit Care 2007;17(3):268–74.
53. Garosi L, McConnell JE, Platt SR, et al. Results of diagnostic investigations and long-term outcome of 33 dogs with brain infarction (2000–2004). J Vet Intern Med 2005;19(5):725–31.
54. Kent M, Delahunta A, Tidwell AS. MR imaging findings in a dog with intravascular lymphoma in the brain. Vet Radiol Ultrasound 2001;42(6):504–10.
55. Bush WW, Throop JL, McManus PM, et al. Intravascular lymphoma involving the central and peripheral nervous systems in a dog. J Am Anim Hosp Assoc 2003; 39(1):90–6.
56. Cachin M, Vandevelde M. Cerebral infarction associated with septic thromboemboli in the dog. Proceedings 8th Annual Meeting of the Veterinary Medicine Forum. Washington, DC: May 10, 1990.

57. Axlund TW, Isaacs AM, Holland M, et al. Fibrocartilaginous embolic encephalo-myelopathy of the brainstem and midcervical spinal cord in a dog. J Vet Intern Med 2004;18(5):765–7.
58. Kotani T, Tomimura T, Ogura M, et al. Cerebral infarction caused by *Dirofilaria immitis* in three dogs. Jpn J Vet Sci 1975;37:379–90.
59. Kalimo H, Kaste M, Haltia M. Vascular diseases. In: Graham DI, Lantos PL, editors. Greenfield's neuropathology. 7th edition. London: Arnold; 2002. p. 233–80.
60. McConnell JF, Garosi L, Platt SR. Magnetic resonance imaging findings of presumed cerebellar cerebrovascular accident in twelve dogs. Vet Radiol Ultrasound 2005;46(1):1–10.
61. Schellinger PD, Fiebach JB, Hacke W. Imaging-based decision making in thrombolytic therapy for ischemic stroke: present status. Stroke 2003;34(2):575–83.
62. Crawley AP, Poublanc J, Ferrari P, et al. Basics of diffusion and perfusion MRI. Appl Radiol 2003;32(4):13–23.
63. Thomas WB, Sorjonen DC, Scheuler RO, et al. Magnetic resonance imaging of brain infarction in seven dogs. Vet Radiol Ultrasound 1996;37(5):345–50.
64. Garosi L, McConnell JF, Platt SR, et al. Clinical and topographic magnetic resonance characteristics of suspected brain infarction in 40 dogs. J Vet Intern Med 2006;20(2):311–21.
65. Garosi LS, McConnell JF. Ischaemic stroke in dogs and humans: a comparative review. J Small Anim Pract 2005;46(11):521–9.
66. Kraft SL, Gavin PR. Intracranial neoplasia. Clin Tech Small Anim Pract 1999; 14(2):112–23.
67. Whitley NT, Corzo-Menendez N, Carmichael NG, et al. Cerebral and conjunctival haemorrhages associated with von Willebrand factor deficiency and canine angiostrongylosis. J Small Anim Pract 2005;46(2):75–8.
68. Bradley WG Jr. MR appearance of hemorrhage in the brain. Radiology 1993; 189(1):15–26.
69. Parizel PM, Makkat S, Van Miert E, et al. Intracranial hemorrhage: principles of CT and MRI interpretation. Eur Radiol 2001;11(9):1770–83.
70. Liang L, Korogi Y, Sugahara T, et al. Detection of intracranial hemorrhage with susceptibility-weighted MR sequences. Am J Neuroradiol 1999;20(8):1527–34.
71. Tidwell AS. Principles of computed tomography and magnetic resonance imaging. In: Thrall DE, editor. Textbook of veterinary diagnostic radiology. 5th edition. St. Louis (MO): Saunders Elsevier; 2007. p. 50–77.
72. Anzalone N, Scotti R, Riva R. Neuroradiologic differential diagnosis of cerebral intraparenchymal hemorrhage. Neurol Sci 2004;25(Suppl 1):S3–5.
73. Williams KJ, Summers BA, de Lahunta A. Cerebrospinal cuterebriasis in cats and its association with feline ischemic encephalopathy. Vet Pathol 1998; 35(5):330–43.
74. Quesnel AD, Parent JM, McDonell W, et al. Diagnostic evaluation of cats with seizure disorders: 30 cases (1991–1993). J Am Vet Med Assoc 1997;210(1): 65–71.
75. White BC, Grossman LI, O'Neil BJ, et al. Global brain ischemia and reperfusion. Ann Emerg Med 1996;27(5):588–94.
76. Timm K, Flegel T, Oechtering G. Sequential magnetic resonance imaging changes after suspected global brain ischaemia in a dog. J Small Anim Pract 2008;49(8):408–12.
77. Panarello GP, Dewey CW, Baroni G, et al. Magnetic resonance imaging of two suspected cases of global brain ischemia. J Vet Emerg Crit Care 2004;14(4): 269–77.

78. Wenger DA, Victoria T, Rafi MA, et al. Globoid cell leukodystrophy in cairn and West Highland white terriers. J Hered 1999;90(1):138–42.
79. Cozzi F, Vite CH, Wenger DA, et al. MRI and electrophysiological abnormalities in a case of canine globoid cell leucodystrophy. J Small Anim Pract 1998;39(8): 401–5.
80. Matsuki N, Yamato O, Kusuda M, et al. Magnetic resonance imaging of GM2-gangliosidosis in a golden retriever. Can Vet J 2005;46(3):275–8.
81. Kaye EM, Alroy J, Raghavan SS, et al. Dysmyelinogenesis in animal model of GM1 gangliosidosis. Pediatr Neurol 1992;8(4):255–61.
82. Koie H, Shibuya H, Sato T, et al. Magnetic resonance imaging of neuronal ceroid lipofuscinosis in a border collie. J Vet Med Sci 2004;66(11):1453–6.
83. Armstrong D, Quisling RG, Webb A, et al. Computed tomographic and nuclear magnetic resonance correlation of canine ceroid-lipofuscinosis with aging. Neurobiol Aging 1983;4(4):297–303.
84. Vite CH, Magnitsky S, Aleman D, et al. Apparent diffusion coefficient reveals gray and white matter disease, and T2 mapping detects white matter disease in the brain in feline alpha-mannosidosis. Am J Neuroradiol 2008; 29(2):308–13.
85. Vite CH, McGowan JC, Braund KG, et al. Histopathology, electrodiagnostic testing, and magnetic resonance imaging show significant peripheral and central nervous system myelin abnormalities in the cat model of alpha-mannosidosis. J Neuropathol Exp Neurol 2001;60(8):817–28.
86. Ellinwood NM, Wang P, Skeen T, et al. A model of mucopolysaccharidosis IIIB (Sanfilippo syndrome type IIIB): N-acetyl-alpha-D-glucosaminidase deficiency in Schipperke dogs. J Inherit Metab Dis 2003;26(5):489–504.
87. Abramson CJ, Platt SR, Jakobs C, et al. L-2-Hydroxyglutaric aciduria in Staffordshire bull terriers. J Vet Intern Med 2003;17(4):551–6.
88. Brenner O, de Lahunta A, Summers BA, et al. Hereditary polioencephalomyelopathy of the Australian cattle dog. Acta Neuropathol 1997;94(1):54–66.
89. Brenner O, Wakshlag JJ, Summers BA, et al. Alaskan husky encephalopathy – a canine neurodegenerative disorder resembling subacute necrotizing encephalomyelopathy (Leigh syndrome). Acta Neuropathol 2000;100(1):50–62.
90. Wakshlag JJ, de Lahunta A, Robinson T, et al. Subacute necrotising encephalopathy in an Alaskan husky. J Small Anim Pract 1999;40(12):585–9.
91. Harkin KR, Goggin JM, DeBey BM, et al. Magnetic resonance imaging of the brain of a dog with hereditary polioencephalomyelopathy. J Am Vet Med Assoc 1999;214(9):1342–4.
92. Torisu S, Washizu M, Hasegawa D, et al. Brain magnetic resonance imaging characteristics in dogs and cats with congenital portosystemic shunts. Vet Radiol Ultrasound 2005;46(6):447–51.
93. Garosi LS, Dennis R, Platt SR, et al. Thiamine deficiency in a dog: clinical, clinicopathologic, and magnetic resonance imaging findings. J Vet Intern Med 2003;17(5):719–23.
94. Singh M, Thompson M, Sullivan N, et al. Thiamine deficiency in dogs due to the feeding of sulphite preserved meat. Aust Vet J 2005;83(7):412–7.
95. Penderis J, McConnell JF, Calvin J. Magnetic resonance imaging features of thiamine deficiency in a cat. Vet Rec 2007;160(8):270–2.
96. Ashrafian H, Davey P. A review of the causes of central pontine myelinosis: yet another apoptotic illness? Eur J Neurol 2001;8(2):103–9.
97. O'Brien DP, Kroll RA, Johnson GC, et al. Myelinolysis after correction of hyponatremia in two dogs. J Vet Intern Med 1994;8(1):40–8.

98. Mariani CL, Clemmons RM, Graham JP, et al. Magnetic resonance imaging of spongy degeneration of the central nervous system in a Labrador retriever. Vet Radiol Ultrasound 2001;42(4):285–90.
99. Tamura S, Tamura Y, Uchida K. Magnetic resonance imaging findings of neuroaxonal dystrophy in a papillon puppy. J Small Anim Pract 2007;48(8): 458–61.
100. Flegel T, Matiasek K, Henke D, et al. Cerebellar cortical degeneration with selective granule cell loss in Bavarian mountain dogs. J Small Anim Pract 2007;48(8): 462–5.
101. Henke D, Bottcher P, Doherr MG, et al. Computer-assisted magnetic resonance imaging brain morphometry in American Staffordshire terriers with cerebellar cortical degeneration. J Vet Intern Med 2008;22(4):969–75.
102. Nibe K, Kita C, Morozumi M, et al. Clinicopathological features of canine neuroaxonal dystrophy and cerebellar cortical abiotrophy in Papillon and Papillon-related dogs. J Vet Med Sci 2007;69(10):1047–52.
103. Olby N, Blot S, Thibaud JL, et al. Cerebellar cortical degeneration in adult American Staffordshire terriers. J Vet Intern Med 2004;18(2):201–8.
104. van der Merwe LL, Lane E. Diagnosis of cerebellar cortical degeneration in a Scottish terrier using magnetic resonance imaging. J Small Anim Pract 2001;42(8):409–12.
105. Olby N, Munana K, De Risio L, et al. Cervical injury following a horse kick to the head in two dogs. J Am Anim Hosp Assoc 2002;38(4):321–6.
106. Adamo PF, Crawford JT, Stepien RL. Subdural hematoma of the brainstem in a dog: magnetic resonance findings and treatment. J Am Anim Hosp Assoc 2005;41(6):400–5.
107. Kitagawa M, Okada M, Kanayama K, et al. Traumatic intracerebral hematoma in a dog: MR images and clinical findings. J Vet Med Sci 2005;67(8):843–6.
108. Thomas WB, Wheeler SJ, Kramer R, et al. Magnetic resonance imaging features of primary brain tumors in dogs. Vet Radiol Ultrasound 1996;37(1):20–7.
109. Kraft SL, Gavin PR, DeHaan C, et al. Retrospective review of 50 canine intracranial tumors evaluated by magnetic resonance imaging. J Vet Intern Med 1997; 11(4):218–25.
110. Troxel MT, Vite CH, Massicotte C, et al. Magnetic resonance imaging features of feline intracranial neoplasia: retrospective analysis of 46 cats. J Vet Intern Med 2004;18(2):176–89.
111. Snyder JM, Lipitz L, Skorupski KA, et al. Secondary intracranial neoplasia in the dog: 177 cases (1986–2003). J Vet Intern Med 2008;22(1):172–7.
112. Snyder JM, Shofer FS, Van Winkle TJ, et al. Canine intracranial primary neoplasia: 173 cases (1986–2003). J Vet Intern Med 2006;20(3):669–75.
113. Stalin CE, Granger N, Jeffery ND. Cerebellar vascular hamartoma in a British shorthair cat. J Feline Med Surg 2008;10(2):206–11.
114. Schoeman JP, Stidworthy MF, Penderis J, et al. Magnetic resonance imaging of a cerebral cavernous haemangioma in a dog. J S Afr Vet Assoc 2002;73(4): 207–10.
115. Lorenzo V, Pumarola M, Munoz A. Meningioangiomatosis in a dog: magnetic resonance imaging and neuropathological studies. J Small Anim Pract 1998; 39(10):486–9.
116. Fluehmann G, Konar M, Jaggy A, et al. Cerebral cholesterol granuloma in a cat. J Vet Intern Med 2006;20(5):1241–4.
117. Sessums KB, Lane SB. Imaging diagnosis: intracranial mucocele in a dog. Vet Radiol Ultrasound 2008;49(6):564–6.

118. Sturges BK, Dickinson PJ, Bollen AW, et al. Magnetic resonance imaging and histological classification of intracranial meningiomas in 112 dogs. J Vet Intern Med 2008;22(3):586–95.

119. Forterre F, Tomek A, Konar M, et al. Multiple meningiomas: clinical, radiological, surgical, and pathological findings with outcome in four cats. J Feline Med Surg 2007;9(1):36–43.

120. Hathcock JT. Low field magnetic resonance imaging characteristics of cranial vault meningiomas in 13 dogs. Vet Radiol Ultrasound 1996;37(4): 257–63.

121. Graham JP, Newell SM, Voges AK, et al. The dural tail sign in the diagnosis of meningiomas. Vet Radiol Ultrasound 1998;39(4):297–302.

122. Johnson LM, Hecht S, Arendse AU, et al. What is your diagnosis? Cystic meningioma. J Am Vet Med Assoc 2007;231(6):861–2.

123. Tamura S, Tamura Y, Nakamoto Y, et al. MR imaging of histiocytic sarcoma of the canine brain. Vet Radiol Ultrasound 2009;50(2):178–81.

124. Sharkey LC, McDonnell JJ, Alroy J. Cytology of a mass on the meningeal surface of the left brain in a dog. Vet Clin Pathol 2004;33(2):111–4.

125. Lipsitz D, Levitski RE, Chauvet AE. Magnetic resonance imaging of a choroid plexus carcinoma and meningeal carcinomatosis in a dog. Vet Radiol Ultrasound 1999;40(3):246–50.

126. Kube SA, Bruyette DS, Hanson SM. Astrocytomas in young dogs. J Am Anim Hosp Assoc 2003;39(3):288–93.

127. Kraft SL, Gavin PR, Leathers CW, et al. Diffuse cerebral and leptomeningeal astrocytoma in dogs: MR features. J Comput Assist Tomogr 1990;14(4):555–60.

128. Lipsitz D, Higgins RJ, Kortz GD, et al. Glioblastoma multiforme: clinical findings, magnetic resonance imaging, and pathology in five dogs. Vet Pathol 2003; 40(6):659–69.

129. Stacy BA, Stevenson TL, Lipsitz D, et al. Simultaneously occurring oligodendroglioma and meningioma in a dog. J Vet Intern Med 2003;17(3):357–9.

130. Dickinson PJ, Keel MK, Higgins RJ, et al. Clinical and pathologic features of oligodendrogliomas in two cats. Vet Pathol 2000;37(2):160–7.

131. Gruber A, Leschnik M, Kneissl S, et al. Gliomatosis cerebri in a dog. J Vet Med A Physiol Pathol Clin Med 2006;53(8):435–8.

132. Westworth DR, Dickinson PJ, Vernau W, et al. Choroid plexus tumors in 56 dogs (1985–2007). J Vet Intern Med 2008;22(5):1157–65.

133. Vural SA, Besalti O, Ilhan F, et al. Ventricular ependymoma in a German Shepherd dog. Vet J 2006;172(1):185–7.

134. MacKillop E, Thrall DE, Ranck RS, et al. Imaging diagnosis – synchronous primary brain tumors in a dog. Vet Radiol Ultrasound 2007;48(6):550–3.

135. McConnell JF, Platt S, Smith KC. Magnetic resonance imaging findings of an intracranial medulloblastoma in a Polish lowland sheepdog. Vet Radiol Ultrasound 2004;45(1):17–22.

136. Kitagawa M, Koie H, Kanayamat K, et al. Medulloblastoma in a cat: clinical and MRI findings. J Small Anim Pract 2003;44(3):139–42.

137. Tzipory L, Vernau KM, Sturges BK, et al. Antemortem diagnosis of localized central nervous system histiocytic sarcoma in 2 dogs. J Vet Intern Med 2009; 23(2):369–74.

138. Higgins RJ, LeCouteur RA, Vernau KM, et al. Granular cell tumor of the canine central nervous system: two cases. Vet Pathol 2001;38(6):620–7.

139. Liu CH, Liu CI, Liang SL, et al. Intracranial granular cell tumor in a dog. J Vet Med Sci 2004;66(1):77–9.

140. Duesberg CA, Feldman EC, Nelson RW, et al. Magnetic resonance imaging for diagnosis of pituitary macrotumors in dogs. J Am Vet Med Assoc 1995;206(5): 657–62.

141. Wood FD, Pollard RE, Uerling MR, et al. Diagnostic imaging findings and endocrine test results in dogs with pituitary-dependent hyperadrenocorticism that did or did not have neurologic abnormalities: 157 cases (1989–2005). J Am Vet Med Assoc 2007;231(7):1081–5.

142. Nagata T, Nakayama H, Uchida K, et al. Two cases of feline malignant craniopharyngioma. Vet Pathol 2005;42(5):663–5.

143. Bagley RS, Wheeler SJ, Klopp L, et al. Clinical features of trigeminal nerve-sheath tumor in 10 dogs. J Am Anim Hosp Assoc 1998;34(1):19–25.

144. Avner A, Dobson JM, Sales JI, et al. Retrospective review of 50 canine nasal tumours evaluated by low-field magnetic resonance imaging. J Small Anim Pract 2008;49(5):233–9.

145. Kitagawa M, Okada M, Yamamura H, et al. Diagnosis of olfactory neuroblastoma in a dog by magnetic resonance imaging. Vet Rec 2006;159(9):288–9.

146. Miles MS, Dhaliwal RS, Moore MP, et al. Association of magnetic resonance imaging findings and histologic diagnosis in dogs with nasal disease: 78 cases (2001–2004). J Am Vet Med Assoc 2008;232(12):1844–9.

147. Moore MP, Gavin PR, Kraft SL, et al. MR, CT and clinical features from four dogs with nasal tumors involving the rostral cerebrum. Vet Radiol 1991;32(1):19–25.

148. Lipsitz D, Levitski RE, Berry WL. Magnetic resonance imaging features of multilobular osteochondrosarcoma in 3 dogs. Vet Radiol Ultrasound 2001;42(1): 14–9.

Cerebrovascular Disease in Dogs and Cats

Laurent S. Garosi, DVM, MRCVS

KEYWORDS

• Stroke • Neurology • Dog • Cat

The term "cerebrovascular disease" is defined as any abnormality of the brain resulting from a pathologic process compromising its blood supply.[1] Pathologic processes of the blood vessel include occlusion of the lumen by a thrombus or embolus, rupture of a blood vessel wall, lesion or altered permeability of the vessel wall, and increased viscosity or other changes in the quality of the blood.[2] Cerebrovascular accident (CVA), also known as stroke, is the most common clinical presentation of cerebrovascular disease, defined as a sudden onset of nonconvulsive and nonprogressive focal brain signs secondary to cerebrovascular disease.[3] By convention, these signs must remain for more than 24 hours to qualify for the diagnosis of CVA, which is usually associated with permanent damage to the brain. If the clinical signs resolve within 24 hours, the episode is called a transient ischemic attack (TIA).[4]

CAUSES AND PATHOPHYSIOLOGY

From a pathologic point of view, the lesions affecting the cerebral blood vessels are divided into 2 broad categories, ischemic stroke and hemorrhagic stroke. Ischemic strokes result from occlusion of a cerebral blood vessel by a thrombus or embolism, depriving the brain of oxygen and glucose. Hemorrhagic strokes result from rupture of a blood vessel wall within the brain parenchyma or subarachnoid space, causing bleeding into or around the brain (**Fig. 1**).[2]

Ischemic Strokes

Ischemic strokes have been reported infrequently in the veterinary medical literature when compared with the human medical literature.[5–23] Most reports have been based on postmortem results in dogs that died or were euthanized as a result of the severity of the ischemic stroke or the suspected underlying cause of the stroke. This limitation may affect the prevalence and type of underlying causes, as it is likely that only the most severely affected dogs, or dogs in which infarction

Davies Veterinary Specialists, Manor Farm Business Park, SG5 3HR Higham Gobion, England, UK
E-mail address: lsg@vetspecialists.co.uk

Vet Clin Small Anim 40 (2010) 65–79
doi:10.1016/j.cvsm.2009.09.001
0195-5616/09/$ – see front matter © 2010 Elsevier Inc. All rights reserved.

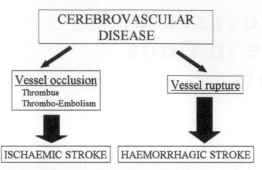

Fig. 1. Causes of cerebrovascular disease in dogs and cats.

occurred secondarily to a disease with a poor prognosis, would die or be euthanized. Suspected underlying causes identified in histopathologically confirmed cases include: septic thromboemboli associated with bacterial endocarditis or other sources of infection[13,24]; atherosclerosis associated with primary hypothyroidism and Miniature Schnauzers with hyperlipoproteinemia[8,9,11,25,26]; aberrant parasite migration (*Cuterebra*)[27,28] or parasitic emboli (*Dirofilaria immitis*)[6,7]; embolic metastatic tumor cells[11]; intravascular lymphoma[17]; fibrocartilaginous embolism[20]; and aortic or cardiac thromboembolism.[22,23]

In the author's study of magnetic resonance imaging (MRI) of dogs with brain infarct, a concurrent medical condition was detected in just over 50% of dogs, most commonly hyperadrenocorticism, chronic kidney disease, hypothyroidism, and hypertension.[22] The most commonly suspected causes of hypertension were chronic kidney disease and hyperadrenocorticism.[22] In human patients, infarcts of unknown cause are referred to as cryptogenic infarcts.[1] No age, sex, or breed predisposition was identified in that study, although Cavalier King Charles Spaniels (CKCS) and Greyhounds were overrepresented.[22]

Reports of ischemic strokes in cats are scarce. The term feline ischemic encephalopathy has been used to describe cases of peracute onset of clinical signs consistent with a unilateral cerebral or brainstem problem caused by ischemia. Although the cause remains unknown in most cases, some of them have been linked to *Cuterebra* migration.[27,28] It is believed that the migrating parasite or the host response leads to vasospasm in the cerebral vasculature, typically the middle cerebral artery.

The pathophysiology of ischemic stroke is based on the principle that with limited energy stores, the brain relies on a constant supply of glucose and oxygen to maintain ionic pump function. When perfusion pressure falls to critical levels, ischemia develops, progressing to infarction if it persists long enough or is severe enough. An infarct is an area of compromised brain parenchyma caused by a focal occlusion of one or more blood vessels. An infarct may be due either to vascular obstruction that develops within the occluded vessels (thrombosis) or to obstructive material that originates from another vascular bed and travels to the brain (thromboembolism).[2] Infarcts can be a consequence of small vessel disease (ie, superficial or deep perforating artery) that gives rise to a lacunar infarct, or large vessel disease (ie, a major artery of the brain or its main branches) that gives rise to a territorial infarct.[1] Two distinct regions can be distinguished, the core where ischemia is severe and infarction develops rapidly, and the surrounding penumbra containing a more moderate decrease of cerebral blood flow (CBF) that allows longer duration of ischemic stress to be tolerated.[29] The relative volume of these 2 regions changes as the infarct evolves. The factors causing the evolution of the penumbra to irreversible injury are multiple and complex, and include the degree of blood flow reduction, the region of the brain involved, and the individual patient. In the penumbra, neurons are still viable but at risk of becoming irreversibly injured.[29] Tissue within the penumbra has the potential for recovery and therefore is the target for therapy in acute ischemic stroke.[30] At the cellular level, the ischemic neuron becomes depolarized as adenosine triphosphate is depleted and the Na^+/K^+ adenosine triphosphate pump and other ionic membrane pumps fail, leading to loss of fluid-electrolyte homeostasis.[31,32] This process results in loss of ionic gradients and a net translocation of water from the extracellular to the intracellular compartment, causing the cell to swell (cytotoxic edema).[33] Over time the ischemic cascade progresses, resulting in cell lysis, increased macrophage activity, and disruption of the blood-brain barrier, leading to vasogenic edema.[34–37] Vasogenic edema typically takes 4 to 6 hours to develop once blood flow decreases to ischemic levels, and may continue to progress for 24 to 48 hours. Because neurons have the highest demand for oxygen, neuronal function is first affected; this is followed, in declining order of vulnerability, by the function of oligodendrocytes, astrocytes, mesodermal microglia, and fibrovascular elements.[34] If sufficient perfusion is not reestablished, severe ischemia results in an area of dead tissue described as an infarct.[38] Ischemia is thus a continuum between normal cellular function and cell death.

Hemorrhagic Stroke

In contrast to the high incidence in man, intracerebral hemorrhage resulting from spontaneous rupture of vessels is considered rare in dogs.[16,39] Secondary hemorrhage has been reported in dogs in association with rupture of congenital vascular abnormalities,[11,40–42] primary and secondary brain tumors,[5,43–45] intravascular lymphoma (malignant angioendotheliomatosis),[46,47] cerebral amyloid angiopathy[48] and inflammatory disease of the arteries and veins (necrotizing vasculitis),[49] brain infarction (hemorrhagic infarction),[10,15] and impaired coagulation (extracranial diseases predisposing for disseminated intravascular coagulation such as neoplasia, von Willebrand disease, or *Angiostrongylus vasorum*).[11,44,50] Nontraumatic subdural or subarachnoid hemorrhage has been reported in dogs[51,52] but remains very rare when compared with its occurrence in man, where aneurysmal rupture is the most common underlying cause.

In hemorrhagic stroke, blood leaks from the vessel directly into the brain, forming a hematoma within the brain parenchyma, or into the subarachnoid space.[19] The mass of clotted blood causes physical disruption of the tissue and pressure on the surrounding brain.[53] This process alters intracranial volume/pressure relationships, and can lead to increased intracranial pressure (ICP) and decreased CBF. Initially, ICP may remain normal due to a system of compensation.[19] Within the closed space of the skull are 3 noncompressable constituents, brain tissue, blood, and cerebrospinal fluid (CSF). A change in the volume of one constituent will be balanced by a compensatory change in another. This principle is called the Monroe-Kellie doctrine. As the hematoma continues to expand, this compensatory system becomes exhausted and ICP starts to increase; this can be clinically associated with herniation. Due to mechanical autoregulation, CBF remains constant even though the cerebral perfusion pressure (CPP) may vary between 40 and 120 mm Hg.[54] The normal autoregulation of CBF may be impaired following cerebrovascular accidents, causing blood flow to damaged regions to become directly dependent on systemic blood pressure. Such animals may be unable to compensate for reductions in mean arterial blood pressure (MABP), causing decreased CPP in the presence of increased ICP.[54] This anomaly emphasizes the importance of maintaining systemic blood pressure. In these circumstances, systemic hypotension can result in inadequate perfusion of the brain, which leads to cerebral ischemia and secondary neuronal injury.

CLINICAL PRESENTATION

In ischemic or hemorrhagic stroke, the denominative feature is the temporal profile of neurologic events.[55] It is the abruptness with which the neurologic deficits develop that is highly suggestive of the disorder as being vascular.[2] This event is then followed by a plateau and then resolution of the neurologic deficit in all except the fatal strokes. Worsening edema can result in progression of neurologic signs for 24 to 72 hours.[19] Intracranial hemorrhage can be an exception and cause rapid progressive onset over a very short period of time. Clinical signs usually improve after 24 to 72 hours due to a decrease in size of the hematoma and edema.[19,56]

Neurologic deficits usually refer to a focal anatomic diagnosis and depend on the neurolocalization of the vascular insult (telencephalon, thalamus, midbrain, pons, medulla, cerebellum).[55] Infarction of an individual brain region is associated with specific clinical signs that reflect the loss of function of that specific region.[21] In its mildest form, the impaired regional CBF causes a TIA. The cause of TIA in humans is usually small emboli from the heart or atherosclerotic plaques in the carotid or vertebrobasilar arteries. Similar paroxysmal events have been reported in dogs with suspected or histologically proven infarction,[16,21,23] but the underlying cause remains undetermined. With hemorrhagic stroke, the clinical picture is different, as the hemorrhage usually involves the territory of more than one artery and pressure effects cause secondary signs. Neurologic signs are largely related to raised ICP, which gives rise to nonspecific signs of forebrain, brainstem, or cerebellar disturbance.[19]

CONFIRMATION OF DIAGNOSIS

Initial evaluation of animals with suspected stroke should focus on the differential diagnosis, including traumatic, metabolic, neoplastic, inflammatory/infectious, and toxic encephalopathies.[57] Fundus examination should be considered in all animals and may reveal tortuous vessels (suggestive of systemic hypertension), hemorrhage (suggestive of coagulopathy or systemic hypertension), or papilledema (suggestive of elevated ICP). Imaging studies of the brain (computed tomography, conventional and functional MRI) are necessary to confirm stroke, define the vascular territory involved, determine the extent of the lesion, and distinguish between ischemic and hemorrhagic stroke. Imaging studies are also necessary to rule out other causes such as tumor, trauma, and encephalitis. Once stroke is confirmed, diagnostic tests focus on identifying an underlying cause (**Boxes 1** and **2**).

Confirmation of the Diagnosis of Stroke

Ischemic stroke

Computed tomography (CT) images are frequently normal during the acute phase of ischemia; therefore the diagnosis of ischemic stroke using CT relies on the exclusion of mimics of stroke. Early CT signs of ischemia can be subtle and difficult to detect even by experienced readers, and include parenchymal hypodensity, loss of gray-white matter differentiation, subtle effacement of the cortical sulci, and local mass effect.[15,58–60]

Conventional MRI can detect ischemic stroke within 12 to 24 hours of onset and can distinguish hemorrhagic lesions from infarction.[21,23] T2-weighted and fluid-attenuated inversion recovery (FLAIR) images are particularly useful in imaging of ischemic stroke to give a more anatomic image of the brain and depict edema, old infarcts,

---

Box 1
Ancillary diagnostic tests in cases of ischemic stroke

- Serial blood pressure measurements
- Complete blood count
- Serum biochemistry profile
- Urinalysis
- Urine protein/creatinine ratio
- Serum antithrombin III activity
- D-dimers
- Endocrine testing for hyperadrenocorticism, thyroid diseases, and pheochromocytoma
- Thoracic radiographs
- Abdominal ultrasound
- Echocardiography and electrocardiography

---

microangiopathic changes, tumors, and other abnormalities. With these sequences, ischemic infarction appears as a hyperintense lesion.[21] Differentiation of the core from the surrounding penumbra is, however, not possible. T2*-weighted (gradient echo) images are used to identify or exclude hemorrhage.[55,61,62] Although infarcts are sometimes difficult to differentiate from other lesions such as inflammatory diseases, they tend to have certain distinguishing characteristics on conventional MR images[21,63]:

- The conformity of an ischemic infarct to a vascular territory is an important element in the diagnosis that helps in distinguishing these lesions from brain tumors, inflammation, and trauma. Because infarcts are caused by occlusion of a blood vessel, they conform to a vascular territory with sharp demarcation from the surrounding normal brain tissue and minimal or no mass effect.
- Ischemic infarcts are caused by failure of perfusion and therefore energy depletion. This depletion results in failure of the Na^+/K^+ pump and accumulation of Na^+ and water within the cell, that is, cytotoxic edema. The MRI changes rely on an increase in tissue water content. The T2-weighted or FLAIR images gradually become more hyperintense because of T2 prolongation that increases signal intensity, particularly over the first 24 hours.

Box 2
Ancillary diagnostic tests in cases of hemorrhagic stroke

- Serial blood pressure measurements
- Complete blood count
- Serum biochemistry profile
- Buccal mucosa bleeding time
- Prothrombin time (PT)
- Activated partial thromboplastin time (APTT)
- Thoracic radiographs
- Abdominal ultrasound

- MRI changes are best appreciated in the gray matter and are well visualized in deep gray matter structures such as the thalamus and basal ganglia, which are more vulnerable to ischemia.
- Contrast-enhancement, associated with reperfusion, is not usually seen until at least 7 to 10 days.

Several functional magnetic resonance imaging (fMRI) techniques improve the early diagnosis of stroke and evaluation of treatment in human patients. These methods include diffusion and perfusion imaging and magnetic resonance angiography (MRA). Diffusion and perfusion MRI are new techniques that monitor water transport in the microenvironment at cellular or capillary levels. These techniques provide complementary information about the pathophysiological processes following cerebral ischemia.[64] Diffusion-weighted imaging (DWI) is used commonly in human patients to improve the sensitivity and specificity of the diagnosis of acute stroke, making it an ideal sequence for positive identification of hyperacute stroke.[65,66] The temporal evolution of the DWI signal also allows the discrimination of acute versus chronic lesions.[21,23] MR perfusion-weighted imaging is employed to depict brain regions of hypoperfusion and identifies the tissue at risk by comparing the results with the findings on DWI.

In addition to its use for tissue evaluation, MRA can noninvasively assess the intracranial vascular status of stroke patients. Two techniques can be used: time-of-flight (TOF) MRA and contrast-enhanced MRA. One of the main limitations of MRA is its lower resolution compared with conventional angiography. This limitation becomes progressively worse as the luminal size decreases.[55] In human patients, angiographic techniques are particularly used for screening of carotid artery stenosis, vascular malformation (such as arteriovenous malformation, venous angioma) and aneurysms. The use of MRA in dogs has been described, and may allow identification of underlying vascular lesions in cases of canine stroke.[17,55]

Hemorrhagic stroke

CT is exquisitely sensitive at detecting acute hemorrhage, which is evident as increased density due to attenuation of X-ray beam by the globin portion of blood.[67] The attenuation gradually decreases until the hematoma is isodense at about 1 month after the onset. The periphery of the hematoma enhances with contrast at 6 days to 6 weeks due to revascularization.[67] Until recently, CT was the preferred imaging modality in human patients to determine the presence of hemorrhage in early stroke. Recent developments in MRI mean that CT now offers no advantage in the diagnosis of ischemic stroke.[67,68]

With conventional MRI, the signal intensity of intracranial hemorrhage is influenced by several intrinsic (time from ictus, source, size and location of hemorrhage) and extrinsic (pulse sequence and field strength) factors.[69] The exact effect of these various factors is difficult to evaluate with clinical studies because it is frequently impossible to ascertain the precise interval between hemorrhage and MR imaging. As the hematoma ages, oxyhemoglobin breaks down sequentially into several paramagnetic products: first deoxyhemoglobin, then methemoglobin, and finally, hemosiderin.[19] The 2 most important biophysical properties are the paramagnetic effects of iron as the hemoglobin oxygenation states change and the integrity of red blood cell membranes that compartmentalize the iron.[69] The earliest detection of hemorrhage depends on the conversion of oxyhemoglobin to deoxyhemoglobin, which occurs after the first 12 to 24 hours.[69] In oxyhemoglobin, iron is shielded from surrounding water molecules and the MR signal is similar to that of normal brain parenchyma. In deoxyhemoglobin, iron is exposed to surrounding water molecules, which creates a signal loss that makes it easy to identify on T2-weighted and susceptibility-weighted sequences.[19] Details of time-related changes on MR images relative to the stage of advancement of hematoma from hyperacute to chronic have been reviewed elsewhere.[16,19,70] Gradient-echo sequences have been proven to be the most accurate of all of the MR pulse sequences, and more accurate than CT in predicting the extent of hemorrhage on pathologic examination in a dog model.[71] Compared with other sequences, gradient-echo scans demonstrate readily detectable hypointensity regardless of the time from ictus, the source and location of hemorrhage, or the field strength. Due to the progressive centripetal increase in the deoxyhemoglobin concentration, the periphery of the hematoma is often initially more hypointense on susceptibility-weighted images than on T2-weighted images.[19] Hypointensity on gradient-echo images is, however, not specific for hemorrhage and may also be seen with calcification, air, iron, foreign bodies, and melanin. However, air, calcification, and many foreign bodies are also hypointense on other pulse sequences.[23]

Cerebrospinal Fluid Analysis

CSF analysis is unlikely to confirm a diagnosis of stroke but may help to rule out inflammatory disease. In most cases of stroke it is either normal, or reflects a mild mononuclear or neutrophilic pleocytosis, occasionally with elevated protein.[18,21,72]

Identification of Underlying Causes of Stroke

Patients with ischemic stroke should be evaluated for hypertension (and its potential underlying causes), endocrine disease (hyperadrenocorticism, hypothyroidism, hyperthyroidism, diabetes mellitus), kidney disease (especially protein-loosing nephropathy), heart disease, and metastatic disease.[22,55] Despite thorough investigations, concurrent medical conditions were not identified in almost half of the dogs with ischemic stroke in one of the author's studies.[22] This finding parallels the prevalence of cryptogenic infarction in human patients.[3] This percentage is only slightly higher than that previously reported for histopathologically confirmed brain infarcts of unknown cause in dogs (39%).[5–8,10–18,20] Antemortem diagnostic investigations, such as angiographic studies of the vertebrobasilar and carotid system, and lipid and hemostatic profiles would be necessary in the future to investigate potential causes of ischemic stroke in dogs.

Diagnostic tests of presumed/confirmed cases of hemorrhagic stroke focus on screening the animal for coagulopathy, hypertension (and potential underlying causes), and metastatic disease (particularly hemangiosarcoma). Recommended ancillary diagnostic tests are listed in **Boxs 1** and **2**.

TREATMENT

Once the diagnosis of a stroke is made, any potential underlying disease is identified and treated accordingly. The general aim is to provide supportive care, maintain adequate tissue oxygenation, and manage neurologic and nonneurologic complications. Nursing management of a recumbent dog is vital to the success of more specific therapies. This management includes prevention of decubital ulceration, aspiration pneumonia, and urine scald, in addition to physical therapy and enteral nutrition. More specific therapies are aimed at preventing further neurologic deterioration.

Ischemic Stroke

Most cases of ischemic stroke recover within several weeks with only supportive care.[22] Potential underlying causes should be investigated and treated accordingly to limit the risk of recurrences. Treatment revolves around 3 principles: (1) monitoring and correction of basic physiologic variables (eg, oxygen level, fluid balance, blood pressure, body temperature); (2) inhibition of the biochemical and metabolic cascades subsequent to ischemia to prevent neuronal death (neuroprotection); and (3) restoration or improvement of CBF by thrombolysis in cases of thrombus.[73] The potentially salvageable penumbra is the target for both thrombolytic and neuroprotective therapy.[74] The time period during which injury may be reversible is called the therapeutic window.[75] This "window of opportunity" is approximately 6 hours before irreversible neurologic damage occurs.

Monitoring and correction of basic physiologic variables

Fortunately, the vast majority of ischemic stroke patients have no major difficulty maintaining adequate airways, breathing, and circulation early in their clinical course.[76] Some controversies exist surrounding the management of hypertension in the setting of an ongoing acute ischemic stroke. As well as being a potential risk factor for stroke, hypertension can occur as a physiologic response to ensure adequate CPP in the penumbra of the infarct for up to 72 hours after onset.[77,78] Maintaining normal systemic arterial blood pressure is essential, and aggressive lowering of blood pressure is avoided during the acute stages unless the patient is at a high risk of end-stage organ damage (systolic blood pressures remaining above 180 mm Hg).[76,79] In such cases, hypertension can often be controlled with an angiotensin-converting enzyme inhibitor such as enalapril (0.25–0.5 mg/kg twice a day) or benazepril (0.25–0.5 mg/kg twice a day), or calcium channel blockers such as amlodipine (0.1–0.25 mg/kg once a day), which tends to be more effective.[73] Treatment with these oral antihypertensives is preferred, but parenteral medications such as nitroprusside, intravenous β-blockers, calcium channel blockers, or diuretics may be necessary in animals that cannot tolerate oral medications.[80]

Neuroprotection

There is no evidence that glucocorticoids provide any benefit in stroke.[81] Aside from the lack of proven benefit in veterinary stroke patients, the use of glucocorticoids may increase the risk of gastrointestinal complications and infection.[82] Treatment strategies for ischemic stroke considered in man using other neuroprotective agents (N-methyl-D-aspartate [NMDA] antagonists, Ca^{2+} channel blockers, sodium channel modulators) or antiplatelets and thrombolytic therapy have not been evaluated clinically in dogs. Although the aforementioned neuroprotective agents have resulted in a dramatic decrease in the size of stroke lesion in experimental animal models, these agents have either failed to prove their efficacy in clinical trials or are awaiting further investigation.[83,84]

Thrombolytic therapy

At present, there are no definitive data in humans or animals to confirm a benefit of thrombolysis using unfractionated heparin in patients with acute ischemic stroke. Despite conflicting results regarding its efficacy, intravenous recombinant tissue plasminogen activator (tPA) is sometimes used in human stroke patients if it can be given within the first 3 hours after the onset.[85] This critical time window makes thrombolytic treatment unrealistic in veterinary neurology. Furthermore, this type of treatment carries a significant risk of intracranial hemorrhage.[86] Antiplatelet therapy with low-dose aspirin (0.5 mg/kg by mouth once a day) can be used prophylactically to prevent clot formation in proven cardiac sources of an embolus.[80,87] No controlled studies in veterinary medicine have assessed these treatments.

Hemorrhagic Stroke

The most important consideration in hemorrhagic stroke is maintaining cerebral perfusion by treating hypotension and elevated ICP, and treating any underlying cause. Management includes stabilization of the patient by protecting the airway and monitoring and correction of vital signs; monitoring neurologic status; identifying and treating any underlying cause; and specific treatments such as managing raised ICP.[73] The risk of neurologic deterioration and cardiovascular instability is highest during the first 24 hours after the onset, as the space-occupying lesion slowly expands and cerebral vasogenic edema develops.[82] The initial focus is extracranial stabilization, closely followed by therapies directed toward intracranial stabilization and treatment of any identified underlying cause. Careful monitoring is essential during the initial period and includes assessment of vital parameters as well as neurologic status.

Extracranial stabilization

Extracranial stabilization involves careful monitoring of vital parameters (oxygen levels, fluid balance, blood pressure, body temperature) and correction of any abnormalities. Hypoxia should be avoided, as with any other intracranial disease. However, there is no evidence in human patients to support the routine use of oxygen for the treatment of hemorrhagic stroke in the absence of hypoxia.

Hypoventilation may occur as a result of damage to the respiratory center in the brainstem following raised ICP. The impaired respiratory drive results in elevated $PaCO_2$ and resultant cerebral vasodilation, which in turn aggravates intracranial hypertension. $PaCO_2$ should be maintained within a normal range and not allowed to exceed 40 mm Hg, including intubation and ventilation if necessary.[82]

Maintaining adequate tissue perfusion is important in any patient with hemorrhagic stroke. The primary goal of fluid therapy is rapid restoration of blood pressure, such that CPP is maintained greater than 70 mm Hg. Hypovolemia should be recognized and treated with volume expansion using artificial colloids or hypertonic saline (7.5%) to achieve rapid restoration of blood volume and pressure while limiting the volume of fluid administered. Hypertonic saline has many properties that may make it a superior resuscitation fluid for patients with intracranial disease such as hemorrhagic stroke. The recommended dose of hypertonic sodium chloride (7%–7.5%) for volume expansion is 3 to 5 mL/kg administered over 10 to 15 minutes. The use of glucose-containing solutions is discouraged, as hyperglycemia has been shown to correlate with poor outcome in human stroke patients.[88] Therefore, blood glucose should be monitored from the time of presentation. Hypotonic fluids should also be avoided.

As for ischemic stroke, attempts to lower and normalize blood pressure should be reserved for animals at a high risk of end-stage organ damage (systolic blood pressures remaining above 180 mm Hg) or animals with severe ocular manifestations of hypertension such as retinal detachment or intraocular hemorrhage.[76,82] However, moderate levels of hypertension should not be treated, as systemic hypertension may be secondary to the intense reflex sympathetic response to intracranial hypertension, which is a compensatory mechanism to maintain cerebral perfusion. Treatment recommendations for lowering blood pressure are detailed in the previous section on the treatment of ischemic stroke.

Intracranial stabilization

Once initial assessment and extracranial stabilization have occurred, medical intervention to address intracranial issues focuses on decreasing ICP.[73] Three principles can be applied: (1) reducing cerebral edema associated with intracranial hemorrhage; (2) optimizing cerebral blood volume; and (3) eliminating space-occupying mass.

Osmotic diuretics such as mannitol are useful for treating cerebral edema and resultant intracranial hypertension associated with disorders such as head trauma, brain tumors, or encephalitis. There is no compelling evidence that mannitol exacerbates intracranial hemorrhage. Although the efficacy is still controversial, osmotic diuretics are routinely used in the control of ICP in human patients with known intracranial hemorrhage.[89] Mannitol (0.25–1.0 g/kg intravenous over 10 to 20 minutes up to every 8 hours) may be used to treat elevated ICP secondary to hemorrhagic stroke.[54] Mannitol's main effect is to enhance CBF by reducing blood viscosity.[54] It should, however, be avoided in hypovolemic patient.

Cerebral blood volume is another intracranial component that contributes to ICP. In a rapidly deteriorating animal, hyperventilation can be used to temporarily reduce ICP with a target $PaCO_2$ of less than 35 mm Hg. The aim of hyperventilation is to reduce cerebral blood volume and hence ICP, by causing cerebral vasoconstriction. However, excessive hyperventilation can be accompanied by a reduction in global CBF, which may drop below ischemic thresholds; therefore it is not recommended unless the $PaCO_2$ is closely monitored with capnography or arterial blood gas analysis.[90]

Elimination of the space-occupying mass within the cranial vault is the third method to reduce ICP. Surgical evacuation of the hematoma can therefore be employed in dogs with large hematomas (mostly subarachnoid) and a deteriorating neurologic status.

PROGNOSIS

The prognosis for ischemic or hemorrhagic stroke depends on the severity of the neurologic deficit, the initial response to supportive care, and the severity of any underlying cause. Fortunately, most cases of ischemic stroke recover within several weeks with only supportive care. In a recent retrospective study of 33 dogs with MRI or necropsy evidence of brain infarction, there was no association between the region of the brain involved (telencephalic, thalamic/midbrain, cerebellum), the type of infarction (territorial or lacunar), and the outcome.[22] However, dogs with a concurrent medical condition had a significantly shorter survival time than those dogs with no identifiable medical condition. Dogs with a concurrent medical condition also were significantly more likely to suffer from subsequent infarcts.[22] Hemorrhagic stroke is far less common than ischemic stroke, but is associated with higher mortality.[23,91]

REFERENCES

1. Kalimo H, Kaste M, Haltia M. Vascular diseases. In: Graham DI, Lantos PL, editors. Greenfield's neuropathology. 7th edition. London: Arnold; 2002. p. 233–80.
2. Adams RD, Victor M. Cerebrovascular diseases. In: Adams RD, Victor M, editors. Principles of neurology. 6th edition. New York: McGraw-Hill Inc; 1997. p. 777–83.
3. Sacco RL. Classification of stroke. In: Fisher M, editor. Clinical atlas of cerebrovascular disorders. London: Wolfe; 1994. p. 2.2–2.25.
4. Carolei A, Marini C, Fieschi C. Transient ischaemic attacks. In: Ginsberg MD, Bogousslavsky J, editors. Cerebrovascular disease: pathophysiology, diagnosis and management. London: Blackwell Science; 1998. p. 941–60.
5. Fankhauser R, Lüginbuhl H, McGrath J. Cerebrovascular disease in various animal species. Ann N Y Acad Sci 1965;127:817–60.

6. Patton C, Garner F. Cerebral infarction caused by heartworms (*Dirofilaria immitis*) in a dog. J Am Vet Med Assoc 1970;156:600–5.
7. Kotani T, Tomimura T, Ogura M, et al. Cerebral infarction caused by *Dirofilaria immitis* in three dogs. Nippon Juigaku Zasshi 1975;37:379–90.
8. Patterson J, Rusely M, Zachary J. Neurologic manifestations of cerebrovascular atherosclerosis associated with primary hypothyroidism in a dog. J Am Vet Med Assoc 1985;186:499–503.
9. Liu SK, Tilley LP, Tappe JP, et al. Clinical and pathologic findings in dogs with atherosclerosis: 21 cases (1970–1983). J Am Vet Med Assoc 1986;189:227–32.
10. Bagley R, Anderson W, de Lahunta A, et al. Cerebellar infarction caused by arterial thrombosis in a dog. J Am Vet Med Assoc 1988;192:785–7.
11. Joseph RJ, Greenlee PG, Carrillo JM, et al. Canine cerebrovascular disease: clinical and pathological findings in 17 cases. J Am Anim Hosp Assoc 1988;24:569–76.
12. Swayne DE, Tyler DE, Batker J. Cerebral infarction with associated venous thrombosis in a dog. Vet Pathol 1988;25:317–20.
13. Cachin M, Vandevelde M. Cerebral infarction associated with septic thromboemboli in the dog. In: Proceedings of the 8th Annual Meeting Veterinary Internal Medicine Forum. Washington, DC: ACVIM; 1990. p. 1136.
14. Norton F. Cerebral infarction in a dog. Prog Vet Neurol 1992;3:120–5.
15. Tidwell AS, Mahony OM, Moore RP, et al. Computed tomography of an acute haemorrhagic cerebral infarct in a dog. Vet Radiol Ultrasound 1994;35:290–6.
16. Thomas WB. Cerebrovascular disease. Vet Clin North Am Small Anim Pract 1996;26:925–43.
17. Kent M, De Lahunta A, Tidwell AS. MR imaging findings in a dog with intravascular lymphoma in the brain. Vet Radiol Ultrasound 2001;42:504–10.
18. Berg JM, Joseph RJ. Cerebellar infarcts in two dogs diagnosed with magnetic resonance imaging. J Am Anim Hosp Assoc 2003;39:203–7.
19. Platt SR, Garosi L. Canine cerebrovascular disease: do dogs have strokes? J Am Anim Hosp Assoc 2003;39:337–42.
20. Axlund TW, Isaacs AM, Holland M, et al. Fibrocartilaginous embolic encephalomyelopathy of the brainstem and midcervical spinal cord in a dog. J Vet Intern Med 2004;18:765–7.
21. Garosi LS, McConnell JF, Platt SR, et al. Clinical characteristics and topographical magnetic resonance of suspected brain infarction in 40 dogs. J Vet Intern Med 2006;20:311–21.
22. Garosi LS, McConnell JF, Platt SR, et al. Results of investigations and outcome of dog brain infarcts. J Vet Intern Med 2005;19:725–31.
23. McConnell JF, Garosi LS, Platt SR, et al. MRI findings of presumed cerebellar cerebrovascular accident in twelve dogs. Vet Radiol Ultrasound 2005;46:1–10.
24. Cook LB, Coates JR, Dewey CW, et al. Vascular encephalopathy associated with bacterial endocarditis in four dogs. J Am Anim Hosp Assoc 2005;41:252–8.
25. Hess RS, Kass PH, Van Winkle TJV. Association between diabetes mellitus, hypothyroidism or hyperadrenocorticism, and atherosclerosis in dogs. J Vet Intern Med 2003;17:489–94.
26. Rogers WA, Donovan EF, Kociba GJ. Lipids and lipoproteins in normal dogs and in dogs with secondary hyperlipoproteinemia. J Am Vet Med Assoc 1975;166:1092–100.
27. Glass EN, Cornetta AM, deLahunta A, et al. Clinical and clinicopathological features in 11 cats with Cuterebra larvae myiasis of the central nervous system. J Vet Intern Med 2008;12:365–8.

28. Williams KJ, Summers BA, de Lahunta A. Cerebrospinal cuterebriasis in cats and its association with feline ischemic encephalopathy. Vet Pathol 1998;35:330–3.
29. Heiss WD, Graf R, Wienhard K, et al. Dynamic penumbra demonstrated by sequential multitracer PET after middle cerebral artery occlusion in cats. J Cereb Blood Flow Metab 1994;14:892–902.
30. Kogure T, Kogure K. Molecular and biochemical events within the brain subjected to cerebral ischaemia (targets for therapeutical intervention). Clin Neurosci 1997; 4:179–83.
31. Siesjo BK, Katsura K, Zhao Q, et al. Mechanisms of secondary brain damage in global and focal ischemia: a speculative synthesis. J Neurotrauma 1995;12: 943–56.
32. Siesjo BK. Pathophysiology and treatment of focal cerebral ischemia. Part I: pathophysiology. J Neurosurg 1992;77:169–84.
33. Ikeda Y, Long DM. The molecular basis of brain injury and brain edema. The role of oxygen free radicals. Neurosurgery 1990;27:1–11.
34. Collins RC, Dobkin BH, Choi DW. Selective vulnerability of the brain: new insights into the pathophysiology of stroke. Ann Intern Med 1989;110:992–1000.
35. Dugan LL, Sensi SL, Canzoniero LM, et al. Mitochondrial production of reactive oxygen species in cortical neurons following exposure to N-methyl-D-aspartate. J Neurosci 1995;15:6377–88.
36. Mody I, MacDonald JF. NMDA receptor-dependent excitotoxicity: the role of intracellular Ca^{2+} release. Trends Pharmacol Sci 1995;16:356–9.
37. Samdani AF, Dawson TM, Dawson VL. Nitric oxide synthase in models of focal ischaemia. Stroke 1997;28:1283–8.
38. Summers BA, Cummings JF, de Lahunta A. Degenerative diseases of the central nervous system. In: Summers BA, Cummings JF, deLahunta A, editors. Veterinary neuropathology. St Louis (MO): Mosby-Year Book; 1985. p. 237–49.
39. Muhle AC, Kircher P, Fazer R, et al. Intracranial haemorrhage in an eight-week-old puppy. Vet Rec 2004;154:338–9.
40. Hause WR, Helphrey ML, Green RW, et al. Cerebral arteriovenous malformation in a dog. J Am Anim Hosp Assoc 1982;18:601–7.
41. Thomas WB, Adams WH, McGavin MD, et al. Magnetic resonance imaging appearance of intracranial hemorrhage secondary to cerebral vascular malformation in a dog. Vet Radiol Ultrasound 1997;38:371–5.
42. Stoffregen D, Kallfelz F, DeLahunta A. Cerebral hemorrhage in an old dog. J Am Anim Hosp Assoc 1985;21:495–8.
43. Long SN, Michieletto A, Anderson TJ, et al. Suspected pituitary apoplexy in a German shorthaired pointer. J Small Anim Pract 2003;44:497–502.
44. Waters DJ, Hayden DW, Walter PA. Intracranial lesions in dogs with hemangiosarcoma. J Vet Intern Med 1989;3:222–30.
45. Dennler M, Lange EM, Schmied O, et al. Imaging diagnosis—metastatic hemangiosarcoma causing cerebral hemorrhage in a dog. Vet Radiol Ultrasound 2007; 48:138–40.
46. McDonough SP, Van Winkle TJ, Valentine BA, et al. Clinicopathological and immunophenotypical features of canine intravascular lymphoma (malignant angioendotheliomatosis). J Comp Pathol 2002;126:277–88.
47. Summers BA, DeLahunta A. Cerebral angioendotheliomatosis in a dog. Acta Neuropathol 1985;68:10–4.
48. Uchida K, Miyauchi Y, Nakayama H, et al. Amyloid angiopathy with cerebral hemorrhage and senile plaque in aged dogs. Nippon Juigaku Zasshi 1990;52: 605–11.

49. Sasaki M, Pool R, Summers BA. Vasculitis in a dog resembling isolated angiitis of the central nervous system in humans. Vet Pathol 2003;40:95–7.
50. Dunn KJ, Nicholls PK, Dunn JK, et al. Intracranial haemorrhage in a Doberman puppy with von Willebrand's disease. Vet Rec 1995;136:635–6.
51. Nykamp S, Scrivani P, DeLahunta A, et al. Chronic subdural hematoma and hydrocephalus in a dog. Vet Radiol Ultrasound 2001;42:511–4.
52. Packer RA, Bergman RL, Coates JR, et al. Intracranial subarachnoid hemorrhage following lumbar myelography in two dogs. Vet Radiol Ultrasound 2007;48:323–7.
53. Auer RN, Sutherland GR. Primary intracerebral hemorrhage: pathophysiology. Can J Neurol Sci 2005;32:3–12.
54. Dewey CW. Head-trauma management. In: Dewey CW, editor. A practical guide to canine and feline neurology. Ames (IA): Iowa State University Press; 2003. p. 179–92.
55. Garosi LS, McConnell JF. Ischaemic stroke in dogs and humans: a comparative review. J Small Anim Pract 2005;46:521–9.
56. Wessmann A, Chandler K, Garosi LS. Ischaemic and haemorrhagic stroke in the dog. Vet J 2009;180:290–303.
57. Hillock SM, Dewey CW, Stefanacci JD, et al. Vascular encephalopathies in dogs: risk factors, pathophysiology, and clinical signs. Compend Contin Educ Pract Vet 2006;28:196–207.
58. Inoue Y, Takemoto K, Miyamoto T, et al. Sequential computed tomography scans in acute cerebral infarction. Radiology 1980;135:655–62.
59. Schriger DL, Kalafut M, Starkman S, et al. Cranial computed tomography interpretation in acute stroke: physician accuracy in determining eligibility for thrombolytic therapy. J Am Med Assoc 1998;279:1293–7.
60. Grotta JC, Chiu D, Lu M, et al. Agreement and variability in the interpretation of early CT changes in stroke patients qualifying for intravenous rtPA therapy. Stroke 1999;30:1528–33.
61. Garosi LS, Platt SR, McConnell JF, et al. Intracranial haemorrhage associated with Angiostrongylus vasorum infection in three dogs. J Small Anim Pract 2005; 46:93–9.
62. Wessmann A, Iu D, Lamb CR, et al. Brain and spinal cord haemorrhage associated with Angiostrongylus vasorum infection in four dogs. Vet Rec 2006;158: 858–63.
63. Thomas WB, Sorjonen DC, Scheuler RO, et al. Magnetic resonance imaging of brain infarction in seven dogs. Vet Radiol Ultrasound 1996;37:345–50.
64. Sartor K, Fiebach JB. Clinical utility of diffusion and perfusion MR imaging in acute stroke. Imaging Decisions MRI 2003;4:4–12.
65. Mullins ME, Schaefer PW, Sorensen AG, et al. CT and conventional and diffusion-weighted MR imaging in acute stroke: study in 691 patients at presentation to the emergency department. Radiology 2002;224:353–60.
66. Heiland S. Diffusion and perfusion-weighted MR imaging in acute stroke: principles, methods, and applications. Imaging Decisions MRI 2003;7:4–12.
67. Hoggard N, Wilkinson ID, Paley MN, et al. Imaging of haemorrhagic stroke. Clin Radiol 2002;57:957–68.
68. Schellinger PD, Jansen O, Fiebach JB, et al. A standardized MRI stroke protocol: comparison with CT in hyperacute intracerebral hemorrhage. Stroke 1999;30: 765–8.
69. Parizel PM, Makkat S, Van Miert E, et al. Intracranial hemorrhage: principles of CT and MRI interpretation. Eur Radiol 2001;11:1770–83.

70. Tamura S, Tamura Y, Tsuka T, et al. Sequential magnetic resonance imaging of an intracranial hematoma in a dog. Vet Radiol Ultrasound 2006;47:142–4.

71. Weingarten K, Zimmerman RD, Deo-Narine V, et al. MR imaging of acute intracranial hemorrhage: findings on sequential spin-echo and gradient echo images in a dog model. AJNR Am J Neuroradiol 1991;12:457–67.

72. Kitagawa M, Okada M, Kanayama K, et al. Traumatic intracerebral hematoma in a dog: MR images and clinical findings. J Vet Med Sci 2005;67: 843–6.

73. Garosi LS, Platt SR. Treatment of cerebrovascular disease. In: Bonagura JD, Twedt DC, editors. Current veterinary therapy XIV. St Louis (MO): Saunders Elsevier; 2009. p. 1074–7.

74. Hakim AM. Ischaemic penumbra: the therapeutic window. Neurology 1998;51: S44–6.

75. Furlan M, Marchal G, Viader F, et al. Spontaneous neurological recovery after stroke and the fate of the ischaemic penumbra. Ann Neurol 1996;40:216–26.

76. Thurman RJ, Jauch EC. Acute ischaemic stroke: emergent evaluation and management. Emerg Med Clin North Am 2002;20:609–30.

77. Yatsu FM, Zivin J. Hypertension in acute ischaemic stroke: not to treat. Arch Neurol 1985;42:999–1000.

78. Droste DW, Ritter MA, Dittrich R, et al. Arterial hypertension and ischaemic stroke. Acta Neurol Scand 2003;107:241–51.

79. Adams HP Jr, Brott TG, Crowell RM, et al. Guidelines for the management of patients with acute ischaemic stroke. A statement for healthcare professionals from a special writing group of the Stroke Council, American Heart Association. Stroke 2004;25:1901–14.

80. Strakman S, Dobkin B. Cerebral vascular emergencies. In: Shoemaker WC, Ayers SM, editors. Textbook of critical care. 4th edition. Philadelphia: WB Saunders; 2000. p. 1539–45.

81. De Reuck J, Vandekerckhove T, Bosma G, et al. Steroid treatment in acute ischaemic stroke. A comparative retrospective study of 556 cases. Eur Neurol 1988;28:70–2.

82. Acierno MJ, Labato MA. Hypertension in dogs and cats. Compendium 2004;26: 336–45.

83. Hickenbottom SL, Grotta J. Neuroprotective therapy. Semin Neurol 1998;18: 485–92.

84. Ovbiagele B, Kidwell CS, Starkman S, et al. Neuroprotective agents for the treatment of acute ischaemic stroke. Curr Neurol Neurosci Rep 2003;3: 9–20.

85. The National Institute of Neurological Disorders and Stroke rt-PA Stroke Study Group. Tissue plasminogen activator for acute ischaemic stroke. N Engl J Med 1995;333:1581–7.

86. The National Institute of Neurological Disorders and Stroke rt-PA Stroke Study Group. Intracerebral haemorrhage after intravenous t-PA therapy for ischaemic stroke. Stroke 1997;28:2109–18.

87. van Kooten F, Ciabattoni G, Patrono C, et al. Platelet activation and lipid peroxidation in patients with acute ischemic stroke. Stroke 1997;28:1557–63.

88. Sieber FE, Martin LJ, Brown PR, et al. Diabetic chronic hyperglycemia and neurologic outcome following global ischemia in dogs. J Cereb Blood Flow Metab 1996;16:1230–5.

89. Bereczki D, Fekete I, Prado GF, et al. Mannitol for acute stroke. Cochrane Database Syst Rev 2007;(18):CD001153.

90. Hillock SM, Dewey CW, Stefanacci JD, et al. Vascular encephalopathies in dogs: diagnosis, treatment, and prognosis. Compend Contin Educ Pract Vet 2006;28: 208–16.
91. Bogousslavsky J, Van Melle G, Regli F. The Lausanne Stroke Registry: analysis of 1000 consecutive patients with first stroke. Stroke 1988;19:1083–92.

Vestibular Disease in Dogs and Cats

John H. Rossmeisl Jr, DVM, MS

KEYWORDS

• Neurology • Canine • Feline • Equilibrium

The vestibular system is the major sensory (special proprioceptive) system that, along with the general proprioceptive and visual systems, maintains balance.[1–4] An individual's sense of balance is best summarized as a normal orientation with respect to the influence of gravitational forces. The vestibular system also functions to coordinate body posture and ocular position in relation to the position or motion of the head. Considering its physiologic roles, the clinical hallmarks of vestibular dysfunction are abnormalities of the gait, head and body posture, and ocular movement.[1,2]

VESTIBULAR NEUROANATOMY

For clinical purposes, the anatomic constituents of the vestibular system are functionally divided into peripheral and central components. The peripheral portions of the vestibular system are located in the inner ear (**Fig. 1**A) and consist of the receptors, ganglion, and peripheral axons of the vestibular division of cranial nerve VIII. The central components (**Fig. 1**B) are the vestibular nuclei in the medulla and the vestibular projections to the cerebellum, spinal cord, and rostral brainstem.[1,2]

Peripheral Vestibular System

The receptors for the vestibular system are colocalized with those for the auditory system in the bony and membranous labyrinths of the petrous temporal bone (inner ear). The bony labyrinth is divided into 3 major contiguous regions: the semicircular canals, the vestibule, and the cochlea. The lumens of each of these structures are filled with perilymph.

Within the bony labyrinth is the membranous labyrinth, which contains 4, endolymph-filled, communicating structures called the (1) semicircular ducts, (2) utricle, (3) saccule, and (4) cochlear duct (see **Fig. 1**A). The semicircular ducts are contained within the semicircular canals, the utricle and saccule within the vestibule, and the cochlear duct within the bony cochlea. Each of the semicircular ducts is oriented at right angles to the others, thus occupying 3 planes.[2] In one end of each of the membranous semicircular ducts is a terminal dilation called the ampulla, and on

Neurology and Neurosurgery, Department of Small Animal Clinical Sciences, Virginia-Maryland Regional College of Veterinary Medicine, Virginia Tech, Blacksburg, VA 24061, USA
E-mail address: jrossmei@vt.edu

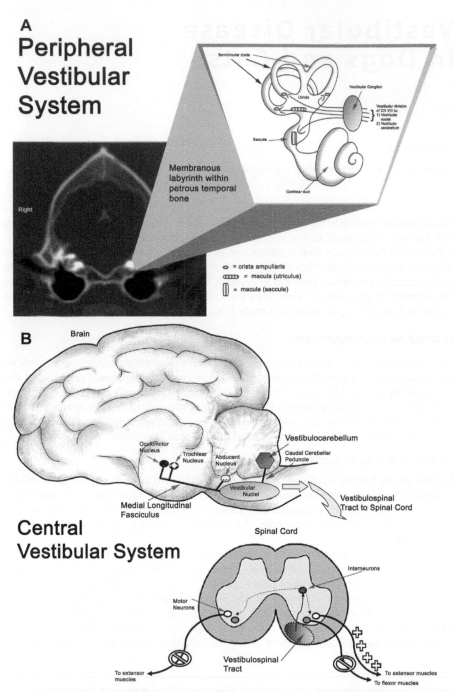

Fig. 1. Schematic neuroanatomy of the peripheral (*A*) and central (*B*) components of the vestibular system. (*Illustrations prepared by* Terry Lawrence, Virginia-Maryland Regional College of Veterinary Medicine, Department of Biomedical Illustration. *Courtesy of* Virginia-Maryland Regional College of Veterinary Medicine, Department of Biomedical Illustration.)

one side of each ampulla are structures called cristae, each of which is lined with ciliated neuroepithelial hair cells. The ampulla and crista collectively within the terminal portion of each semicircular duct is termed the crista ampullaris. The neural activity within these hair cells is continuously tonic, such that movement of the head in any direction of angular rotation subsequently results in displacement of endolymphatic fluid, altering the tonic neural influence of the semicircular ducts by deflection of the hair cells in the corresponding crista ampullaris. Dendrites of neurons from the vestibular portion of cranial nerve VIII synapse on these hair cells, and the deflection of the hair cells stimulates vestibular neurons. The 3 cristae ampullares receptors primarily respond to acceleration, deceleration, and rotation (ie, dynamic equilibrium), but are not activated at constant velocities.[1,2] The semicircular canals are organized in such a fashion that movement in a plane that activates vestibular neurons in the crista ampullaris of one semicircular duct simultaneously inhibits neurons in the synergistic duct on the opposite side of the head. This paired and reciprocal system of ductal innervation functions to instantaneously activate the appropriate postural antigravity muscles following the detection of head rotation, thus preventing the development of an abnormal posture.[4]

The maculae are the receptors located in the membranous utriculus and saccule (see **Fig. 1**A). The macula of the saccule is oriented in a vertical plane, whereas the macula of the utriculus is in a horizontal plane. The surface of each macula is covered with neuroepithelial hair cells, which project cilia into an otolithic membrane that covers the neuroepithelial surface of each macula. Movement of the otolithic membrane causes deflection of the cilia of the macular hair cells, and subsequently triggers an action potential in the dendritic zone of the vestibular neurons that synapse in each macula.[2,3] The macular receptors of the utricle and saccule provide continual tonic nervous input, whose net functional effect is to maintain static equilibrium (sensation of static head position relative to gravity), as well as respond to linear acceleration, which participates in the preservation of a normal, upright head and body posture.[3]

The vestibular division of cranial nerve VIII has dendritic connections with the cristae and the maculae, and its axons project through the internal acoustic meatus. The cell bodies of bipolar vestibular axons are located in the vestibular ganglion (see **Fig. 1**A), which is located in the petrous temporal bone.[5]

Central Vestibular System

After leaving the internal acoustic meatus, vestibular axons project to the lateral aspect of the medulla where the majority terminate in the vestibular nuclei (see **Fig. 1**B), while a smaller fraction course into the flocculonodular lobe of the cerebellar cortex and cerebellar medulla by way of the caudal cerebellar peduncle.[2,5] There are 4 vestibular nuclei on either side of the midline adjacent to the lateral wall of the fourth ventricle that form the vestibular trigone. The neurons in these nuclei are interneurons that generally provide excitatory influences to local interneurons in other parts of the central nervous system. The clinically relevant central vestibular nuclear projections have 3 primary targets, which are neurons of the (1) spinal cord, (2) rostral brainstem, or (3) cerebellum.[2,3]

Spinal cord projections

The vestibulospinal tract is the primary spinal cord projection that descends from the vestibular nuclei in the medulla to all segments of the spinal cord in the ipsilateral ventral funiculus, and exerts the following influences over motor neurons, which are mediated via segmental interneurons: ipsilateral extensor muscles are facilitated, ipsilateral flexor muscles are inhibited, and contralateral extensor muscles are inhibited (see **Fig. 1**B). Therefore, the overall effect of vestibular system activation is an ipsilateral increase in antigravity muscle tone and contralateral inhibition of tone and stretch reflexes.[2,3] These pathways contribute to coordination of motor activity to the limbs, neck, and trunk in response to movement of the head. A vestibular lesion that unilaterally abolishes or diminishes the normally tonic neural vestibular input results in the unopposed stimulation of the vestibulospinal tract of the unaffected side, which effectively causes the head and body to lean toward the side of the lesion.

Brainstem projections
Medial longitudinal fasciculus The medial longitudinal fasciculus (MLF) (see **Fig. 1**B) ascends from vestibular nuclei in the medulla to synapse on lower motor neurons in the motor nuclei of cranial nerves III, IV, and VI,[3,5] This pathway provides coordinated, conjugate ocular movements as the head changes position. The MLF is also part of the pathway that is responsible for the observation of physiologic nystagmus that is induced when testing the vestibulo-ocular reflex.

Reticular formation and vomiting center Axons from the vestibular nuclei project to the vomiting center within the reticular formation. This pathway accounts for the vomiting that can be associated with motion sickness/vestibular disease. Vomiting is uncommonly seen in veterinary vestibular diseases, when compared with human equivalents.[1,3,4]

Conscious perception of balance Conscious perception of balance and equilibrium are obviously important, based on the verbal descriptions of abnormalities in cortical spatial perceptions often provided by humans with vestibular disorders.[3,4] The afferent pathways for conscious perception of vestibular dysfunction are currently poorly understood, but are believed to ascend through thalamic relay centers to the temporal cerebral cortex.[4]

Cerebellar projections
Vestibular axons from the vestibular nuclei and vestibular ganglion project to the vestibulocerebellum (flocculonodular lobe and fastigial nucleus) via the caudal cerebellar peduncle.[2,6] These axons maintain coordination of the eyes, neck, trunk, and limbs in relation to movements of the head, as well as when the head is in a static position.

CLINICAL SIGNS OF VESTIBULAR DYSFUNCTION

Diseases of the vestibular system cause varyingly severe balance and postural disturbances along with vestibular ataxia. Clinical signs may be a result of dysfunction of the peripheral or central components of the vestibular apparatus (see **Fig. 1**A and B). Clinical signs of vestibular dysfunction are typically reflective of a unilateral disease process, but may occasionally be bilateral.

Common Clinical Features of Vestibular Disease

Diseases that affect the peripheral or central components of the vestibular system are accompanied by a set of cardinal clinical features that are often outwardly visible or easily evoked during the neurologic examination (**Table 1**).

Head tilt
A head tilt (**Fig. 2**) is the postural abnormality that results from the unilateral loss of antigravity muscular tone in the neck region. The degree of ventral deviation of the ear can vary from a few degrees to 45°. The ventrally deviated ear is directed toward

Table 1
Clinical signs common to central and peripheral vestibular diseases

Clinical Sign	Description and Comments
Head postural abnormality	Head tilt; deviation of one ear ventrally; the ventrally deviated ear is usually directed toward the lesion
Pathologic nystagmus	Jerk nystagmus present with distinct fast and slow phases; abnormal ocular movement can occur in a horizontal, rotary, or vertical direction
Vestibular strabismus	Positional ventral to ventrolateral strabismus (dropped globe) present ipsilateral to a vestibular lesion and usually apparent only when extending the head and neck
Vestibular ataxia	Flexing of the neck and trunk with the concavity toward the lesion; leaning, falling, rolling, or circling toward the side of the lesion

the side of the vestibular lesion in most cases, except when a paradoxic central vestibular lesion is present (see later discussion).

Nystagmus
Nystagmus is an involuntary and rhythmic movement of the eyes. Nystagmus can be physiologic or pathologic in nature. The most common forms of both inducible physiologic and pathologic nystagmus seen in veterinary practice are characterized by unequal directional eye movements and are thus termed jerk-types of nystagmus.[1,2] Jerk nystagmus is characterized as having distinct fast and slow phases of ocular movement. When describing jerk nystagmus, it is conventional to define it according to the axis of movement (horizontal, vertical, rotary) of the globe as well as the direction of the fast phase.

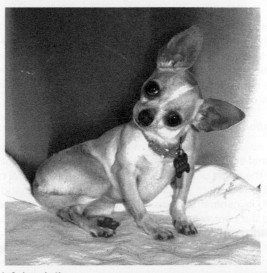

Fig. 2. Dog with a left head tilt.

Physiologic nystagmus In a normal animal, rotation of the head will result in the induction of a jerk nystagmus in the plane of rotation, with the fast phase occurring in the same direction as the movement. A distinct slow phase of ocular movement will occur in the direction opposite of the head rotation. The purpose of this physiologic response, which is termed the vestibulo-ocular reflex, is to preserve image stability on the retina to optimize performance of the visual system.[3] For this system to function, afferent initiating stimuli from the semicircular canals ascend to the vestibular nuclei. The vestibular nuclei are interconnected with the somatic motor nuclei that control extraocular muscle movement in the brainstem (the oculomotor [CN III], trochlear [CN IV], and abducent nuclei [CN VI]) via the MLF (see **Fig. 1**B). Movement of the head results in reciprocating afferent stimuli from the paired semicircular canals in the plane of movement to the vestibular nuclei and then through the MLF in such a fashion that allows for coordinated and conjugate eye movements to occur.[1,2]

Pathologic nystagmus Pathologic nystagmus that can be observed when the head is at rest or in a neutral position is termed spontaneous or resting nystagmus. Pathologic nystagmus may also be inducible in the absence of resting nystagmus when the head is moved into certain positions, such as placing the animal in dorsal recumbency; this is termed positional (pathologic) nystagmus.[1,2] Pathologic nystagmus results from a unilateral disturbance in the normal bilaterally tonic influences provided by vestibular neurons to the motor nuclei of the extraocular muscles (CN III, IV, VI). Spontaneous nystagmus may be a very short-lived abnormality, as it can often be rapidly compensated for by voluntary visual fixation,[1,3,4] especially when the spontaneous nystagmus is the result of a peripheral vestibular lesion.

Vestibular (positional) strabismus
Vestibular strabismus is a positional phenomenon that manifests as a ventral to ventrolateral deviation of the globe, resulting in an increased exposure of the sclera dorsally when the head and neck are extended during testing of the tonic neck reaction. Vestibular strabismus subsequently resolves when the head is returned to a neutral position. Vestibular strabismus occurs on the side ipsilateral to a vestibular lesion.

Vestibular ataxia
The hallmark of vestibular ataxia is its asymmetric nature. Affected animals tend to lean, fall, roll, or circle toward the side of the lesion. Vestibular dysfunction typically results in circling characterized by a tight turning radius. The head and trunk may sway, and animals can assume a base-wide stance. The asymmetry of vestibular ataxia results from the altered physiologic influences normally provided via the vestibulospinal tract, as described earlier (see **Fig. 1**B).

Clinical Differentiation of Central and Peripheral Vestibular Lesions

Once any of these common features has been identified (head tilt, nystagmus, vestibular ataxia, positional strabismus), the priority of the examining clinician should be to attempt to identify the origin of the problem in either the peripheral or central components of the vestibular system (**Table 2**). Definitive diagnosis and management of central lesions will, in general, require more expensive and aggressive diagnostics and therapies, and the common causes of central vestibular disease are often associated with guarded prognoses. With the exception of malignant aural neoplasms, peripheral vestibular lesions are usually associated with good prognoses, and can be usually be diagnosed with equipment and techniques that are available and familiar to veterinary practitioners.

Table 2
Differentiating clinical features of peripheral and central vestibular disease

Clinical Sign	Peripheral Vestibular Lesion	Central Vestibular Lesion
Head tilt	Toward lesion	To either side
Pathologic nystagmus	− Direction not altered by head position − Horizontal or rotary − Fast phase away from lesion	− Direction may change with head position − Horizontal, rotary, or vertical
Postural reactions	Normal	Deficits ipsilateral to lesion
Conscious proprioception	Normal	Deficits ipsilateral to lesion
Cranial nerve deficits	±Ipsilateral CN VII	±CNN V-XII ipsilateral to lesion
Horner syndrome	±Postganglionic	±Preganglionic (rare)
Consciousness	Normal • Disorientation if acute	Normal to comatose

Clinical signs of peripheral vestibular disease

Peripheral vestibular disease does not affect strength or general proprioception; thus, peripheral disease results in an asymmetric ataxia and loss of balance, in the notable absence of detectable paresis or proprioceptive deficits. Spontaneous or positional horizontal or rotary jerk nystagmus can occur with peripheral vestibular lesions, and the fast phase will be away from the side of the lesion. Any pathologic nystagmus noted will not change direction as the head position is changed. Although debatable, it is the general consensus that vertical nystagmus is rarely (or never) associated with peripheral vestibular disease.[2,7] Peripheral vestibular lesions can also affect the facial nerve and postganglionic sympathetic innervation (Horner syndrome) to the head. Both of these neural structures are closely associated with the inner ear and vestibular receptors.

Bilateral Peripheral Vestibular Disease

Bilateral peripheral vestibular disease is occasionally seen, and is clinically character-ized by the absence of a head tilt and pathologic nystagmus, and an absent vestibulo-ocular reflex due to bilateral interruption of input from vestibular receptors. Affected animals will usually crouch low to the ground, walk tentatively, and may fall to both sides. The animal also will usually display wide lateral excursions of the head from side to side in an attempt to maintain visual fixation. This condition occurs more commonly in cats, and they often will have little apparent disturbance in equilibrium.[1,2]

Clinical Signs of Central Vestibular Disease

Lesions in the pontomedullary region most often exert a regional affect rather than being limited to a specific nerve or nucleus. Thus, lesions in the area of the vestibular nuclei also incorporate the reticular formation, which includes ascending general proprioceptive (GP) and descending upper motor neuron (UMN) white matter tracts, the reticular activating system (RAS), and cranial nerve V-XII lower motor neurons. Therefore, vestibular signs associated with a depressed level of consciousness (RAS), spastic hemiparesis (descending UMN tract deficit), cranial nerve V-XII deficits, or general proprioceptive deficits (ascending GP tracts) on the same side as the vestibular deficits should be considered to indicate a central vestibular disorder.[2,7] Identification of hemi- or tetraparesis in an animal with vestibular signs is the most reliable indicator of the presence of a central vestibular lesion.[2,7] In addition, spontaneous vertical nystagmus or pathologic nystagmus that changes direction (ie, from horizontal to vertical on changing head position) indicates the presence of central vestibular disease.[1,2]

Paradoxic (Central) Vestibular Disease

A head tilt and balance loss will occasionally be appreciated in a patient that simultaneously has postural reaction deficits that are contralateral to the direction of the head tilt. When these specific clinical signs are noticed, the lesion must involve the caudal cerebellar peduncle or the flocculonodular lobe of the cerebellum on the side of the body opposite that of the head tilt.[2,6] This condition is called paradoxic vestibular disease, and it is always indicative of central vestibular dysfunction. Because the head tilt does not fit the expected pattern for central disease, it is a paradox.

VESTIBULAR DISEASES OF THE DOG AND CAT
Peripheral Vestibular Disorders

In addition to a detailed history and neurologic examination, diagnostics that are helpful to assess the peripheral vestibular apparatus include otoscopic examination, bulla radiographs, bulla ultrasound, microbiology, myringotomy, fine-needle aspirate, serology, and biopsy procedures (**Fig. 3**). Performance of these diagnostics is greatly facilitated by heavy sedation or general anesthesia. Computed tomography (CT) and magnetic resonance imaging (MRI) are also valuable for the diagnosis and morphologic characterization of peripheral vestibular diseases,[8–13] but most disorders that cause peripheral vestibular dysfunction can be identified and managed without these imaging techniques. **Table 3** provides a summary of common origins of peripheral vestibular dysfunction.

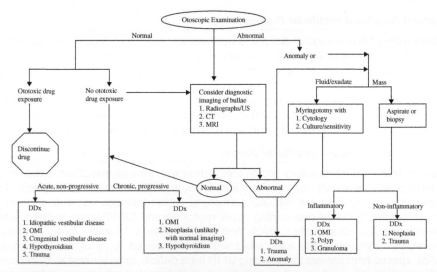

Fig. 3. Diagnostic algorithm for peripheral vestibular disease. CT, computed tomography; DDx, differential diagnoses; MRI, magnetic resonance imaging; OMI, otitis media interna; US, ultrasonography.

Table 3			
Common causes of peripheral vestibular disease by species			
DAMNIT Category	Specific Diseases	Canine	Feline
Anomalous	Congenital vestibular disease	X	X
Metabolic	Hypothyroidism	X	
Neoplastic	Primary aural neoplasia	X	X
	Vestibular neurofibroma		
Infectious/Inflammatory	Otitis media interna (OMI)	X	X
	Naso- and otopharyngeal polyps	X	X
Idiopathic	Idiopathic vestibular disease (vestibular neuronitis)	X	X
Trauma	Inner ear trauma	X	X
Toxic	Ototoxic drugs (systemic and topical)	X	X

Congenital vestibular disease

Congenital vestibular dysfunction has been reported in multiple purebred dogs, including Dobermans, Beagles, Cockers, Akitas, and primarily oriental breeds of cats such as Siamese, Tonkanese, and Burmese.[14,15] Clinical signs are usually apparent at birth or develop within the first few weeks of life, the cause is usually unknown, and there is no therapy. Bilateral vestibular dysfunction has been occasionally reported in some breeds. Signs resolve spontaneously in some animals, whereas others may have residual and permanent head tilts. Affected animals are usually able to compensate well for the vestibular dysfunction. This condition is variably associated with deafness or other congenital malformations. Therefore, performance of brainstem auditory evoked responses (BAER) to evaluate hearing may be indicated in these cases.

Hypothyroidism

Hypothyroidism has been implicated as a possible cause of peripheral cranial mono- and oligoneuropathies that affect CN VIII, and often CN VII concurrently.[16,17] Affected dogs may also have accompanying signs of flaccid limb weakness, suggestive of a more generalized polyneuropathy. Hypothyroidism may result in peripheral cranial neuropathies as a result of myxomatous compression of cranial nerves as they exit their respective skull foraminae. The onset of hypothyroid implicated vestibular disease may be acute or chronic in nature.[16] Diagnosis is based on documentation of low T4, free T4, and elevated thyroid-stimulating hormone (TSH) concentrations. Thyroid hormone supplementation usually results in improvement within a few months.

Aural neoplasia

Primary aural neoplasms can arise from constituents of the pinna, external canal, or middle and inner ear. Aural neoplasms may cause peripheral vestibular disease via direct compression or infiltration of the labyrinthine or neural components of the peripheral vestibular systems, or are indirectly associated with the inflammatory responses they initiate. Ceruminous adenoma/adenocarcinoma, sebaceous adenoma/adenocarcinoma, carcinomas of undetermined etiology, squamous cell carcinoma, and feline lymphoma are the most common primary aural tumors of small animals that are associated with peripheral vestibular dysfunction.[18,19] Vestibular neurofibromas (schwannomas) may also primarily arise from the vestibulocochlear nerve itself, but are uncommon. The majority (85%) of aural neoplasms in cats represent malignant phenotypes, whereas approximately 60% of canine aural tumors are malignant.[18,19] Diagnosis of these neoplasms is often obvious on visual inspection of the ear or otoscopic examination, appearing as irregular, pedunculated, polypoid, or ulcerated masses on the pinna or within the external ear canal or tympanic bulla (**Fig. 4**). The neoplasms will also occasionally result in visible and palpable soft tissue swellings external to the ear (see **Fig. 4**A and B). Otoscopic-assisted biopsy will confirm the diagnosis. CT and MR imaging may be considered to determine the extent of the lesion before cytoreductive surgery or radiation therapy, as these neoplasms may locally invade the adjacent soft tissues of the head (**Fig. 5**), skull, or brainstem.[20] Diagnostic imaging features of lytic bone disease involving the bulla or petrous temporal bone is more often associated with aural neoplasia than inflammatory disease. Thus, if osteolysis is present on radiographs, CT, or MRI, aural neoplasia should be a primary differential diagnostic consideration. Aggressive surgical excision of aural neoplasia is the treatment of choice, although primary or adjunctive radiotherapy may also be of benefit.[19] Prednisone (0.5–1 mg/kg/d by mouth) may transiently palliate some of the clinical signs.

Otitis media interna
Otitis media interna (OMI) is the most common cause of peripheral vestibular disease seen in dogs and cats, and may account for nearly 50% of all cases of canine peripheral vestibular disease.[14,21] It is important to recognize that otitis media alone will not result in vestibular signs. If deficits compatible with peripheral vestibular dysfunction are detected, inner ear involvement is confirmed.[1,22] OMI is the most common cause of combinations of simultaneously occurring ipsilateral deficits of the peripheral portions of cranial nerves VII, VIII, and the postganglionic sympathetic neuron (Horner syndrome) to the head.[2,22] In animals with OMI, peripheral vestibular signs may also be accompanied or preceded by nonneurologic signs referable to infection of the external or middle ears, such as head shaking, temporomandibular pain, bulla pain, or otic discharge.[21,22] Otitis media has been shown to be a common complication of chronic otitis externa, occurring in 50% to 80% of dogs with chronic otitis externa.[23]

A thorough otoscopic examination, bulla imaging, and myringotomy are the primary tools used to diagnose OMI. Otoscopic diagnosis of OMI can be complicated by

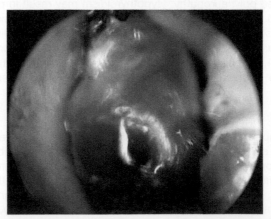

Fig. 4. Otoendoscopic view of a pedunculated mass obliterating the lumen of the external ear canal from a dog with peripheral vestibular disease. The histologic diagnosis was a carcinoma of undetermined origin.

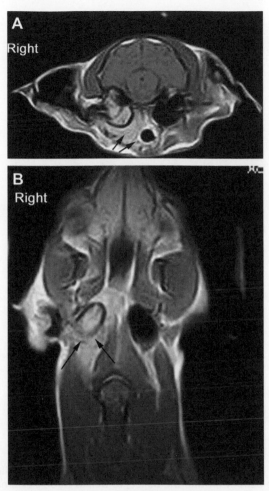

Fig. 5. Postcontrast, axial (A) and dorsal planar (B) T1-weighted MR images from the level of the tympanic bullae from a cat with right peripheral vestibular signs and a palpable soft tissue swelling at the base of the right ear (arrows). Both the material in the right tympanic bulla and the periaural soft tissues demonstrate contrast enhancement. Biopsy of these lesions revealed lymphosarcoma.

chronic remodeling of the external ear canal (hyperplasia, stenosis) that impedes visualization of the tympanum and sampling of the middle ear cavity. In addition, the presence of an intact or grossly normal tympanic membrane or normal appearing external ear canal does not exclude the possibility that OMI may be present. It has been reported that 70% of dogs with OMI had an intact tympanum.[23] Bulla radiographs, CT, and MRI provide supportive diagnostic information by revealing fluid or soft tissue accumulations within the bullae, and often secondary reactive or remodeling changes of the middle and external ear (**Fig. 6**A and B; sclerosis, thickening, or lysis of the bullae, calcification or stenosis of external ear canal), depending on the chronicity of the lesion.[10–12] CT imaging has been reported to be more sensitive than radiography for evaluation of the bullae in cases of OMI.[10,12,13] When performing a radiographic bulla series, obtaining rostrocaudal open-mouth and oblique views in addition to

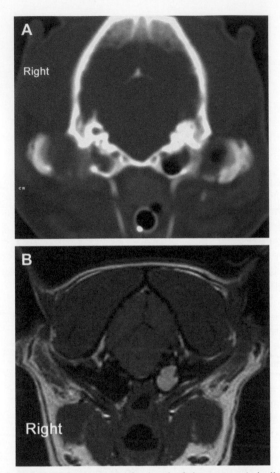

Fig. 6. Axial CT (*A*) and MR (*B*) images at the level of the tympanic bullae from dogs with OMI. (*A*) Soft tissue densities within the bullae, as well as chronic external ear remodeling (calcification, canal stenosis) are apparent. (*B*) Postcontrast T1-weighted image demonstrating hyperintense material within the left bulla.

standard lateral and dorsoventral views is helpful. Ultrasonographic imaging techniques that are effective in the identification of fluid within the bullae have also been described.[13] Ultrasonography offers advantages over radiography, CT, and MRI in that the bullae can usually be satisfactorily imaged without anesthesia.

Myringotomy samples should be submitted for cytologic evaluation and culture. Commonly cultured organisms include staphylococcal species, *Pseudomonas, Streptococcus, Proteus, Malassezia,* and *Candida.* The emergence of multidrug-resistant *Pseudomonas* and staphylococcal species in veterinary medicine has confirmed the importance of culture and sensitivity in the management of chronic or recurrent OMI. The presence of anatomic conformational defects, otic foreign bodies, keratinization disorders, ectoparasites, and allergic disease may predispose the animal to otitis externa and therefore OMI. A primary secretory otitis media (PSOM) has been also described, primarily in Cavalier King Charles Spaniels, to commonly cause vestibular signs. In PSOM, the debris in the middle ear consists of a viscous mucous plug.[24]

Medical treatment of OMI and PSOM consists in thorough cleansing and flushing of any exudates and debris from the affected ear under anesthesia, 4 to 8 weeks of broad-spectrum, systemically administered antimicrobial therapy, ideally based on culture and sensitivity, identification and treatment of predisposing factors, and anti-inflammatory (topical or systemic) therapy.[21,24,25] When cleansing the ear, exercise caution when considering the instillation of any solution or drug that is potentially ototoxic. Sterile physiologic (0.9%) saline or sterile water are readily available, nontoxic, inexpensive, and sufficient for most ear-cleansing applications.

Otogenic infections arising from the external or middle ears can extend into the calvarium, causing brain abscessation and bacterial meningoencephalitis.[26] Clinical signs in these cases indicate central vestibular lesions, but may be preceded by peripheral vestibular signs. Aggressive surgical debridement and parenteral antibiotic therapy are required in these cases.

Bulla osteotomy or total ear canal ablation procedures should be considered in animals that do not respond to medical treatment, experience a relapse of clinical signs despite appropriate therapy, or have chronic, end-stage remodeling of the ear anatomy. In general, animals with OMI that are successfully treated will compensate for residual vestibular dysfunction and recover, but facial paresis may be permanent and can be a complication of surgery.

Naso- and otopharyngeal polyps

Inflammatory polyps arise from the mucosal lining of the tympanum, auditory tube, or pharynx, and are much more common in cats than dogs. Inflammatory polyps are usually unilateral, and are typically seen in young cats (1–5 years of age). Vestibular signs may be preceded by signs of chronic upper respiratory, pharyngeal, or otic disease. Polyps are usually easily diagnosed with otoscopic and oral examinations (**Fig. 7**). Radiographs, CT, or endoscopy may occasionally be required for diagnosis, or to document the presence of middle ear involvement when planning treatment. Removal of the polyp via traction polypectomy through the mouth or external ear canal

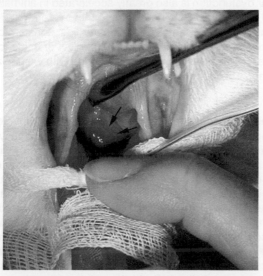

Fig. 7. Intraoral photograph from a cat with peripheral vestibular signs from an otopharyngeal polyp (*arrows*). The soft palate is retracted with a spay hook.

is usually successful and sufficient if there is no involvement of the tympanic cavity, but is associated with a 30% to 40% recurrence rate. Surgical removal via a bulla osteotomy/ear canal ablation has a recurrence rate of less than 10%.[27] Vestibular signs, Horner syndrome, and facial nerve paresis, which are usually transient, can occur as sequelae of surgical polypectomy.[19]

Canine and feline idiopathic peripheral vestibular disease; geriatric vestibular disease; vestibular neuritis

Canine idiopathic peripheral vestibular disease is the second most common cause of peripheral vestibular dysfunction in dogs,[21] and is a common etiology for unilateral peripheral vestibular dysfunction of peracute onset (head tilt, ataxia, horizontal or rotary nystagmus) in dogs and cats. Although this disease may be seen in any aged dog, geriatric canines appear to be predisposed, and it is very atypical to be seen in dogs younger than 5 years old. In both dogs and cats, idiopathic peripheral vestibular disease results in clinical signs referable to dysfunction of the peripheral vestibular system only; affected animals do not have concurrent facial nerve paralysis or postganglionic Horner syndrome. In the acute setting the clinical signs can be severe (rolling, falling) and some animals may vomit.

Feline idiopathic peripheral vestibular disease differs slightly in that it can occur in cats of any age, has a higher incidence in outdoor cats in the summer and fall months in the northeastern and mid-Atlantic regions of the United States, and will occasionally result in bilateral peripheral vestibular signs.[1,2,28] Idiopathic vestibular disease is diagnosed by excluding other causes of peripheral vestibular dysfunction. Diagnostic imaging studies of the peripheral vestibular apparatus are usually normal in animals with this disease. The cause of this disease is unknown, although it is often compared with vestibular neuronitis in humans, which may be triggered by viral antigens.[3,4]

Diazepam can be administered for its anxiolytic effects. An empiric course of systemic broad-spectrum antibiotic therapy is reasonable to treat occult OMI. Initial signs of improvement occur within 3 to 5 days, and recovery is noted within 2 to 3 weeks. A residual head tilt may persist. Therapy is mainly supportive, and compensation for vestibular dysfunction is also greatly accelerated in animals that are encouraged and assisted to walk. There is no evidence that symptomatic medical therapy, such as anti-inflammatory treatment with corticosteroids, nonsteroidal anti-inflammatories, or antihistamine motion sickness drugs expedites or influences recovery from this disease process. Nausea and vomiting associated with vestibular disease can be treated as necessary. This condition may occasionally recur.

Ototoxicity

Numerous therapeutic substances, including aminoglycoside antibiotics, furosemide, platinum-containing antineoplastic agents, salicylates, and many detergents and alcohol-based solutions have been demonstrated to have ototoxic potential when administered parenterally or topically in the presence of a compromised tympanic membrane.[29] The ototoxicity of most compounds results from induction of damage to or death of the neuroepithelial (hair-cell) receptors within the membranous labyrinth. The clinical manifestations of ototoxicity are drug dependent and wide ranging in severity, and can include both sensorineural deafness and vestibular dysfunction. In the majority of cases, deafness that results is permanent, while vestibular signs may improve or resolve. It is prudent to recognize that the majority of commercially marketed otic antimicrobial and cleansing solutions approved for topical applications contain one or more potentially ototoxic ingredients. Any therapeutic agent with ototoxic potential should be avoided in cases in which the tympanum is known or suspected to be perforated. It may be necessary to perform a BAER to confirm acquired sensorineural deafness.

Central Vestibular Disorders

Clinical localization of the lesion to the central vestibular system is generally an indication for the performance of more aggressive and invasive diagnostics (intracranial cross-sectional imaging such as MRI and CT, CSF analysis, serologic and genetic assays, and BAER). MRI is the preferred diagnostic imaging modality for patients with central vestibular dysfunction. In a retrospective review of canine vestibular disease, brain morphologic abnormalities were detected in 100% of dogs with clinical evidence of central vestibular dysfunction in which MRI was performed.[8] With few exceptions, many of the common causes of central vestibular disease (**Table 4**) can be associated with rapid and severe neurologic deterioration or death if not identified and treated promptly.

Hypothyroidism

Central vestibular and vestibulocerebellar signs can rarely be associated with canine hypothyroidism.[30,31] Many dogs (70%) with central vestibular complications of hypothyroidism have no other extraneural clinical evidence of hypothyroidism.[30] However, serum biochemical profiles from affected dogs commonly demonstrate hypercholesterolinemia or hypertriglyceridemia. The cause of hypothyroid-associated central vestibular disease is likely multifactorial, and includes ischemic infarction associated with atherosclerotic vascular disease and central nervous system (CNS) demyelination.[30,32] Intracranial imaging studies from these dogs may be normal or reveal evidence of infarction. Diagnosis is based on documentation of low T4, free T4, and elevated TSH concentrations, excluding other possible causes of central vestibular

Table 4	
Central vestibular diseases of the dog and cat	
DAMNIT Category	**Specific Diseases**
Anomalous	Quadrigeminal arachnoid-like cysts
	Caudal occipital malformation syndrome
	Hydrocephalus
Metabolic	Hypothyroidism[a] (±infarction)
Nutritional	Thiamine deficiency
Neoplasia	Primary intracranial neoplasms[a]
	• Meningioma, glioma, medulloblastoma, choroid plexus tumors, lymphoma
	Metastatic neoplasms
Infectious/Inflammatory	*Viral*—Canine distemper virus, feline infectious peritonitis
	Bacterial—Abscess, Rocky Mountain spotted fever, ehrlichiosis, bartonellosis
	Protozoal—Toxoplasmosis, neosporosis
	Mycotic—Cryptococcosis, blastomycosis, others
	Noninfectious meningoencephalitides—Granulomatous meningoencephalitis, necrotizing meningoencephalitides
Trauma	Brainstem trauma
Toxic	Metronidazole[a]
Vascular	Cerebrovascular disease[a]

[a] Discussed in this article.

dysfunction. Thyroid hormone supplementation results in rapid improvement within a few days.

Intracranial neoplasia

Meningiomas, which are the most common primary intracranial tumor in both dogs and cats, have a propensity to develop along the lateral and ventral surfaces of the cerebellopontomedullary region.[33] Choroid plexus tumors also commonly develop at the cerebellopontomedullary angle and within the fourth ventricle.[34] Gliomas may develop anywhere within the brainstem parenchyma. In these cases, central vestibular signs are common, and may develop as a result of increased intracranial pressure, compression or invasion of vestibular nuclei, obstructive hydrocephalus, or a brain herniation due to a neoplasm causing mass effect from any location within the brain.

The preferred method of presumptive antemortem diagnosis of intracranial neoplasia is MRI, as CT causes beam-hardening artifact that may preclude visualization of small lesions in the cerebellum, pons, and medulla. The MRI characteristics of common canine and feline intracranial neoplasms have been well defined (**Fig. 8**), and often allow for accurate and noninvasive prediction of the histologic tumor type.[35–37] However, definitive diagnosis of intracranial neoplasia requires tumor biopsy. Although analysis of CSF typically reflects nonspecific abnormalities, exfoliated neoplastic cells may detected in animals with choroid plexus carcinomas and CNS lymphoma.[34]

In cases of infratentorial neoplasia, the prognosis is likely dependent on the histologic type of the tumor, the severity of tumor-associated neurologic dysfunction, the neuroanatomic location and extent of the neoplasm, and the type of treatments administered. Although there are few evidence-based data in the literature that provide objective prognostic information pertaining to infratentorial tumors, the prognosis is generally considered unfavorable compared with that of supratentorial tumors. Intra-axial tumors (gliomas) are typically associated with a worse prognosis than extra-axial tumors (meningioma, choroid plexus tumor; **Fig. 9**), and the severity of neurologic dysfunction is also considered to be negatively correlated with outcome.

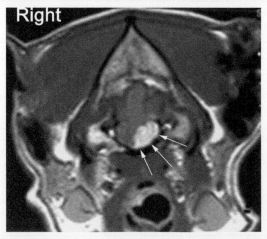

Fig. 8. Axial T1-weighted, postcontrast MRI scan obtained from a dog with left head tilt, vertical nystagmus, and left hemiparesis. A uniformly enhancing, extra-axial mass lesion is present in the left ventrolateral aspect of the medulla (*arrows*). A transitional meningioma was confirmed at necropsy.

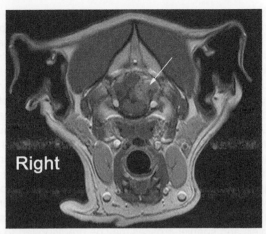

Fig. 9. Axial, T1-weighted, postcontrast MRI scan obtained from a dog with paradoxic central vestibular signs consisting of a right head tilt, rotary nystagmus, and left hemiparesis. An extra-axial, hyperintense mass (choroid plexus tumor) is present in left cerebellopontomedullary region (*arrow*).

In the infratentorial region, cytoreductive surgery is usually limited to cases with extra-axial neoplasia. Primary or postoperative adjunctive external beam radiotherapy (fractionated or stereotactic) has been shown to be beneficial for improving the quality of life and prolonging survival in animals with brain tumors.[38] Palliative treatment with corticosteroids (0.5–1.0 mg/kg/d by mouth) may temporarily improve clinical signs.

Meningoencephalitis
Multiple infectious agents and noninfectious inflammatory diseases (see **Table 4**) can involve the central vestibular system. Depending on the causative agent, central vestibular signs may be the predominant clinical manifestation, part of a multifocal CNS presentation, or a component of a polysystemic clinical disease. The pathogenesis, diagnosis, and management of the meningoencephalitides are covered in detail in this issue and elsewhere.[1,2,39]

Metronidazole toxicosis
Metronidazole administration can cause central vestibular disease or vestibulocerebellar signs, particularly in dogs.[40,41] Neurologic toxicity has usually been reported to occur following subacute to chronic administration of metronidazole doses that exceed 60 mg/kg/d.[40–43] However, individual animal susceptibilities to the toxic effects of this drug are apparently variable, as toxicity has been observed at lower doses in both dogs and cats. Felines may commonly present with neurologic signs referable to forebrain dysfunction, such as seizures, blindness, or alterations in consciousness.[42,43] The exact mechanism of toxicity is unknown, but is theorized to be modulated by γ-aminobutyric acid receptors in the vestibulocerebellum.[41] Diagnosis is based on an appropriate history of exposure and clinical signs. Treatment should include cessation of metronidazole therapy and supportive care. The recovery time with nonspecific, supportive therapies is 1 to 2 weeks. It has been demonstrated that administration of diazepam (0.5 mg/kg intravenous once; then 0.5 mg/kg by mouth every 8 hours for 3 days) greatly expedited improvement and recovery from metronidazole toxicity in dogs.[41] Dogs treated with diazepam recovered in 1.5 days versus 11 days for dogs receiving supportive care only.

Cerebrovascular disease

Ischemic infarctions and transient ischemic attacks (TIAs) have been increasingly recognized as a cause of acute-onset, focal, and nonprogressive central and paradoxic vestibular signs in dogs, and to a lesser extent, cats.[30,44,45] TIAs are characterized by an abrupt onset, brief (<24 hours), focal neurologic disturbance that results from functional ischemia.[30,45] TIAs may precede infarctions visible on imaging studies. Central vestibular dysfunction resulting from ischemic infarcts can result from infarction of the medullary components of the central vestibular apparatus or the vestibulocerebellum. Cerebellar ischemic infarcts typically appear wedge-shaped and are hypoattenuating on CT images. With MRI, ischemic infarcts demonstrate T1 iso- to hypointensity, T2 and fluid-attenuated inversion recovery hyperintensity, and mild to absent contrast enhancement depending on the timing of imaging in relation to the onset of clinical signs. Cerebellar infarctions often topographically appear as territorial lesions that occur within the distribution of the rostral cerebellar artery.[45] Diagnosis of infarctions is greatly supported by performing diffusion-weighted and T2* gradient-echo images. Spaniels and spaniel-crosses may be predisposed to cerebellar infarctions.[45] In cases in which infarcts are suspected, the animal should be evaluated for underlying hypertension, hyperadrenocorticism, hypothyroidism, and cardiac or renal disease.[30,44] Many animals with infarcts in this area will improve with time and supportive care. The future risk for infarction and neurologic-associated mortality is significantly higher in dogs with infarcts in which a predisposing medical condition is identified.[44]

SUMMARY

The vestibular system is the primary sensory modality that participates in the maintenance of balance. Clinical signs of vestibular disease include asymmetric ataxia, head tilt, and pathologic nystagmus. Neuroanatomic localization of observed vestibular signs to either the peripheral or central components of the vestibular system is paramount to the management of the patient with vestibular dysfunction, as the causes, diagnostic approaches, and prognoses are dependent on the neuroanatomic diagnosis. This article reviews functional vestibular neuroanatomy, as well as the diagnosis and treatment of common causes of small animal vestibular disease.

REFERENCES

1. Thomas WB. Vestibular dysfunction. Vet Clin North Am 2000;30(1):227–49.
2. deLahunta A, Glass E. Vestibular system: special proprioception. In: Veterinary neuroanatomy and clinical neurology. 3rd edition. St. Louis (MO): Saunders/Elsevier; 2009. p. 319–47.
3. Angelaki DE, Cullen KE. Vestibular system: the many facets of a multimodal sense. Annu Rev Neurosci 2008;31:125–50.
4. Brandt T, Strupp M. General vestibular testing. Clin Neurophysiol 2005;116:406–26.
5. Evans HE, Kitchell RL. Cranial nerves and cutaneous innervation of the head. In: Evans HE, editor. Miller's anatomy of the dog. 3rd edition. Philadelphia: WB Saunders; 1993. p. 953–87.
6. King AS. Physiological and clinical anatomy of the domestic mammals. In: Central nervous system. vol. 1. New York: Oxford University Press; 1994. p. 171–82.
7. Troxel MT, Drobtaz KJ, Vite CH. Signs of neurologic dysfunction in dogs with central versus peripheral vestibular disease. J Am Vet Med Assoc 2005;227(4):570–4.

8. Garosi LS, Dennis R, Penderis J, et al. Results of magnetic resonance imaging in dogs with vestibular disorders: 85 cases (1996–1999). J Am Vet Med Assoc 2001; 218(3):385–91.

9. Allgoewer I, Lucas S, Schmitz SA. Magnetic resonance imaging of the normal and diseases feline middle ear. Vet Radiol Ultrasound 2000;41(5):413–8.

10. Love NE, Kramer RW, Spodnick GJ, et al. Radiographic and computed tomographic evaluation of otitis media in the dog. Vet Radiol Ultrasound 1995;36(5): 375–9.

11. Owen MC, Lamb CR, Lu D, et al. Material in the middle ear of dogs having magnetic resonance imaging for investigation of neurologic signs. Vet Radiol Ultrasound 2004;45(2):149–55.

12. Rohleder JJ, Jones JC, Duncan RB. Comparative performance of radiography and computed tomography in the diagnosis of middle ear disease in 31 dogs. Vet Radiol Ultrasound 2006;47(1):45–52.

13. Dickie AM, Doust R, Cromarty L, et al. Comparison of ultrasonography, radiography, and a single computed tomography slice for the identification of fluid within the canine tympanic bulla. Res Vet Sci 2003;75:209–16.

14. Schunk KL. Disorders of the vestibular system. Vet Clin North Am 1988;18: 641–55.

15. Forbes S, Cook JR Jr. Congenital peripheral vestibular disease attributed to lymphocytic labyrinthitis in two related litters of Doberman pinscher pups. J Am Vet Med Assoc 1991;198(3):447–9.

16. Jaggy A. Neurologic manifestations of canine hypothyroidism. In: Bonagura JD, editor. Kirk's current veterinary therapy XIII. Philadelphia: WB Saunders; 2000. p. 974–5.

17. Jaggy A, Oliver JE, Ferguson DC, et al. Neurologic manifestations of hypothyroidism: a retrospective study of 29 dogs. J Vet Intern Med 1994;8:328–36.

18. London CA, Dubilzeig RR, Vail DM, et al. Evaluation of dogs and cats with tumors of the ear canal: 145 cases (1978–1992). J Am Vet Med Assoc 1996;208(9): 1413–8.

19. Fan TM, de Lorimier LP. Inflammatory polyps and aural neoplasia. Vet Clin North Am 2004;34(2):489–509.

20. Lucroy MD, Vernau KM, Samii VF, et al. Middle ear tumours with brainstem extension treated by ventral bulla osteotomy and craniectomy in two cats. Vet Comp Oncol 2004;2(4):234–42.

21. Schunk KL, Averill DR. Peripheral vestibular syndrome in the dog: a review of 83 cases. J Am Vet Med Assoc 1983;182:1354–7.

22. Shell LG. Otitis media and otitis interna—etiology, diagnosis, and medical management. Vet Clin North Am 1988;18(4):885–99.

23. Cole LK, Kwochka KW, Kowalski JJ, et al. Microbial flora and antimicrobial sensitivity patterns of isolated pathogens from the horizontal ear canal and middle ear in dogs with otitis media. J Am Vet Med Assoc 1998;212(4):534–8.

24. Stern-Stertholtz W, Sjostrom L, Wallan Hakanson N. Primary secretory otitis media in the Cavalier King Charles Spaniel: a review of 61 cases. J Small Anim Pract 2003;44(6):253–66.

25. Palmiero BS, Morris DO, Wiemelt SP, et al. Evaluation of outcome of otitis media after lavalge of the tympanic bulla and long-term antimicrobial treatment in dogs: 44 cases (1998–2002). J Am Vet Med Assoc 2004;225(4):548–53.

26. Sturges BK, Dickinson PJ, Kortz GD, et al. Clinical signs, magnetic resonance imaging features, and outcome after surgical and medical treatment of otogenic

intracranial infection in 11 cats and 4 dogs. J Vet Intern Med 2006;20(3): 648–56.

27. Trevor PB, Martin RA. Tympanic bulla osteotomy for the treatment of middle-ear disease in cats: 19 cases (1984–1991). J Am Vet Med Assoc 1993;202(1): 123–9.

28. Burke EE, Moise NS, deLahunta A, et al. Review of idiopathic feline vestibular syndrome in 75 cats. J Am Vet Med Assoc 1985;187:941–3.

29. Merchant SR. Ototoxicity. Vet Clin North Am 1994;24(5):971–9.

30. Higgins MA, Rossmeisl JH, Panciera DL. Hypothyroid-associated central vestibular disease in 10 dogs: 1999–2005. J Vet Intern Med 2006;20(6):1363–9.

31. Bichsel P, Jacobs G, Oliver JE. Neurologic manifestations associated with hypothyroidism in 4 dogs. J Am Vet Med Assoc 1988;192:1745–7.

32. Hess RS, Kass PH, Van Winkle TJ. Association between diabetes mellitus, hypothyroidism or hyperadrenocorticism, and atherosclerosis in dogs. J Vet Intern Med 2003;17:489–94.

33. Snyder JM, Shofer FS, Van Winkle TJ, et al. Canine primary intracranial neoplasia: 173 cases (1986–2003). J Vet Intern Med 2006;20:669–75.

34. Westworth DR, Dickinson PJ, Vernau W, et al. Choroid plexus tumors in 56 dogs (1985–2007). J Vet Intern Med 2008;22:1157–65.

35. Cherubini GB, Mantis P, Martinez TA, et al. Utility of magnetic resonance imaging for distinguishing neoplastic from non-neoplastic brain lesions in dogs and cats. Vet Radiol Ultrasound 2005;46(5):384–7.

36. Thomas WB, Wheeler SJ, Kramer R, et al. Magnetic resonance imaging of primary brain tumors in dogs. Vet Radiol Ultrasound 1996;37(1):20–7.

37. Troxel MT, Vite CH, Massicotte C, et al. Magnetic resonance imaging features of feline intracranial neoplasia: retrospective analysis of 46 cats. J Vet Intern Med 2004;18:176–89.

38. Evans SM, Dayrell-Hart B, Powlis W, et al. Radiation therapy of canine brain masses. J Vet Intern Med 1993;7:216–9.

39. Munana KR. Encephalitis and meningitis. Vet Clin North Am 1996;26(4):857–74.

40. Dow SW, LeCouteur RA, Poss ML, et al. Central nervous system toxicosis associated with metronidazole treatment of dogs: 5 cases (1984–1987). J Am Vet Med Assoc 1989;195:365–8.

41. Evans J, Levesque D, Knowles K, et al. Diazepam as a treatment for metronidazole toxicosis in dogs: a retrospective study of 21 cases. J Vet Intern Med 2003; 17(3):304–10.

42. Caylor KB, Cassimatis MK. Metronidazole neurotoxicosis in 2 cats. J Am Anim Hosp Assoc 2001;37(3):258–62.

43. Saxon B, Magne ML. Reversible central nervous system toxicosis associated with metronidazole therapy in three cats. Prog Vet Neurol 1993;4:25–7.

44. Garosi L, McConnell J, Platt S, et al. Results of diagnostic investigations and long-term outcome of 33 dogs with brain infarction (2000–2004). J Vet Intern Med 2005;19:725–31.

45. McConnell JF, Garosi L, Platt SR. Magnetic resonance imaging findings of presumed cerebellar cerebrovascular accident in twelve dogs. Vet Radiol Ultrasound 2005;46:1–10.

Idiopathic Granulomatous and Necrotizing Inflammatory Disorders of the Canine Central Nervous System

Scott J. Schatzberg, DVM, PhD

KEYWORDS

- Central nervous system
- Granulomatous meningoencephalomyelitis
- Necrotizing meningoencephalitis

Granulomatous meningoencephalomyelitis (GME), necrotizing meningoencephalitis (NME), and necrotizing leukoencephalitis (NLE) are common inflammatory conditions of the canine central nervous system (CNS). Although each disease has unique histopathological features, these canine disorders collectively seem to be aberrant immune responses directed against the CNS. Despite having been recognized for several decades, the etiopathogeneses for these disorders remain elusive, and gold standard treatment protocols have yet to be established.

The antemortem diagnosis of the specific variants of canine meningoencephalitis (ME) is challenging, because histopathological confirmation is required for a definitive diagnosis. In most cases, a presumptive antemortem diagnosis is achieved via a multimodal approach that includes: assessment of case signalment, neurologic signs and neuroanatomic localization, cerebrospinal fluid (CSF) analysis, cross-sectional imaging of the CNS, and infectious disease testing. The antemortem diagnosis often is complicated by an overlap in the neurodiagnostic profiles among GME, NME, and NLE. Therefore, the terminology meningoencephalitis of unknown etiology (MUE) may be preferable on an antemortem basis in cases of idiopathic ME where histopathology is lacking.[1-3]

Department of Small Animal Medicine and Surgery, College of Veterinary Medicine, University of Georgia, 501 DW Brooks Drive, Athens, GA 30602, USA
E-mail address: schatz13@uga.edu

Vet Clin Small Anim 40 (2010) 101–120
doi:10.1016/j.cvsm.2009.09.003

A review of the neurologic signs and general neurodiagnostic approach to canine ME is followed by an overview of the specific clinical and neuropathological features of GME, NME, and NLE. The etiopathogenesis of each disorder is explored, including potential genetic, immunologic, and environmental factors along with the current and prospective immunomodulatory therapies for MUE.

MENINGOENCEPHALITIS: CLINICAL SIGNS AND NEURODIAGNOSTIC APPROACH
Clinical Signs

The clinical presentation of ME is variable and typically reflects the arrangement and location of the CNS lesions. Although the spinal cord may be affected by CNS inflammation, the clinical signs associated with brain inflammation are considered primarily here. Meningoencephalitis commonly is acute in onset, progressive in nature, and associated with a multifocal to diffuse neuroanatomic localization. Extraneural signs are rare; however, pyrexia and systemic leukocytosis occasionally accompany CNS inflammation.

Neurodiagnostic Approach

The differential diagnosis for dogs presented for an acute onset of multifocal CNS signs includes genetic abnormalities, metabolic derangements, infectious and idiopathic ME, neoplasia, and toxin exposure. To differentiate among these disorders may be challenging; diagnostic testing typically includes: a minimum database (complete blood cell count (CBC), chemistry panel, and urinalysis), survey radiographs of the thorax (plus or minus abdominal ultrasound) to rule down systemic disease and metastatic neoplasia, advanced cross-sectional imaging via computed tomography (CT) scan or magnetic resonance imaging (MRI), and cerebrospinal fluid (CSF) collection and analysis. Although more often used for suspected brain tumors, CT-guided brain biopsy and histopathological evaluation of brain tissue may be considered in cases of suspected ME.[4]

CSF analysis
CSF analysis routinely includes cytologic evaluation, differential cell counts, and total protein measurement. Although pleocytosis commonly is present in cases of ME, cytology rarely provides definitive differentiation among idiopathic, infectious, and neoplastic disorders. The CSF white blood cell differential, however, when combined with cross-sectional imaging of the CNS, may help the clinician to narrow the differential diagnosis. It is unclear whether the pleocytosis associated with ME is derived from an influx of systemic inflammatory cells or secondary to local production by the CNS macrophage phagocytic system.[5] Regardless of the origin, inflammatory cells accumulate in the Virchow-Robin spaces surrounding blood vessels that penetrate the brain. The magnitude of CSF pleocytosis does not predict survival time, and in rare cases of ME, CSF cell counts may be misleadingly normal.[6] Elevated CSF total protein also is typical in ME and may be secondary to increased permeability of the blood CSF barrier, intrathecal immunoglobulin production, or both.[7] Antibody titers and polymerase chain reaction (PCR) testing for infectious diseases should be considered when CSF analysis and neuroimaging are consistent with ME.

Cross-sectional imaging
Although CT scan may have diagnostic utility in some cases of inflammatory brain disease, MRI is the gold standard imaging modality for ME. MRI may be especially helpful for differentiating among the idiopathic meningoencephalitides, as it often discloses lesions that are reflective of the gross neuropathologies associated with

each disorder. Although there are overlapping clinical and histopathological features among the meningoencephalitides, the topographic distribution of the lesions (eg, NME vs NLE) and presence or absence of necrosis (eg, GME vs NLE) may be imaging features that help direct a presumptive antemortem diagnosis. MRI also has several advantages over CT scan, as it provides excellent anatomic detail (especially of the caudal fossa) and allows for acquisition of images in multiple planes (sagittal, transverse, dorsal).

Despite the limited soft tissue detail provided by CT scan, when coupled with CSF analysis, it may help to provide evidence of ME. The imaging features for several inflammatory brain diseases have been described[8,9]; however, the CT appearance of ME is variable and nonspecific. The presence or absence of contrast enhancement with inflammatory brain disease depends upon the degree of blood–brain barrier (BBB) breakdown.[8,10] Despite the fact that it cannot differentiate definitively among disease processes, CT may be especially useful for localizing lesions before brain biopsy. An important limitation of CT is that it produces a beam-hardening artifact (because of preferential absorption of low-energy radiograph beams), most notably adjacent to the petrous parts of the temporal bones. This artifact may obscure the clinician's ability to interpret brainstem and cerebellar lesions.

GME
Background

In 1962, Koestner used the nomenclature reticulosis for a canine ME that is histopathologically consistent with GME.[11,12] This term was introduced in human neuropathology in the 1950s, but went out of favor by 1980, with the reclassification of reticulosis as a primary CNS B-cell lymphoma.[13] The terminology CNS reticulosis persisted in veterinary medicine despite a lack of similarity to the human lesion.[13] In 1972, Fankhauser and colleagues[14] divided CNS reticulosis in dogs into three categories: inflammatory, neoplastic, and microgliomatosis. Histopathologically, the inflammatory form of reticulosis consists of histiocytic cells mixed with lymphocytes, plasma cells, and occasionally other leukocytes. Monomorphic leukocytes predominate in the neoplastic form.[15] Inflammatory reticulosis of the brain and spinal cord has since been reclassified as GME.[15-19] Neoplastic reticulosis was reclassified as CNS lymphosarcoma (LSA) or malignant histiocytosis.[20] Microgliomatosis has been reported only rarely in dogs.[20]

Clinical Features

GME is difficult to distinguish from the various forms of ME on clinical grounds, but it may represent up to 25% of canine CNS disease.[21] Typically, GME presents as an acute-onset, progressive, multifocal neurologic disease that may be fatal if left untreated.[7,15,22] Females and toy and terrier breeds are overrepresented for GME, however, both ocxes and all breeds may be affected. The mean age of onset of neurologic signs is 55 months (range: 6 to 144 months).[23] Clinical signs reflect focal or multifocal CNS disease, and they depend on the lesion location within the neuraxis. Neurologic deficits referable to the caudal cranial fossa (vestibulocerebellar signs) and cervical spinal cord, in addition to seizures and visual deficits have been reported most frequently.[15] Leptomeningeal involvement may result in mild to severe CSF mononuclear pleocytosis and a total protein elevation; however, the CSF occasionally is normal.

Three forms of GME have been described based on both morphologic and clinical neurologic abnormalities: disseminated, focal and ocular.[24] The disseminated form is most common, and it typically manifests as an acute onset of rapidly progressive multi-focal neurologic signs involving the cerebrum, caudal brainstem, cerebellum, or cervical spinal cord.[7] Neurologic signs associated with the uncommon, focal form of GME may be acute or slowly progressive, and they are suggestive of a single space-occupying mass lesion.[7,16] In the focal form of GME, solitary granuloma-like lesions may form in the cerebrum, brainstem, carebellum or spinal cord.[15] Cerebrothalamic signs were reported most frequently with focal GME in one study.[7] Focal GME must be differentiated from CNS malignant histiocytosis and primary CNS LSA. The ocular form of GME manifests with an acute onset of visual impairment, variable pupillary changes (commonly dilated and unresponsive), variable degrees of optic disc edema, and occasionally chorioretinitis, especially in the nontapetal fundus.[15,16,25] Dogs with ocular GME concurrently may have or progress to develop disseminated CNS lesions.

Neuroimaging

Although not specific for GME, the most common MRI findings for the disseminated form include multiple hyperintensities on T2-weighted or fluid-attenuated inversion recovery (FLAIR) sequences scattered throughout the CNS white matter.[26,27] These lesions typically assume an infiltrative appearance and have irregular margins. Despite the predilection of the GME for white matter, MRI lesions often are distributed throughout both gray and white matter (**Fig. 1**). The lesions have variable intensity on T1-weighted images and varlable degrees of contrast enhancement.[26] Vasogenic edema in the white matter is commonly present on T2-weighted images and appears hyperintense to cerebral parenchyma. Meningeal enhancement is uncommon. Mild NME, infectious ME, CNS LSA, and less commonly glial and metastatic neoplasms, may present with similar clinical and MRI findings to disseminated GME, and discriminating among these differentials may be challenging.

The focal form of GME may be identified on CT or MRI as a nonspecific single space-occupying mass lesion.[10,28] In ocular GME, the optic nerves may be isointense on T2-weighted images, and may enhance on T1-weighted image with contrast medium.[29] The optic chiasm also may appear enlarged, reflecting the gross pathology that may be associated with this form (**Fig. 2**).

Although CT scan is not as sensitive as MRI in delineating parenchymal and meningeal lesions, it may provide evidence of brain inflammation.[8] Both focal and disseminated forms of GME may be associated with contrast enhancement on CT, and mass effect may be observed by displacement of surrounding brain tissue. Disseminated GME is typified by multiple foci of poorly defined, enhancing lesions of the parenchyma and meninges. Some lesions may be associated with hypoattenuating vasogenic edema and mass effect.[8]

Neuropathology

GME is an angiocentric, nonsuppurative, mixed lymphoid inflammatory process predominately affecting the white matter of the brain and spinal cord.[11,17] Disseminated GME consists of widely scattered, blood vessel-orientated lesions in the cerebrum, caudal brainstem, cerebellum, spinal cord, and meninges. The focal form of GME is a true mass lesion resulting from the coalescence of perivascular cellular infiltrates, involving a large number of blood vessels in one region.[15] The ocular form of GME also consists of perivascular cellular infiltrates primarily localized to the retinal or postretinal aspects of the optic nerve and optic chiasm (see **Fig. 2**).[15,25]

On gross examination, GME lesions may appear as discolored yellow-to-gray areas that infiltrate the normal brain parenchyma. Typical histopathological lesions include the concentric proliferation of inflammatory cells around blood vessels (see **Fig. 1**).[15]

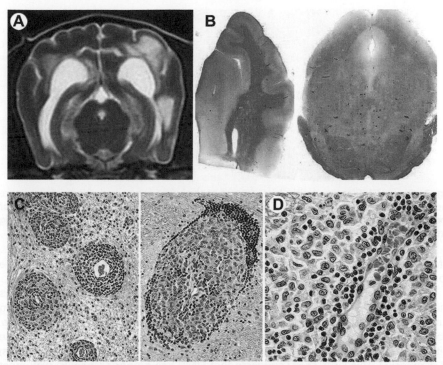

Fig. 1. Disseminated GME. (*A*) Transverse, T2-weighted MRI image at the level of the midbrain and cerebral hemispheres. Multiple, infiltrative hyperintensities are scattered throughout the central white matter. These hyperintense lesions likely represent a combination of edema and inflammation. (*B*) Subgross GME lesions seen here in the cerebrum and midbrain. (*C*) The cells in the perivascular cuffs include lymphocytes, plasma cells, and large, pale histiocytic cells. The left panel shows coalescing cuffs. Despite the density of the cuffs, there is little tendency for cells to infiltrate the parenchyma. (*D*) High-magnification view of lymphocytes and large histiocytoid cells in a perivascular cuff. Plasma cells, rare in this image, also may be present.

These so-called perivascular cuffs commonly are composed of histiocytes or lymphocytes in addition to varying numbers of monocytes and plasma cells arranged in reticulin fibers. Conventional wisdom is that GME lesions result from the migration and maturation of blood-derived monocytes or histiocytes[15]; however, the origin of the CNS inflammation (intrathecal vs systemic) has not been investigated rigorously. Occasionally, a few neutrophils and multinucleate giant cells also are present. Chronic granulomatous lesions may compress and invade adjacent CNS parenchyma, leading to necrosis and vasogenic edema formation.[15,16] In areas of chronic edema, the surrounding neuropil may contain astrogliosis.

Prognosis

Anecdotally, the prognosis for GME is considered to be poor without aggressive immunosuppression. Immunosuppressive therapies, of which corticosteroids form the cornerstone, are thought to markedly improve the prognosis of GME.[1,3,30] Most dogs with idiopathic ME, however, are treated following a presumptive diagnosis of

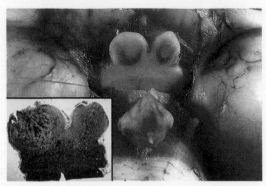

Fig. 2. Ocular GME/optic neuritis. Involvement of the optic nerves and chiasm can produce the clinical deficits of optic neuritis. Note the brownish discoloration of the cut surface of each optic nerve. The inset displays a subgross histologic view of the optic chiasm revealing extensive perivascular infiltrates.

GME, so the true efficacy of the various treatment options is unknown. Treatments are considered collectively for GME, NME, and NLE in the MUE section.

The largest study of histopathologically confirmed GME cases included 42 dogs with survival times ranging from 1 to more than 1215 days.[7] The major factors affecting survival were neuroanatomic localization and focal versus multifocal neurologic signs. Dogs with focal GME were reported to survive longer (median 114 days) than those with the disseminated form, which die within a few days to weeks (median 8 days) of diagnosis.[7] This large study suggests that GME has a poor prognosis, with most dogs succumbing to the disorder or euthanized within a few weeks to months after diagnosis, despite steroid treatment. The study, however, was limited to postmortem confirmed disease, so survival times and the associated prognosis may be biased toward dogs with severe GME.

Etiopathogenesis

Despite its recognition as a clinical entity for over 40 years, the etiopathogenesis for GME remains unclear. Genetic, autoimmune, infectious, neoplastic, and even toxic causes have been theorized. Previous work has demonstrated that females are predisposed to GME; this finding is similar to other autoimmune demyelinating diseases including multiple sclerosis (MS) and experimental allergic encephalitis (EAE).[7,31,32] The pathogenesis of the female predisposition for autoimmune CNS diseases is unclear; however, a connection between sex steroid-associated alterations in T-helper cytokines, suppression of regulatory cytokines, and X-chromosome susceptibility alleles may be involved.[31,32]

Kipar and colleagues[5] have suggested that GME is a delayed-type hypersensitivity reaction with an autoimmune basis, supported by a predominance of major histocompatability complex class 2 and CD3 antigen-positive T-lymphocytes. Suzuki and colleagues[33] subsequently confirmed a predominance of CD3-positive T-lymphocytes and a complete absence of the CD79 (B-cell marker) immunoreactivity in four cases of GME. The same group, however, was unable to demonstrate statistical differences in the number of CD3-positive cells between GME and NME or GME and central malignant histiocytosis.[33,34] Immunophenotyping studies are in progress and preliminarily suggest a consistent pattern among disseminated GME cases.[13] Antiastrocytic antibodies also have been identified in the CSF of dogs with GME.[35] The complete immunologic profile of GME, and whether CNS autoantibodies are the cause or consequence of inflammation, remain to be elucidated.

Despite the conventional view that GME is a disorder of immune dysregulation, some veterinary neuropathologists suggest that GME is a lymphoproliferative disorder with features of both inflammation and neoplasia (Brian Summers, personal communication, 2003). Focal GME is particularly similar to neoplasia, as lymphocytes within the perivascular cuffs often have variable degrees of pleomorphism and mitotic indices.[14] Interestingly, CSF from disseminated GME cases occasionally contains lymphoblasts (Schatzberg, personal observation). It is unclear whether the abnormal lymphocytes within brain lesions or CSF are reactive inflammatory cells or representative of a true neoplastic population.

Potential infectious triggers for GME have been considered in recent years.[36,37] Borna virus was reported in several dogs with ME in Japan and Switzerland and has been proposed as a causative agent for GME.[38,39] Borna virus, however, is unlikely to be a common etiology for GME, given its predilection for CNS gray matter. Schwab and colleagues[37] have demonstrated positive immunohistochemistry (IHC) for West Nile, canine parainfluenza, and encephalomyocarditis viruses in severe GME lesions. The significance of these observations is unclear, as the positive IHC may be caused by antibody cross-reactivity with endogenous proteins, as has been described with measles infections.[40] Alternatively, these results may support the theory that GME is a nonspecific inflammatory response to various antigens, of which pathogens comprise an important subset.

To date, molecular investigations at the University of Georgia College of Veterinary Medicine have failed to disclose consistent infectious agents associated with GME; however, work is ongoing to investigate an extremely diverse group of potential viral, bacterial, and rickettsial triggers.[2] Recently, the author's group identified Bartonella spp and Mycoplasma spp in sporadic, confirmed cases of disseminated GME (Barber, unpublished data, 2009). The author's view is that GME is most likely a nonspecific immunologic response, and multiple environmental triggers (pathogens, vaccinations) and genetic factors are likely to play roles in the etiopathogenesis.

THE NECROTIZING ENCEPHALITIDES: NECROTIZING MENINGOENCEPHALITIS (NME) AND NECROTIZING LEUKOENCEPHALITIS (NLE)
Background

NME and NLE are CNS inflammatory disorders with similarly elusive etiopathogeneses to that of GME. Historically referred to as Pug dog encephalitis and necrotizing encephalitis of Yorkshire terriers, respectively, these idiopathic meningoencephalitides have been reported in various toy breeds including the Pug, Maltese, Chihuahua, Yorkshire Terrier, Pekingese, West Highland White Terrier, Boston Terrier, Japanese Spitz, and Miniature Pinscher.[13,41–46] To avoid confusion associated with the breed-specific terminology, these inflammatory disorders are described best with the neuropathological nomenclature reflective of the topographies of the brain lesions associated with each (eg, NME and NLE). Because of the overlap in clinical signs and neuropathology, the encompassing term necrotizing encephalitis (NE) may be preferable on an antemortem basis.

Clinical Features

The onset of neurologic signs associated with NME varies from 6 months to 7 years of age, and most commonly occurs in young dogs, with a mean age of 29 months.[43,47] NLE typically manifests between 4 months to 10 years of age, with a mean age of onset of 4.5 years.[48] Dogs with both NME and NLE commonly manifest cerebrothalamic signs because of the predominance of lesions in the prosencephalon; NLE also commonly causes mid-to-caudal brainstem signs.[6] Because of the multifocal nature of inflammatory disease, however, variations may occur with either disorder, and clinical signs are primarily reflective of the lesion locations. The signs associated with NE typically are rapidly progressive and most commonly include seizures, depression, circling, vestibulocerebellar signs, visual deficits, and ultimately death.

Neuroimaging

The characteristic distribution of lesions observed in NME and NLE may aid in the cross-sectional imaging diagnoses (see neuropathology section). Typical MRI lesions associated with NME include asymmetric, multifocal prosencephalic lesions affecting the gray and white matter, with variable contrast enhancement on T1-weighted imaging.[49] Loss of gray/white matter demarcation also may be discernible (**Fig. 3**A).[49,50] Lesions appear hyperintense on T2-weighted images and isointense to slightly hypointense on T1-weighted images, with slight contrast enhancement. In NLE, multiple, asymmetric bilateral prosencephalic lesions mainly affecting the subcortical white matter have been described.[51] The NLE lesions are hyperintense on T2-weighted and FLAIR images and often include multiple cystic areas of necrosis (**Fig. 4**A). These lesions are hypointense or isointense on T1-weighted images, and contrast enhancement is variable. MRI findings may increase the clinician's confidence in a presumptive diagnosis of NE.

CT scan may also support a diagnosis of NE. In the acute stages of either NME or NLE, focal hypodense lesions may be appreciated in the prosencephalon.[9] The lesions may or may not enhance with contrast. In chronic NE, the primary lesions on CT scan are characterized by necrosis and cystic changes.[9]

Neuropathology

The histopathological hallmarks of both NME and NLE include nonsuppurative ME and bilateral, asymmetric cerebral necrosis. NME commonly affects the cerebral hemispheres and subcortical white matter, with profound inflammation extending from the leptomeninges through the cerebral cortex into the corona radiata (**Fig. 3**B).[15] The anatomic demarcation between gray and white matter often is lost, a feature identified reliably on gross histopathological examination (see **Fig. 3**A, C).[6] Meningeal infiltrates, characterized by plasma cells, lymphocytes, and occasionally histiocytes, are most abundant in the cerebral sulci and fissures (**Fig. 3**D). Areas of malacia, necrosis with liquefaction, and cavitation (similar to those seen in NLE) may be present in NME. Chronic, protracted cases may demonstrate neuronal loss and gemistocyte infiltration.

In contrast, NLE is relatively sparing of the cerebral cortex and meninges, and predominately affects periventricular cerebral white matter including the centrum semiovale, thalamocortical fibers, internal capsule, and thalamus (**Fig. 4**C).[15] Lesions also may occur in the brainstem. The degree of necrosis associated with NLE is related directly to the duration and severity of the disease. Areas of necrosis often coalesce to form larger, more dramatic areas of cavitation with NLE as compared with NME. Within the affected white matter, numerous swollen and necrotic axons, gemistocytes, gitter cells (local macrophages), reactive microglial, and occasional perivascular infiltrates may be present (**Fig. 4**B, D).[15] Interestingly, neurons in the gray matter appear unaffected despite the surrounding inflammation. Small numbers of lymphocytes and plasma cells may be present in the leptomeninges; however, meningeal inflammation typically is minimal.

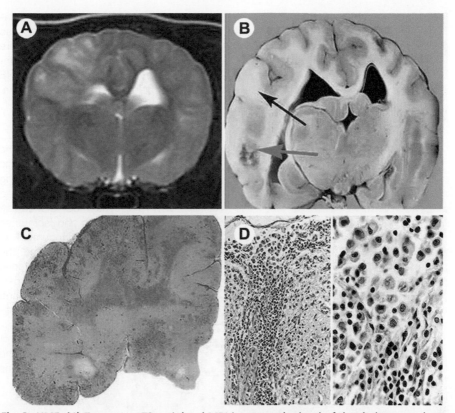

Fig. 3. NME. (*A*) Transverse, T2-weighted MRI image at the level of the thalamus and cerebral hemispheres. Note the asymmetric, hyperintense, infiltrative lesions affecting the cerebral hemispheres at the level of the thalamus. The demarcation between gray and white matter is obscured, and no evidence of cavitation is seen. (*B*) Transverse sections of the brain at the level of the diencephalon. Inflammation dulls the white matter and characteristically effaces the junction of gray and white matter in the cerebrum (*black arrows*). Note also asymmetric swelling, midline shift, slight ventricular enlargement, and focal cavitation (*green arrow*). (*C*) Occipital lobe of a Pomeranian dog. A diffuse infiltrative lesion is present extending from the cortical surface through the gray matter and multifocally entering the white matter. This was a substantially unilateral disease. (*D*) Cerebral cortex. Meningeal mixed inflammatory infiltrates that include large and small mononuclear cells and plasma cells.

Etiopathogenesis

The etiopathogeneses for NME and NLE are poorly understood. Recently, Greer and colleagues evaluated pedigree information on a large cohort of Pugs and demonstrated a strong familial inheritance pattern for NME.[52] Although these transmission data are not surprising, a simple Mendelian inheritance pattern could not be demonstrated. The latter suggests that NME is a multifactorial disorder. A multifactorial pathogenesis recently has been demonstrated for acute necrotizing encephalopathy (ANE) in children, which occurs secondary to influenza and parainfluenza infections.[53] Missense mutations in the nuclear pore gene RANBP2 have been demonstrated to be susceptibility alleles for familial and recurrent cases of ANE. A similar combination

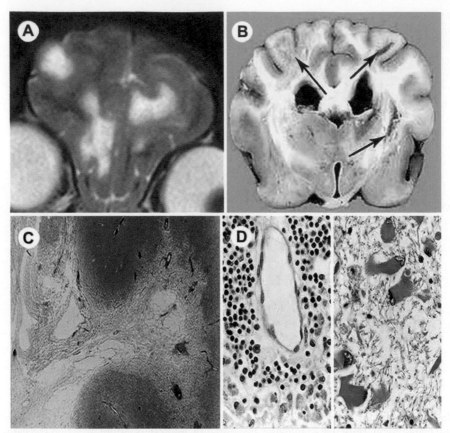

Fig. 4. NLE. (*A*) Transverse, T2-weighted MRI at the level of the fronto-parietal lobes. Multiple, asymmetric bilateral forebrain lesions mainly affecting the subcortical white matter are present. (*B*) Asymmetric, cavitating lesions in the corona radiata, internal capsule, and thalamo-cortical fibers *(arrows)*. (*C*) Low-magnification view. Corona radiata with intense edema, dissolution of white matter, early cavitations and residual perivascular cuffing. (*D*) Corona radiata, high magnification. Left pane—lymphoid and histiocytoid cells cuffing a vessel. Right panel—large reactive astrocytes (gemistocytes).

of genetics and infectious or other environmental triggers may be responsible for canine NE. Molecular studies are ongoing to assess for genetic susceptibility loci and a diverse group of potential infectious triggers that may lead to immune dysregulation in NME and NLE.

Although it is tempting to consider NME and NLE as distinct entities, these disorders may represent a spectrum of CNS injury with similar pathogeneses. Interestingly, neuropathologists have evaluated the brains from Pugs, several Maltese terriers, and Chihuahuas with lesions that typify NLE (rather than NME as reported in these breeds)[13] (de Lahunta and Summers, personal communication, 2003) Conversely, the author has studied histopathologically confirmed NME in a Yorkshire Terrier (Schatzberg and Summers, unpublished data, 2006). Autoimmune encephalomyelitis (EAE) models in rats may provide insights into such variations in lesion topographies within and among different dog breeds. Minor modifications of MHC haplotypes in

EAE rats result in different but reproducible patterns of brain inflammation following exposure to a myelin-oligodendrocyte-glycoprotein.[54] Similarly, the histopathologic differences among the NEs may result from minor genetic differences among breeds, modifying genes, or variations in antigenic exposures.

An autoimmune pathogenesis has been suggested for NME based on the presence of antiastrocytic and glial fibrillary acid protein (GFAP) autoantibodies in CSF of affected dogs.[35,55,56] Similar antibody levels, however, occur in the CSF of dogs with GME, brain tumors, and even some clinically normal dogs.[55,57] Whether GFAP autoantibodies are the inciting cause of NME, representative of a breed-specific fragility of astrocytes, or the consequence of prolonged tissue destruction secondary to infectious disease, requires further investigation.

Because of the neuropathological similarities to the viral meningoencephalitides in other species, viral etiologies have been considered for NE.[36,43] The histopathologic lesions associated with canine NME are especially similar to those present in human herpesvirus ME.[43,58] As canine herpes virus-1 (CHV-1) may cause encephalitis in neonates,[58–60] it is conceivable that NE is triggered by a recrudescence of a latent herpesvirus infection. Interestingly, the isolation of a herpes-like virus was reported in the NME report by Cordy and Holliday in 1989,[43] but the viral isolate was not retained.

Further attempts at viral isolation from dogs with NME have been unsuccessful (Summers, personal communication); however, Mx proteins, interferon-induced Guanosine triphosphotases associated with viral and inflammatory diseases, have been demonstrated in brain tissues from Pugs with NME.[61] To date, broadly reactive PCR assays for herpesviruses have been negative on a large number of paraffinized and freshly frozen NME brains.[36,52] Moreover, PCR screening of NME brains for an extremely diverse group of DNA and RNA viruses has failed to identify viral nucleic acids (Schatzberg, unpublished data, 2009). Although the lack of viral nucleic acids in NME brains argues against a directly acting, neurotropic virus, these PCR data do not exclude the possibility of a viral trigger for NE via molecular mimicry.[62–64] Another possibility is that a pathogen is present (but at undetectable levels) in the presence of a self-perpetuating immune response, a phenomenon that has been described for flavivirus infections.[65] Investigations are ongoing to pursue direct-acting neuropathogens as well as para- and post-infectious pathogeneses for autoimmune inflammation in canine NE.

MENINGOENCEPHALITIS OF UNKNOWN ETIOLOGY
Background and Perspectives

Most retrospective studies evaluating immunosuppressive treatment protocols for canine idiopathic ME include very few cases with confirmed histopathological diagnoses. The various combination protocols published in small cases series have been applied predominantly to cases of MUE.[1,3,30,66] Because MUE represents a broad spectrum of disease, it is unlikely that a gold standard therapy will be identified. Further complicating the interpretation of published cases is a paucity of prospective data on steroid monotherapy for MUE. As such, the utility of secondary immunomodulation is difficult to evaluate objectively. Standardized corticosteroid protocols also are lacking within and among published reports. Occasionally, standardized dosing and intervals for the adjunctive immunotherapy under investigation are lacking, and exit strategies have not been designed for patients that are non-responsive to treatment. In summary, the true efficacy of the various immunosuppressive agents for confirmed GME and NE is unknown.

Treatment Protocols

At present, immunosuppression is the mainstay of therapy for MUE. Most clinicians treat MUE with corticosteroids (prednisone or dexamethasone). Depending on the severity of signs and the index of suspicion for infectious disease, some specialists will initiate therapy with anti-inflammatory steroids (0.5 mg/kg to 1.0 mg/kg once daily prednisone) and await serology and PCR results for regional infectious diseases. If the index of suspicion is extremely high for idiopathic inflammatory disease (eg, Pug with MRI lesions consistent with NME), the author typically initiates immunosuppressive therapy directly. Response to corticosteroids is variable and may be temporary, but dogs often have a favorable initial response to steroid monotherapy. Additional immunosuppression is considered on a case-by-case basis, but the author typically uses secondary immunomodulatory agents upon review of negative serology and PCR results. At such time, the prednisone protocol presented in **Box 1** is used (Schatzberg, unpublished data, 2009), often in combination with one or more of the immunomodulatory drugs. Cytosine arabinoside, procarbazine, cyclosporine, lomustine, leflunomide, and mycophenolate mofetil (MMF) have been reported retrospectively as adjunctive therapies.

As mentioned previously, steroid monotherapy has not been investigated prospectively as a treatment for MUE. With disseminated GME, 23 cases were reported retrospectively, with a survival range of 8 to 41 days.[7] In a clinical setting, steroid monotherapy may resolve signs associated with MUE in some dogs, but insufficiently or only transiently provides resolution in others. Moreover, long-term, high-dose corticosteroid therapy often causes adverse effects including polyuria–polydipsia, polyphagia, weight gain, hepatotoxicity, gastrointestinal (GI) ulceration, pancreatitis, and iatrogenic hyperadrenocorticism. These combined factors have led to a recent focus on complementary immunomodulatory drugs to treat MUE.

Cytosine Arabinoside

Cytosine arabinoside is a chemotherapeutic agent used to treat several neoplastic conditions in both human and veterinary medicine. Over the past several years, cytosine arabinoside has been used for its immunosuppressive properties as an adjunctive therapy for MUE.[3,66] Cytosine arabinoside is a synthetic nucleoside analog that crosses the BBB in dogs, undergoes enzymatic activation, competes for incorporation into nucleic acids, and competitively inhibits DNA polymerase in mitotically active cells.[67] CA also causes topoisomerase dysfunction, prevents DNA repair, and inhibits ribonucleotide reductase and glycoprotein synthesis.[68,69] Cytosine arabinoside is metabolized via deamination in the liver, plasma, granulocytes, and GI tract. Adverse effects are dose-dependent and include myelosuppression, vomiting, diarrhea, and hair loss.[67]

Box 1
Prednisone protocol
1.5 mg/kg twice daily for 3 weeks
1.0 mg/kg twice daily for 6 weeks
0.5 mg/kg twice daily for 3 weeks
0.5 mg/kg once daily for 3 weeks
0.5 mg/kg every other day indefinitely (may reduce to 0.25 mg/kg EOD)

Cytosine arabinoside typically is administered as a subcutaneous injection at a dose of 50 mg/m^2 every 12 hours for 2 consecutive days and repeated every 3 to 6 weeks, indefinitely.[3] Previous reports of cytosine arabinoside treatment regimes for MUE showed survival ranges of 4 to 1025 days[3] and 78 to 603 days.[66] The authors commonly use cytosine arabinoside as an adjunctive therapy for MUE in combination with prednisone as described previously. Typically, a CBC is performed 10 to 14 days after the first course of cytosine arabinoside therapy and then periodically throughout the course of treatment. In the author's experience, adverse effects have been minimal, and dogs with MUE have a fair long-term prognosis with combined cytosine arabinoside/prednisone therapy.

With combined cytosine arabinoside/prednisone therapy, the cytosine arabinoside dosing interval is increased gradually over several months, and the steroids are tapered to the lowest dose possible, which often ameliorates clinical signs and minimizes systemic adverse effects.[3] Recurrence of clinical signs with steroid dose reductions may occur, so the authors gradually taper steroids as described previously. After 4 months of a steroid taper, dogs typically are maintained indefinitely on 0.5 mg/kg prednisone by mouth once daily or every other day depending on the resolution of neurologic signs. Relapses are treated aggressively, as they may be refractory to treatment. Recently, intravenous rescue cytosine arabinoside protocols (intravenous constant rate infusion of cytosine arabinoside at 200 mg/m^2 over 48 hours) have been described for the initial treatment of severe MUE, which at University of Georgia College of Veterinary Medicine also has proven useful for severe relapses.[70] With relapses, some dogs additionally may require tertiary immunomodulatory drugs for the control of clinical signs.

Procarbazine

Procarbazine is an antineoplastic, alkylating agent with multiple sites of action, and it has been used extensively to treat MUE. It is lipid-soluble; additionally, it crosses the BBB and alkylates DNA at the O6 position of guanine, inhibiting insertion of essential DNA precursors. Procarbazine also disrupts RNA and protein synthesis. For treatment of MUE, procarbazine is given by mouth at a dose of 25 to 50 mg/m^2/d. Adverse effects include myelosuppression, nausea, vomiting, hepatic dysfunction, and neurotoxicity.

Procarbazine has been used as an adjunctive therapy with corticosteroids and as a sole immunomodulatory agent for MUE. The use of procarbazine and prednisone as combination therapy was investigated in 20 dogs with MUE and compared with an untreated group of 11 dogs with confirmed GME.[30] The prednisone dose was reduced or discontinued in 17 dogs, and the median survival time was 15 months. The authors recommended monitoring a CBC once weekly for the first month of therapy and monthly thereafter. If improvement is noted after the first month, the procarbazine dose can be reduced to every other day, provided that relapses are not observed.

Cyclosporine

Cyclosporine is an immunosuppressive agent that can be used as a monotherapy but more typically is combined with prednisone or ketoconazole to achieve remission in cases of MUE.[1] Cyclosporine acts by directly suppressing T-lymphocyte activation and proliferation.[71] In addition, cyclosporine prevents synthesis of several cytokines including interleukin (IL)-2, indirectly inhibiting T-cell proliferation. The rationale for its use in the treatment of MUE/presumptive GME is based on the suggestion that GME has T-cell mediated delayed-type hypersensitivity.[5] Although cyclosporine has poor BBB permeability, ME may allow the drug access to the CNS compartment. Moreover, cyclosporine likely concentrates effectively in the cerebral endothelial cells and choroid plexi.[72] Lesions associated with GME and NE are primarily perivascular; therefore, a therapeutic concentration of cyclosporine likely reaches the intracellular compartments of the lymphocytes and macrophages in affected areas of the CNS in these disorders.[73]

Cyclosporine works rapidly and reaches effective steady-state blood levels within 24 to 48 hours of initiation of therapy.[73] When used as the sole therapeutic agent for MUE, a starting dose of 6 mg/kg by mouth every 12 hours of cyclosporine has been recommended to achieve therapeutic serum concentrations.[1] The microemulsified form (Neoral), or its generic equivalent (cyclosporine modified), is recommended, as a uniform blood level is attained at lower doses compared with Cyclosporine USP, Sandimmune.[74] The most common adverse effects include diarrhea, anorexia, and vomiting, all of which typically subside when the dose is divided more evenly throughout the day. Occasionally, gingival hyperplasia, papillomatosis, hirsutism, excessive shedding, and insulin resistance may occur, requiring discontinuation of therapy.[75] Rare adverse effects include nephrotoxicity and/or hepatotoxicity.

Cyclosporine is metabolized by cytochrome P-450; thus, phenobarbital will decrease cyclosporine blood levels as it induces the P-450 enzyme.[75] If the use of cyclosporine is cost-prohibitive, it may be combined with ketoconazole. Ketoconazole significantly lowers the dose of cyclosporine needed to achieve effective blood levels by inhibiting the cytochrome P-450 enzymes and decreasing the systemic clearance of the drug. The recommended combined doses for combination therapy are 5mg/kg by mouth SID cyclosporine and 8mg/kg by mouth SID ketoconazole.[1] Adverse effects associated with ketoconazole include anorexia, vomiting, and diarrhea. Hepatotoxicity has been reported rarely, and it is noteworthy that ketoconazole is teratogenic.

In 2007, Adamo and colleagues retrospectively evaluated the utility of cyclosporine for the treatment of MUE.[1] Ten cases of MUE were evaluated including dogs treated with cyclosporin monotherapy and cyclosporin in combination with corticosteroids and/or ketoconazole. The overall median survival time for all dogs in the study was 930 days (range, 60 to more than 1290 days). Adverse effects were minimal and included excessive shedding, gingival hyperplasia, and hypertrichosis.

Lomustine

Lomustine is an antineoplastic agent with potent immunosuppressive properties that relate to its toxic effect on lymphocytes. Lomustine is a highly lipid soluble, nitrosourea compound. It readily crosses the BBB and alkylates both DNA and RNA. Bone marrow suppression (leukopenia and delayed thrombocytopenia) and GI upset (vomiting and diarrhea) are the most common adverse effects. Hepatotoxicity also has been reported in dogs when used at very high doses (90 mg/m^2 every 3 to 4 weeks concurrently with other hepatotoxic drugs).[76] Serum chemistry monitoring is recommended after the first treatment, then every 3 months thereafter. Although the use of lomustine for MUE is common, and anecdotally effective, (Allen Sisson, personal communication, 2009), there are no peer-reviewed manuscripts that have evaluated its utility in this application.

In 2007, investigators on two separate abstracts reported that when combined with low-dose prednisone to treat MUE (23 cases total), lomustine resulted in longer survival times compared with prednisone alone.[77,78] Flegel and colleagues[79] reported a dose of 60 mg/m^2 by mouth every 6 weeks to be effective, with minimal adverse effects. Further evaluation of lomustine as an adjunctive therapy for MUE is needed.

Mycophenolate Mofetil

MMF is a lymphocyte-specific immunomodulatory drug that decreases the recruitment of inflammatory cells and has been reported preliminarily in five dogs as an adjunctive therapy for MUE.[79] An initial dose of 20 mg/kg by mouth twice daily was recommended; after 1 month of treatment, the dose was decreased to 10 mg/kg twice daily. Adverse effects included hemorrhagic diarrhea, which subsided with dose reduction or discontinuation of the drug. Neither bone marrow suppression nor hepatotoxicity were reported in the limited number of dogs treated. Although initial responses are encouraging, the authors concluded that larger, prospective studies are needed to evaluate the efficacy of MMF in the treatment of MUE.

Leflunomide

Leflunomide is an immunomodulatory drug that has efficacy in experimental models of autoimmune diseases.[80] The active metabolite of this drug, teriflunomide (A77), inhibits T- and B-cell proliferation, suppresses immunoglobulin production, and interferes with cell adhesion. In addition to its immunosuppressive effects, leflunomide has both in vitro and in vivo antiviral properties.[81] The recommended dose range of leflunomide is 1.5 to 4 mg/kg by mouth SID; however, this dose may be adjusted, based on A77 blood level measured 24 hours after administration.[80] In people, A77 reaches peak blood levels in 6 to 12 hours, has a long half-life of approximately 2 weeks, and can take up to 2 months to reach steady state. Dose adjustments should be made to keep blood levels in a safe, therapeutic range (20 to 40 μg/mL). Adverse effects are seemingly rare in dogs; however, they may include thrombocytopenia and hemorrhagic colitis.

In 1998, Gregory and colleagues[80] reported on five dogs with MUE that were treated with leflunomide because of a poor response or adverse effects associated with prednisolone therapy. All dogs, treated over 4 to 11 months, had good to excellent improvement in their neurologic status with no reported adverse effects. Post-treatment MRI of two dogs showed partial to marked resolution of cortical lesions. Further studies are needed to critically evaluate the potentially useful role of leflunomide in MUE.

CANINE MUE: TREATMENT PERSPECTIVES

A blinded, controlled, randomized, prospective study is needed desperately to assess current and prospective (eg, plasma exchange, intravenous immunoglobulins) therapeutic regimes for canine MUE. A multi-institutional study likely will be required to obtain sufficient case numbers to perform head-to-head comparisons of the various therapies. If histopathology is lacking, prospective studies for MUE will require rigorous inclusion criteria, aimed at the inclusion of predominantly GME and NE cases. Without such criteria, it will be impossible to evaluate therapeutic intervention. The impracticality of obtaining antemortem histopathology (eg, brain biopsy) in many cases complicates differentiating prognoses among GME, NE, infectious ME, and neoplasia. Until more rigorous studies are performed, however, the best therapies and prognoses for the specific disorders will remain unknown.

It is noteworthy that Schwab and colleagues[37] recently evaluated CNS tissues for the presence of pathogens in 53 dogs with MUE. On an antemortem basis, most of these cases would have fit the author's criteria for immunosuppressive therapy. Interestingly, the investigation revealed a causative agent in 26% of MUE cases, including porcine herpes virus-1, Escherichia coli, a new disease pattern of parvovirus infection, West Nile virus, canine parainfluenza virus, and encephalomyocarditis virus. Recent pan-viral PCR studies have identified bunya- and polyomaviruses in CSF from cases of canine MUE (Schatzberg, unpublished data, 2009). It is possible that antiviral therapies ultimately will play a role in the empiric treatment of canine MUE.

SUMMARY

Despite having been recognized for decades, GME and NE continue to challenge the veterinary community. These idiopathic meningoencephalitides seem to be CNS disorders of immune dysregulation, each with relatively unique neuropathologies. From a treatment perspective, it is unclear whether one should continue to focus on the similarities or shift attention to the differences among these disorders. Optimal treatments for the individual disorders remain unknown, because most cases are treated with empiric immunosuppression without definitive diagnoses. At present, although treatments vary by institution, most cases of MUE within individual specialty hospitals are treated similarly to one another. The prognosis for canine ME, in general, seemingly has improved with adjunctive immunomodulatory therapies. A more basic understanding of the etiopathogeneses (eg, genetic, immunologic, and pathogenic components) remains critical for targeted therapies and ultimately for improving survival times for these elusive and often life-threatening disorders.

ACKNOWLEDGMENTS

A special note of thanks to Drs Clive Huxtable, Brian Summers, and Alexander de Lahunta for sharing many of the neuropathology slides that can be found on the online veterinary neuropathology atlas: (http://web.vet.cornell.edu/public/oed/neuropathology/index.asp). The author also would like to thank Dr Lauren Talarico for her help with the preparation of this issue.

REFERENCES

1. Adamo PF, Rylander H, Adams WM. Cyclosporin use in multidrug therapy for meningoencephalomyelitis of unknown aetiology in dogs. J Small Anim Pract 2007; 48(9):486–96.
2. Schatzberg S. Polymerase chain reaction for viral, bacterial, and rickettsial nucleic acid detection in dogs with meningoencephalitis of unknown etiology. In: 20th Annual Symposium of the European College of Veterinary Neurology. Bern (Switzerland): 2007. p. 63–4.
3. Zarfoss M, Schatzberg S, Venator K, et al. Combined cytosine arabinoside and prednisone therapy for meningoencephalitis of unknown aetiology in 10 dogs. J Small Anim Pract 2006;47:588–95.
4. Koblik PD, LeCouteur RA, Higgins RJ, et al. CT-guided brain biopsy using a modified Pelorus Mark III stereotactic system: experience with 50 dogs. Vet Radiol Ultrasound 1999;40:434–40.
5. Kipar A, Baumgartner W, Vogl C, et al. Immunohistochemical characterization of inflammatory cells in brains of dogs with granulomatous meningoencephalitis. Vet Pathol 1998;35:43–52.
6. de Lahunta A, Glass E. Veterinary neuroanatomy and clinical neurology. 3rd edition. St. Louis (MO): Saunders Elsevier; 2009.
7. Munana KR, Luttgen PJ. Prognostic factors for dogs with granulomatous meningoencephalomyelitis: 42 cases (1982–1996). J Am Vet Med Assoc 1998;212: 1902–6.

8. Plummer SB, Wheeler SJ, Thrall DE, et al. Computed tomography of primary inflammatory brain disorders in dogs and cats. Vet Radiol Ultrasound 1992;33:307–12.
9. Thomas WB. Inflammatory diseases of the central nervous system in dogs. Clin Tech Small Anim Pract 1998;13:167–78.
10. Speciale J, Van Winkle TJ, Steinberg SA, et al. Computed tomography in the diagnosis of focal granulomatous meningoencephalitis: retrospective evaluation of three cases. J Am Anim Hosp Assoc 1992;28:327–32.
11. Cordy DR. Canine granulomatous meningoencephalomyelitis. Vet Pathol 1979; 16:325–33.
12. Koestner A. Primary lymphoreticuloses of the nervous system in animals. Acta Neuropathol Suppl 1975;6:85–9.
13. Higgins RJ, LeCouteur RA. GME, NME, and breed-specific encephalitis and allied disorders: variations of the same theme or different diseases? A clinical and pathological perspective. In: 20th Annual Symposium of the European College of Veterinary Neurology. Bern (Switzerland): 2007. p. 35–37.
14. Fankhauser R, Fatzer R, Luginbuhl H. Reticulosis of the central nervous system (CNS) in dogs. Adv Vet Sci Comp Med 1972;16:35–72.
15. Summers BA, Cummings JF, De Lahunta A. Veterinary neuropathology. St. Louis (MO): Mosby; 1995.
16. Braund KG. Granulomatous meningoencephalitis. J Am Vet Med Assoc 1985; 186:138–41.
17. Braund KG, Vandevelde M, Walker TL. Granulomatous meningoencephalomyelitis in six dogs. J Am Vet Med Assoc 1978;172:1195–200.
18. Sorjonen DC. Cerebrospinal fluid electrophoresis. Use in canine granulomatous meningoencephalomyelitis. Veterinary Medicine Report 1989;1:399–403.
19. Thomas JB, Eger C. Granulomatous meningoencephalomyelitis in 21 dogs. J Small Anim Pract 1989;30:287–93.
20. Vandevelde M, Fatzer R, Fankhauser R. Immunohistological studies on primary reticulosis of the canine brain. Vet Pathol 1981;18:577–88.
21. Tipold A. Diagnosis of inflammatory and infectious diseases of the central nervous system in dogs: a retrospective study. J Vet Intern Med 1995;9:304–14.
22. Sorjonen DC. Clinical and histopathological features of granulomatous meningoencephalomyelitis in dogs. J Am Anim Hosp Assoc 1990;26:141–7.
23. Munana KR. Encephalitis and meningitis. Vet Clin North Am Small Anim Pract 1996;26:857–75.
24. Cuddon P, Smith-Maxie L. Reticulosis of the central nervous system in the dog. Compen Contin Educ Pract Vet 1984;6:23–32.
25. Nuhsbaum MT, Powell CC, Gionfriddo JR, et al. Treatment of granulomatous meningoencephalomyelitis in a dog. Vet Ophthalmol 2002;5:29–33.
26. Cherubini G, Platt S, Anderson T, et al. Characteristics of magnetic resonance images of granulomatous meningoencephalomyelitis in 11 dogs. Vet Rec 2006; 159:110–5.
27. Cherubini GB, Platt SR, Howson S, et al. Comparison of magnetic resonance imaging sequences in dogs with multi-focal intracranial disease. J Small Anim Pract 2008;49(12):634–40.
28. Kitagawa M, Kanayama K, Satoh T, et al. Cerebellar focal granulomatous meningoencephalitis in a dog: clinical findings and MR imaging. J Vet Med A Physiol Pathol Clin Med 2004;51:277–9.
29. Kitagawa M, Okada M, Watari T, et al. Ocular granulomatous meningoencephalomyelitis in a dog: magnetic resonance images and clinical findings. J Vet Med Sci 2009;71:233–7.

30. Coates JR, Barone G, Dewey CW, et al. Procarbazine as adjunctive therapy for treatment of dogs with presumptive antemortem diagnosis of granulomatous meningoencephalomyelitis: 21 cases (1998–2004). J Vet Intern Med 2007;21:100–6.
31. Herrera BM, Cader MZ, Dyment DA, et al. Multiple sclerosis susceptibility and the X chromosome. Mult Scler 2007;13:856–64.
32. Hoffman GE, Le WW, Murphy AZ, et al. Divergent effects of ovarian steroids on neuronal survival during experimental allergic encephalitis in Lewis rats. Exp Neurol 2001;171:272–84.
33. Suzuki M, Uchida K, Morozumi M, et al. A comparative pathological study on granulomatous meningoencephalomyelitis and central malignant histiocytosis in dogs. J Vet Med Sci 2003;65:1319–24.
34. Suzuki M, Uchida K, Morozumi M, et al. A comparative pathological study on canine necrotizing meningoencephalitis and granulomatous meningoencephalomyelitis. J Vet Med Sci 2003;65:1233–9.
35. Matsuki N, Fujiwara K, Tamahara S, et al. Prevalence of autoantibody in cerebrospinal fluids from dogs with various CNS diseases. J Vet Med Sci 2004;66:295–7.
36. Schatzberg SJ, Haley NJ, Barr SC, et al. Polymerase chain reaction screening for DNA viruses in paraffin-embedded brains from dogs with necrotizing meningoencephalitis, necrotizing leukoencephalitis, and granulomatous meningoencephalitis. J Vet Intern Med 2005;19:553–9.
37. Schwab S, Herden C, Seeliger F, et al. Nonsuppurative meningoencephalitis of unknown origin in cats and dogs: an immunohistochemical study. J Comp Pathol 2007;136(2–3):96–110.
38. Okamoto M, Kagawa Y, Kamitani W, et al. Borna disease in a dog in Japan. J Comp Pathol 2002;126:312–7.
39. Weissenbock H, Nowotny N, Caplazi P, et al. Borna disease in a dog with lethal meningoencephalitis. J Clin Microbiol 1998;36:2127–30.
40. Sheshberadaran H, Norrby E. Three monoclonal antibodies against measles virus F protein cross-react with cellular stress proteins. J Virol 1984;52:995–9.
41. Aresu L, D'Angelo A, Zanatta R, et al. Canine necrotizing encephalitis associated with antiglomerular basement membrane glomerulonephritis. J Comp Pathol 2007;136:279–82.
42. Cantile C, Chianini F, Arispici M, et al. Necrotizing meningoencephalitis associated with cortical hippocampal hamartia in a Pekingese dog. Vet Pathol 2001;38:119–22.
43. Cordy DR, Holliday TA. A necrotizing meningoencephalitis of pug dogs. Vet Pathol 1989;26:191–4.
44. Stalis IH, Chadwick B, Dayrell-Hart B, et al. Necrotizing meningoencephalitis of Maltese dogs. Vet Pathol 1995;32:230–5.
45. Timmann D, Konar M, Howard J, et al. Necrotising encephalitis in a French bulldog. J Small Anim Pract 2007;48:339–42.
46. Tipold A, Fatzer R, Jaggy A, et al. Necrotizing encephalitis in Yorkshire terriers. J Small Anim Pract 1993;34:623–8.
47. Levine JM, Fosgate GT, Porter B, et al. Epidemiology of necrotizing meningoencephalitis in Pug dogs. J Vet Intern Med 2008;22:961–8.
48. Kuwamura M, Adachi T, Yamate J, et al. Necrotising encephalitis in the Yorkshire terrier: a case report and literature review. J Small Anim Pract 2002;43:459–63.
49. Young B, Levine JL, Fosgate A, et al. Magnetic resonance imaging characteristics of Necrotizing meningoencephalitis in Pug dogs. J Vet Intern Med 2009;23(3):527–35.

50. Flegel T, Henke D, Boettcher I, et al. Magnetic resonance imaging findings in histologically confirmed Pug dog encephalitis. Vet Radiol Ultrasound 2008;49:419–24.
51. von Praun F, Matiasek K, Grevel V, et al. Magnetic resonance imaging and pathologic findings associated with necrotizing encephalitis in two Yorkshire terriers. Vet Radiol Ultrasound 2006;47:260–4.
52. Greer KA, Schatzberg SJ, Porter BF, et al. Heritability and transmission analysis of necrotizing meningoencephalitis in the Pug. Res Vet Sci 2008;86(3):438–42.
53. Neilson DE, Adams MD, Orr CM, et al. Infection-triggered familial or recurrent cases of acute necrotizing encephalopathy caused by mutations in a component of the nuclear pore, RANBP2. Am J Hum Genet 2009;84:44–51.
54. Storch MK, Bauer J, Linington C, et al. Cortical demyelination can be modeled in specific rat models of autoimmune encephalomyelitis and is major histocompatability complex (MHC) haplotype-related. J Neuropathol Exp Neurol 2006;65: 1137–42.
55. Shibuya M, Matsuki N, Fujiwara K, et al. Autoantibodies against glial fibrillary acidic protein (GFAP) in cerebrospinal fluids from Pug dogs with necrotizing meningoencephalitis. J Vet Med Sci 2007;69:241–5.
56. Uchida K, Hasegawa T, Ikeda M, et al. Detection of an autoantibody from Pug dogs with necrotizing encephalitis (Pug dog encephalitis). Vet Pathol 1999;36: 301–7.
57. Toda Y, Matsuki N, Shibuya M, et al. Glial fibrillary acidic protein (GFAP) and anti-GFAP autoantibody in canine necrotising meningoencephalitis. Vet Rec 2007; 161:261–4.
58. Whitley RJ, Gnann JW. Viral encephalitis: familiar infections and emerging pathogens. Lancet 2002;359:507–13.
59. Adams J, Corsellis J, Duchen L. Active infective encephalitis: herpes simplex encephalitis. In: Graham DI, Lantos PL, editors. Greenfield's neuropathology. 4th edition. New York: John Wiley & Sons; 1984. p. 273–80.
60. Percy DH, Munnel JF, Olander HJ, et al. Pathogenesis of canine herpesvirus encephalitis. Am J Vet Res 1970;31:145–56.
61. Porter BF, Ambrus A, Storts RW. Immunohistochemical evaluation of mx protein expression in canine encephalitides. Vet Pathol 2006;43:981–7.
62. Evans CF, Horwitz MS, Hobbs MV, et al. Viral infection of transgenic mice expressing a viral protein in oligodendrocytes leads to chronic central nervous system autoimmune disease. J Exp Med 1996;184:2371–84.
63. Oldstone MB. Molecular mimicry and immune-mediated diseases. FASEB J 1998;12:1255–65.
64. Theil DJ, Tsunoda I, Rodriguez F, et al. Viruses can silently prime for and trigger central nervous system autoimmune disease. J Neurovirol 2001;7:220–7.
65. Krueger N, Reid HW. Detection of louping ill virus in formalin-fixed, paraffin wax-embedded tissues of mice, sheep, and a pig by the avidin-biotin-complex immunoperoxidase technique. Vet Rec 1994;135:224–5.
66. Menaut P, Landart J, Behr S, et al. Treatment of 11 dogs with meningoencephalomyelitis of unknown origin with a combination of prednisolone and cytosine arabinoside. Vet Rec 2008;162:241–5.
67. Scott-Moncrieff JC, Chan TC, Samuels ML, et al. Plasma and cerebrospinal fluid pharmacokinetics of cytosine arabinoside in dogs. Cancer Chemother Pharmacol 1991;29:13–8.
68. Garcia-Carbonero R, Ryan DP, Chabner BA. Cytidine analogs. In: Chabner BA, Longo DL, editors. Cancer chemotherapy and biotherapy: principles and practice. Philadelphia: Lippincott Williams and Wilkins; 2001. p. 265–77.

69. Griffin F, Munroe D, Major P, et al. Induction of differentiation of human myeloid leukemia cells by inhibitors of DNA synthesis. Exp Hematol 1982;10:774–81.

70. de Stefani A, De Risio L, Matiasek K. Intravenous cytosine arabinoside in the emergency treatment of 9 dogs with central nervous system inflammatory disease of unknown etiology. In: 20th Annual Symposium of the European College of Veterinary Neurology. Bern (Switzerland): 2007. p. 508.

71. Bennett WM, Norman DJ. Action and toxicity of cyclosporine. Annu Rev Med 1986;37:215–24.

72. Begley DJ, Squires LK, Zlokovic BV, et al. Permeability of the blood-brain barrier to the immunosuppressive cyclic peptide cyclosporin A. J Neurochem 1990;55: 1222–30.

73. Adamo FP, O'Brien RT. Use of cyclosporine to treat granulomatous meningoen-cephalitis in three dogs. J Am Vet Med Assoc 2004;225:1211–6, 1196.

74. Gregory CR. Immunosuppressive agents. In: Bonagura JD, editor. Kirk's current veterinary therapy in small animal practice. Philadelphia: Saunders; 2000. p. 509–13.

75. Robson D. Review of the pharmacokinetics, interactions and adverse reactions of cyclosporine in people, dogs and cats. Vet Rec 2003;152:739–48.

76. Kristal O, Rassnick KM, Gliatto JM, et al. Hepatotoxicity associated with CCNU (lomustine) chemotherapy in dogs. J Vet Intern Med 2004;18:75–80.

77. Flegel T, Bottcher I, Matiasek K, et al. Treatment of immune-mediated noninfec-tious encephalitis: alternative lomustine. In: 20th Annual Symposium of the Euro-pean College of Veterinary Neurology. Bern (Switzerland): 2007. p. 508.

78. Uriarte JL, Thibaud K, Gnirs S. Lomustine treatment in noninfectious meningoen-cephalitis in 8 dogs. In: 20th Annual Symposium of the European College of Veter-inary Neurology. Bern (Switzerland): 2007. p. 508.

79. Feliu-Pascual AL, Matiasek K, de Stefani A, et al. Efficacy of mycophenolate mo-fetil for the treatment of presumptive granulomatous meningoencephalomyelitis: preliminary results. In: 20th Annual Symposium of the European College of Veter-inary Neurology. Bern (Switzerland): 2007. p. 509.

80. Gregory CR, Stewart A, Sturges B, et al. Leflunomide effectively treats naturally occurring immune-mediated and inflammatory diseases of dogs that are unre-sponsive to conventional therapy. Transplant Proc 1998;30:4143–8.

81. Chong AS, Zeng H, Knight DA, et al. Concurrent antiviral and immunosuppres-sive activities of leflunomide in vivo. Am J Transplant 2006;6:69–75.

Congenital Diseases of the Craniocervical Junction in the Dog

Sofia Cerda-Gonzalez, DVM[a],*, Curtis W. Dewey, DVM, MS[b]

KEYWORDS

- Craniocervical junction • Atlantooccipital • Atlantoaxial
- Chiarilike malformation • Syringomyelia
- Occipitoatlantoaxial malformation

ANATOMY OF THE CRANIOCERVICAL JUNCTION

The craniocervical junction (also known as the craniovertebral junction) consists of the occipital bone, foramen magnum, atlas, axis, and the ligaments of the atlantoaxial and atlantooccipital junctions.[1–4] It functions as a single unit to provide support and movement of the head in relation to the body.[1] The craniocervical junction is united by a single, continuous, joint cavity, which includes the atlantooccipital and atlantoaxial junctions and a fluid-filled cavity separating the dens and the body of the atlas (**Fig. 1**).[5] The atlantooccipital junction is further stabilized by dorsal and ventral atlantooccipital membranes, bilateral lateral atlantooccipital ligaments, and ligaments extending from the body of the atlas to the foramen magnum. This junction allows lateral and dorsoventral movement of the head in relation to the cervical spine.[1] The atlantoaxial junction, in turn, is stabilized by the dorsal atlantoaxial ligament and the transverse atlantal ligament. The apical and alar ligaments extend cranially from the dens to the occiput, spanning the atlantoaxial and atlantooccipital junctions.[5,6] The atlantoaxial junction primarily permits rotational movement of the head.[1]

The occipital bone is divided into 3 components: the supraoccipital bone, the exocciput, and the basiocciput. The supraoccipital bone surrounds the foramen magnum, the occipital condyles arise from the exoccipital bone, and the basiocciput forms the base of the skull.[1]

[a] Department of Clinical Sciences, Cornell University College of Veterinary Medicine, T6 002B Vet Res Tower, Ithaca, NY 14850, USA
[b] Department of Clinical Sciences, Cornell University College of Veterinary Medicine, T6 002C Vet Res Tower, Ithaca, NY 14850, USA
* Corresponding author.
E-mail address: sc224@cornell.edu (S. Cerda-Gonzalez).

Vet Clin Small Anim 40 (2010) 121–141
doi:10.1016/j.cvsm.2009.10.001
0195-5616/09/$ – see front matter © 2010 Elsevier Inc. All rights reserved.

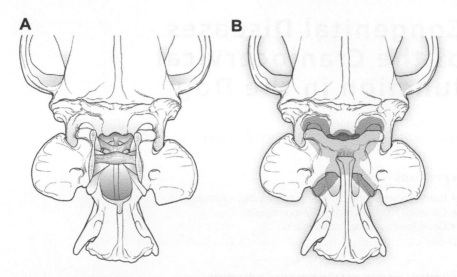

Fig. 1. The bony and ligamentous anatomy of the craniocervical junction (*A*) and the single joint space (*shaded area*) encompassing the atlantooccipital and atlantoaxial junctions (*B*).

CHIARI-LIKE MALFORMATION AND SYRINGOMYELIA

Chiari-like malformation (also called caudal occipital malformation syndrome) is a disorder of the craniocervical junction caused by overcrowding of the neural structures within the caudal fossa caused by congenital hypoplasia of the supraoccipital bone.[7,8] In affected dogs the caudal fossa is small relative to the entire cranial cavity, although the neural structures contained within are of normal size.[7,9,10] This discrepancy leads to cerebellar indentation and herniation into or through the foramen magnum, kinking of the medulla, and obliteration of the dorsal subarachnoid space at the craniocervical junction.[10–14] A dural/fibrous band may also develop at the craniocervical junction and contribute to compression of the subarachnoid space at this level (see dural/fibrous band, later in this article).[15–19]

Impingement of the subarachnoid space at the foramen magnum impairs laminar flow of cerebrospinal fluid (CSF) through this area.[20,21] CSF normally flows between the subarachnoid space of the cranial cavity and that of the spinal cord in a cyclical manner following the cardiac cycle; it exits the cranial cavity during systole and returns during diastole, moving in a direction opposite to blood flow into the cranial cavity. Movement of cilia on ependymal cells lining the ventricular system may also contribute to CSF flow.[22,23] Obstruction to flow at the craniocervical junction secondary to a Chiari-like malformation leads to the formation of a gradient of flow between the foramen magnum and cervical spine, along with turbulence and focal high velocity flow jets within the subarachnoid space at the craniocervical junction.[10,20,21,24–28] There is also excess caudal movement of the brainstem and cerebellum toward the foramen magnum during systole.[20] These changes in CSF flow can lead to accumulations of fluid within the spinal cord parenchyma, called syringomyelia (also termed syringohydromyelia, syrinx).[20,21,29] Hydromyelia, or a dilation of the spinal cord's central canal, may alternatively develop.[22,30] Various theories on the mechanism of syrinx formation have been postulated, and are described in detail elsewhere.[10,24–27,30–33]

The presence and severity of syringomyelia in dogs with Chiari-like malformations is not correlated with a single morphologic abnormality at the craniocervical junction (ie, cerebellar herniation, indentation, and so forth), making its pathogenesis likely multifactorial.[7,21] Syringomyelia may also develop secondary to disorders of the caudal fossa and craniocervical junction unrelated to Chiari-like malformations, such as tumors or cysts within the fourth ventricle, Dandy-Walker syndrome, inflammation, or head trauma.[17,22,32,34–40] Because syringomyelia is not a primary disorder, if it is present the caudal fossa and craniocervical junction should be evaluated to identify its primary cause.[30]

Chiari-like malformations and syringomyelia are most common in toy and small-breed dogs; in particular, Cavalier King Charles spaniels (CKCS) and griffon Bruxellois are predisposed.[41–43] This disorder is inherited in CKCS; an autosomal recessive mode of inheritance with incomplete penetrance is suspected.[42,44–46] Dogs of all ages may present with a Chiari-like malformation or syringomyelia, although clinical signs most frequently develop in young to middle-aged dogs. There does not seem to be a sex predisposition for Chiari-like malformations or syringomyelia.[29,47,48]

Clinical Signs

Affected dogs most frequently demonstrate abnormal pain and tactile sensations, primarily of the neck and flank, including hyperesthesia (pathologic sensitivity of normal skin to touch, light pressure, or moderate temperature changes), allodynia (pain brought on by a stimulus that would not normally produce pain), and paresthesia (a sensation of creeping, tingling, or pricking of the skin that arises spontaneously).[30,49,50] These abnormal sensations most frequently manifest as a history of pain on palpation of the neck, shoulders, and axillae and characteristic paroxysms of "phantom scratching" (ie, scratching without making contact with the skin) of this region, which can range from infrequent episodes to near-constant scratching. Dogs with a Chiari-like malformation or syringomyelia may vocalize when the neck and shoulders are touched during play, or spontaneously without apparent stimulation. Sensory abnormalities may also manifest as rubbing of the face and ears on the floor and on furniture, intolerance to grooming and neck collars, and decreased interaction with people and other dogs. These signs tend to be more frequent during periods of stress or excitement.[7,13,29,37,45,50,51]

Clinical signs are most common in dogs with syringomyelia but they may also occur in dogs with a Chiari-like malformation not accompanied by syringomyelia.[7,9,52] In addition, the severity of signs correlates to syrinx height and width in CKCS.[7,53] In 1 study 95% of dogs with syringomyelia that was 0.64 cm or wider demonstrated clinical signs.[53]

In dogs with syringomyelia, clinical signs are believed to arise primarily from abnormal processing of sensory information secondary to destruction of gray matter within the dorsal horn or compression of spinothalamic tracts throughout the spinal cord.[13,51–53] However, syringomyelia may also be present in asymptomatic dogs; it has been found in up to 44% of clinically normal CKCS screened using magnetic resonance (MR) imaging.[7,40] In these cases the syrinx tends to be smaller in size, symmetric, and less frequently deviated into the dorsal horn of the spinal cord.[7,9,53] In dogs with a Chiari-like malformation alone (without syringomyelia), hyperalgesia and paresthesia may be caused by interruptions in the normal medullary antinociceptive influence on the trigeminal nucleus caudalis and spinal cord dorsal horn.[52] Alternatively, clinical signs may be caused by compression of the brainstem or first cervical nerve at the foramen magnum.[54,55]

Dogs with Chiari-like malformations and syringomyelia may also develop scoliosis.[7,13,17,37,56] Scoliosis can result from damage to lower motor neurons within the ventral gray matter of the spinal cord, leading to paraspinal muscle atrophy and asymmetric cervical muscle tone.[13,17,30,37] Scoliosis may also be a sensory phenomenon.[47] Alternatively, spinal cord damage may manifest as a cervical myelopathy, with tetraparesis, sensory ataxia, and abnormal proprioceptive placing in all limbs. These signs, in particular weakness and muscle atrophy, may be more prominent in the thoracic versus the pelvic limbs (ie, central cord syndrome) in dogs with syringomyelia.[13,30,51] Lastly, cerebellovestibular signs, seizures, and cranial nerve involvement may be seen in dogs with a Chiari-like malformation, with facial paralysis being most common.[9,13,18,47,51]

Diagnosis

MR imaging is the preferred imaging modality for diagnosing this disorder. Findings consistent with a Chiari-like malformation include cerebellar herniation through the foramen magnum, cerebellar indentation by the supraoccipital bone, and crowding of the foramen magnum with obliteration of the subarachnoid space at the craniocervical junction (**Fig. 2**).[7,9,29,47] Kinking of the medulla may also be present.[7,13,51] Ventriculomegaly and occipital dysplasia are frequently seen but are considered a normal variation rather than a pathologic finding and are unrelated to the presence or severity of clinical signs.[7,31,47,48,57,58]

Syringomyelia is seen as a linear hyperintensity within the spinal cord parenchyma, most apparent on T2-weighted sagittal and transverse MR images (**Fig. 3**). Differential diagnoses for this finding include spinal cord edema, inflammation, neoplasia, and hemorrhage.[30] T1-weighted pre- and postcontrast MR imaging sequences and single-shot turbo spin-echo pulse sequences can be used to differentiate these disorders.[59] Syringomyelia develops primarily within the cervical spinal cord, beginning at the level of, or caudal to, the atlantoaxial junction. The fluid-filled cavity most frequently involves the dorsal aspect of the spinal cord, particularly within the dorsal

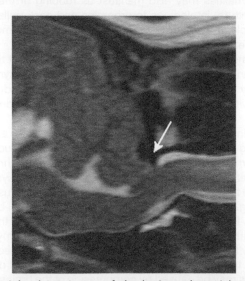

Fig. 2. Sagittal T2-weighted MR image of the brain and cranial cervical spinal cord in a young CKCS with a history of neck pain and scratching of the neck and shoulder region. Cerebellar crowding, indentation, and herniation are present, along with medullary kinking and obliteration of the subarachnoid space at the foramen magnum (*arrow*). These abnormalities are consistent with a Chiari-like malformation.

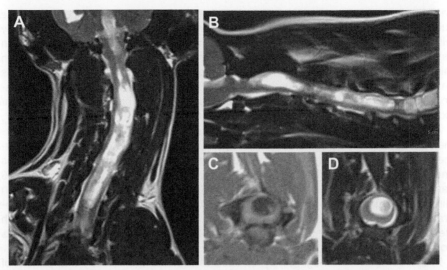

Fig. 3. One-year-old male intact Chihuahua with severe head and neck pain and mild lumbar pain. (*A*) Dorsal T2-weighted MR image of the brain and cervical spinal cord. Syringomyelia (seen as hyperintensity within the spinal cord parenchyma) is present throughout the cervical spinal cord, as is scoliosis (the dog's neck could not be straightened, despite anesthesia). (*B*) Sagittal T2-weighted MR image of the brain and cervical spinal cord. Syringomyelia is present throughout the length of the cervical spinal cord. (*C, D*) Transverse T1-weighted (*C*) and T2-weighted (*D*) MR images of the cervical spinal cord. Note the T1-hypointense and T2-hyperintense areas within the spinal cord, consistent with syringomyelia.

gray matter.[47,48,53,60] It can vary widely in its severity, from spanning a single cervical vertebra to spanning the entire length of the spinal cord (holocord syringomyelia) (**Fig. 4**).

The incidence of anomalies of the craniocervical junction consistent with a Chiari-like malformation is high in toy and small-breed dogs and, in particular, CKCS and griffon Bruxellois.[7,9,13,43,48,61] However, these abnormalities, including the presence

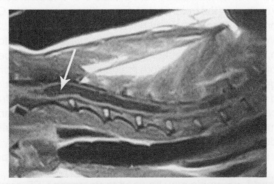

Fig. 4. Sagittal T1-weighted MR image of the cervical spinal cord demonstrating syringomyelia (*arrow*) beginning caudal to the atlantoaxial junction and extending throughout the length of the cervical and cranial thoracic spinal cord. Syringomyelia continued through the thoracolumbar spinal cord (holocord syringomyelia).

and extent of cerebellar herniation, cerebellar indentation, obstruction of the subarachnoid space at the foramen magnum, and occipital dysplasia correlate poorly with clinical status.[7,9] Chiari-like malformations and syringomyelia may be found in asymptomatic dogs, complicating diagnosis and treatment decisions for dogs with this disorder.[7,9,47,48,61] In addition, up to 43% of dogs with Chiari-like malformations have concurrent, unrelated, neurologic disorders, often with similar clinical manifestations, including pseudomembranous otitis media and intervertebral disc protrusion/extrusion.[2,3,8,10,15,47,62–65]

Alternative methods of determining the clinical significance of a Chiari-like malformation or syringomyelia have been investigated to help alleviate this problem. In volumetric studies, clinical signs have been associated with occipital hypoplasia in dogs and people.[7,11] A ratio of caudal fossa size to total cranial cavity volume of 13.3% has a sensitivity of 70% and specificity of 92% when used to differentiate between clinically affected and asymptomatic CKCS with a Chiari-like malformation.[7] Radiographic measurements determining the ratio of caudal fossa height to its length were used to predict the presence of a Chiari-like malformation in griffon Bruxellois dogs with a sensitivity of 87% and a specificity of 78%.[43]

Phase-contrast MR imaging may be used to evaluate the velocity and pattern of CSF flow in dogs with abnormalities of the craniocervical junction, and determine whether flow is impaired at this level in dogs with Chiari-like malformations.[20,21] This imaging modality may be used to confirm the clinical significance of a Chiari-like malformation and to monitor clinical progression, particularly when other disorders of the brain or cervical spine are present.[20,21] Ultrasonography may also be used at the craniocervical junction to identify cerebellar herniation and indentation, medullary kinking, and syringomyelia. However, its sensitivity is low, particularly because syringomyelia most frequently begins caudal to the atlantoaxial junction.[48,60] In dogs with syringomyelia, electromyography of the paraspinal and thoracic limb muscles can show spontaneous activity consistent with denervation changes, although motor nerve conduction velocities remain normal, suggesting axonal loss.[13] CSF analysis is typically normal in dogs with Chiari-like malformations or syringomyelia, although mild-to-moderate mixed cell, lymphocytic, and neutrophilic pleocytoses and elevated protein levels have also been reported.[22,51,56,66,67]

Treatment

Medical and surgical treatment modalities are available for this disorder. There is considerable controversy regarding the treatment of dogs with asymptomatic Chiari-like malformations or syringomyelia. Treatment may not be necessary in these cases, or in those with mild, nonprogressive clinical signs.[30] In dogs with a Chiari-like malformation or syringomyelia, the brain, craniocervical junction, and cervical spine should be evaluated for an alternative cause of the clinical signs before making treatment decisions.

Medical management has dual goals of pain control/modulation of abnormal sensory input and a reduction in CSF production. Affected dogs frequently require multimodal medical management to control their signs, rather than treatment with a single class of medication.[16,50] Although medical management generally improves clinical signs in dogs with Chiari-like malformations or syringomyelia, it does not prevent disease progression and tends to have only a temporary beneficial effect.[19,47,68]

Acetazolamide and furosemide may be used to decrease CSF production.[16,51,56,68] Glucocorticoids are frequently prescribed for their antiinflammatory effects, their ability to limit sympathetically mediated pain, and their effect on CSF production.[68–70] Gabapentin is typically recommended for managing neuropathic pain in dogs. Recently, pregabalin has emerged as an alternative to gabapentin, although limited information is available regarding the use of this medication in dogs.[16,71–73] Cyclooxygenase 2 inhibitors, such as carprofen and meloxicam, may help manage neuropathic pain also.[70,74]

Ketamine (N-methyl-D-aspartate [NMDA] antagonist) and lidocaine (sodium channel blocker) have also been used as a means of reducing central nervous system sensitization in dogs with chronic neuropathic pain, particularly perioperatively.[70,75] Opioid analgesics such as fentanyl and butorphanol may be used perioperatively to treat sensory abnormalities in dogs with Chlari-like malformations or syringomyelia.[7,13,56,70] Antiseizure drugs may be necessary if seizures are present.[56,70] Acupuncture has been used for the treatment of neuropathic pain in these dogs.[70,76]

A suboccipital craniectomy is the surgery of choice for this disorder, coupled with a dorsal laminectomy of the first or second cervical vertebra if compression of the subarachnoid space extends beyond the atlantooccipital junction. A durotomy overlying the atlantooccipital or atlantoaxial junctions is frequently necessary to help restore CSF flow.[16,19,47] Surgery is advised as a more definitive, longer-term, treatment option, and is particularly recommended for dogs that do not respond well to medical management or show progressive neurologic signs. Reports of postoperative outcomes differ widely in their success rate.[16,18,19,56] Earlier surgical intervention may improve postoperative resolution of clinical signs.[19,56]

Although postoperative clinical improvement is typically seen in the form of reduced pain levels or improved neurologic signs, sensory disturbances such as scratching infrequently resolve, and affected dogs often continue receiving medical management for their sensory disturbances following surgery.[76] Resolution of syringomyelia is also infrequent.[16,19,56] Delayed deterioration and a recurrence of signs can occur in up to 47% of cases months to years after surgery.[16,56] This may result from inadequate restoration of CSF flow at the craniocervical junction despite surgery in combination with underrecognition of associated disorders of the craniocervical junction in these patients, such as atlantooccipital overlapping.[15,16,18,21] In addition, scar-tissue formation at the surgery site may reobstruct CSF flow at the foramen magnum and lead to a recurrence of signs. In these cases, a second surgery to remove scar tissue has led to clinical improvement.[16,19,32,50,56] Placement of a dural graft patch and marsupialization of the incised meninges have been used to reduce postoperative scar formation.[16,77] Cranioplasty and placement of a titanium mesh may also help to reduce the formation of this tissue and improve long-term outcomes.[76]

OCCIPITOATLANTOAXIAL MALFORMATIONS

Occipitoatlantoaxial malformations (OAAMs) occur infrequently in dogs; they are not described in cats. In reported cases abnormal embryologic development led to a shifting of the craniocervical junction caudally by 1 vertebral segment, such that the atlantoaxial junction resembles the atlantooccipital junction (see **Fig. 4**). At the atlantooccipital junction the atlas is typically fused to the occipital bone bilaterally. It may also be asymmetrically hypoplastic, with smaller or thickened transverse processes and a shortened body.[78,79] The axis, in turn, may be rotated or fused to the atlas; it may have abnormally large transverse processes and a hypoplastic, aplastic, or deviated dens.[78–80] Displacement of the axis into the foramen magnum has also been reported in a dog with OAAMs, as have fragmentation of the atlas and axis into multiple bony elements according to their centers of ossification. Enlargement and narrowing of the foramen magnum may be seen.[79] OAAMs frequently lead to variable degrees of spinal cord and brainstem compression either by malformed vertebral segments or because of atlantoaxial instability/subluxation. Narrowing of the vertebral canal by up to 50% has been reported with this disorder.[79] A cause for OAAMs has not yet been identified in dogs, although exposure to teratogenic substances has been proposed.[78]

Most affected dogs develop clinical signs within the first year of life; reports of cases as old as 18 months of age are described.[79] OAAMs have been reported in large- and small-breed dogs, including Saint Bernard, CKCS, German shepherd, Jack Russell terrier, French bulldog, and Newfoundland.[78,79] Spinal cord compression secondary to the malformation results in a cervical myelopathy, with clinical signs ranging from ambulatory tetraparesis and ataxia to tetraplegia. Neck pain and scoliosis may also be seen.[78,79]

A bony malformation may be palpable at the craniocervical junction.[78] OAAMs are detectable on lateral and ventrodorsal radiographs of the craniocervical junction. Myelography, postmyelogram computed tomography (CT), and MR imaging can provide information regarding degree of spinal cord compression and allow detection of nonbony areas of compression. CT, in particular when combined with 3-dimensional reconstruction software, can best define bony abnormalities (**Fig. 5**). Care must be taken in positioning these dogs for diagnostic imaging as flexion may exacerbate spinal cord compression if atlantoaxial instability is present. Surgical stabilization of the craniocervical junction has been described in 2 dogs with OAAMs.[81]

ATLANTOOCCIPITAL OVERLAPPING

Nontraumatic atlantooccipital overlapping can be seen in toy and small-breed dogs. In these cases there is a decreased distance between the dorsal arch of the atlas and the supraoccipital bone, with the rostral aspect of the atlas either located immediately ventral to the foramen magnum or within the caudal fossa. The atlas may indent the caudal aspect of the cerebellum and obliterate the cerebellomedullary cistern.

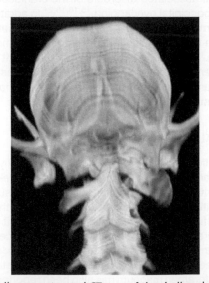

Fig. 5. Three-dimensionally reconstructed CT scan of the skull and cranial cervical vertebrae of a 2-year-old border terrier with a left ear droop and a left-sided head tilt. An OAAM is present, manifesting as a misshapen and hypoplastic left occipital condyle and a fragmented atlas with fusion of its right wing to the right occipital condyle and fusion of its left wing to the axis. Although not apparent on this image, the body of the atlas was fused to the body of the axis.

Atlantooccipital overlapping can also lead to kinking or dorsal displacement of the medulla at its junction with the cervical spinal cord.[15] In contrast to cases of traumatic atlantooccipital overlapping, neither fractures of the occipital bone nor rotation of the atlas are present in dogs with atlantooccipital overlapping.[82–84] These cases also differed from dogs with OAAMs in that atlantooccipital fusion was absent and, excluding dens abnormalities, the first 2 cervical vertebrae did not seem to be malformed.[15,78,79,81]

Atlantooccipital overlapping resembles the human disorder basilar invagination/ basilar impression (these terms have been used interchangeably), in which there is displacement of the first 2 cervical vertebrae toward or through the foramen magnum, either as a congenital abnormality or secondary to a disorder of connective tissue or bone.[85–90] The pathophysiology of atlantooccipital overlapping in dogs is unknown, although evidence of connective tissue disorders has not been detected.[15] In the 4 reported cases, this disorder was found along with other abnormalities of the craniocervical junction, including Chiari-like malformations, atlantoaxial instability, and abnormalities of the dens.[15] Likewise, basilar impression/invagination in people is associated with Chiari malformations, atlantoaxial subluxation, dorsal angulation of the dens, and platybasia.[64,85–88,90] Occipital dysplasia is also present in the human and canine disorder and may have a permissive effect, allowing displacement of the atlas through the foramen magnum.[1]

Syringomyelia was found in a subset of dogs with atlantooccipital overlapping. In these cases, the overlapping was suspected to contribute to syringomyelia by obstructing CSF flow at the craniocervical junction or impairing blood flow through the basilar artery, as in people with basilar impression/invagination.[3,27,39,63] However, this relationship has not been confirmed in dogs.

Clinical signs consist of head and neck pain and a cervical myelopathy, although it remains unclear whether these are related to atlantooccipital overlapping or to concurrent abnormalities of the craniocervical junction. Clinical signs consistent with medullary and cerebellar involvement can also occur.[15]

Atlantooccipital overlapping may be inconspicuous on cervical radiographs; advanced imaging is necessary to identify this disorder. MR imaging best demonstrates overlapping of the dorsal arch of the atlas with the supraoccipital bone, secondary kinking and compression of the medulla and cervical spinal cord at the craniocervical junction, indentation of the cerebellum, and obliteration of the cerebellomedullary cistern. This imaging modality is ideally coupled with a CT scan obtained while the craniocervical junction is in neutral and mildly extended positions, as atlantooccipital overlapping can be a dynamic disorder. Overlapping of the atlas with the occipital bone may be less conspicuous when the craniocervical junction is in a neutral position and more apparent on extension (**Fig. 6**).[15,65,88]

As with other disorders of the craniocervical junction, medical management can help to control neck and head pain in these cases (see section on Chiari-like malformation, treatment).[15] Surgery to stabilize the atlantooccipital junction is reported in a single case of atlantooccipital overlapping.[91] Stabilization of the atlantoaxial junction may also be necessary if concurrent instability is present.[92–95]

ATLANTOAXIAL INSTABILITY (ATLANTOAXIAL SUBLUXATION)

Atlantoaxial instability, also referred to as atlantoaxial subluxation, refers to instability of the atlantoaxial joint that leads to dorsal displacement of the axis in relation to the atlas and, consequently, spinal cord compression. It is most common among small- and toy-breed dogs, with miniature and toy poodle, Yorkshire terrier, Chihuahua,

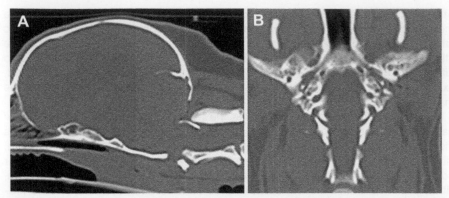

Fig. 6. CT scan of a 6-year-old female spayed Pomeranian with bilateral peripheral vestibular disease, and head and cervical pain. Bilateral otitis media was found as the cause of the dog's vestibular signs. Intervertebral disc disease was also present. (*A*) Sagittal reconstruction showing overlapping of the arch of the atlas with the supraoccipital bone when the craniocervical junction is in extension. (*B*) Dorsal reconstruction of the craniocervical junction reveals normal occipital condyles and cranial articular fovea of the atlas and normal alignment of the atlantooccipital junction.

Pekingese, and Pomeranian breeds being most frequently affected.[6,96–98] Congenital atlantoaxial instability has also been reported in large-breed dogs, including the rottweiler and Doberman pinscher.[99,100] Affected dogs typically develop clinical signs within the first 2 years of life, with 52% to 70% being less than 1 year of age at the time of onset. There is no apparent sex predilection.[6,96,97,101]

Pathophysiology

Congenital atlantoaxial instability most frequently results from aplasia or hypoplasia of the dens; nonunion of the dens with the axis and absence of the transverse ligament of the atlas have also been implicated.[6,102,103] The first 2 cervical vertebrae may also be abnormal in their shape and size.[97,104] Instability leads to dorsal displacement of the axis in relation to the atlas, with subsequent spinal cord compression. The degree of displacement and neural impingement depends on the degree of laxity of the atlantoaxial joint[97] and can be more severe if the dens is intact.[6]

Clinical Signs

Gait dysfunction is present in most cases, seen as upper motor neuron/general proprioceptive ataxia, tetraparesis, or, rarely, tetraplegia. Neck pain is also a frequent finding, reported in 53% to 77% of dogs with atlantoaxial instability.[6,97,102] Clinical signs are exacerbated by neck flexion and can develop following minor trauma such as running into objects head first, falls from furniture, and dog fights. In severe cases respiratory paralysis and sudden death can result.[96,101]

Diagnosis

Cervical radiographs frequently provide a preliminary diagnosis of atlantoaxial instability, showing dorsal displacement of the axis relative to the atlas with increased distance between the spinous process of the axis and the dorsal arch of the atlas and abnormalities of the dens (**Fig. 7**). The atlas may also be abnormally short.[97] If evidence of instability is not seen with the neck in a neural position it may be mildly

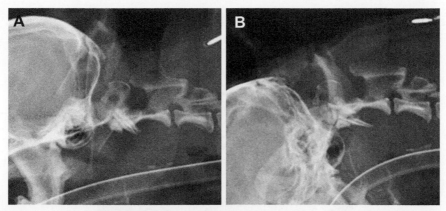

Fig. 7. Left lateral radiographs of the craniocervical junction in a 5-month-old miniature poodle with cervical pain, tetraparesis, and an upper motor neuron/general proprioceptive ataxia in all limbs. The craniocervical junction seems normal when in a neutral position (*A*). With the neck in mild flexion (*B*) dorsal displacement of the axis is seen in relation to the atlas, with increased distance between the dorsal arch of the atlas and the spinous process of the axis.

flexed, ideally using fluoroscopy to minimize the degree of flexion needed to identify instability. Uncooperative patients may necessitate radiographs taken during anesthesia.[6,99] In some cases radiographs may not show the atlantoaxial instability[15] and, when taken alone, radiographs do not demonstrate the degree of neural compression. Additional imaging is therefore recommended in dogs suspected of having atlantoaxial instability to evaluate the degree of spinal cord compression and determine whether other disorders of the craniocervical junction are present alongside atlantoaxial instability/subluxation, such as atlantooccipital overlapping, syringomyelia, dorsal angulation of the dens, or hypoplasia or aplasia of the dens (**Fig. 8**).[15,96,105,106] Myelography may also be used to assess the degree of spinal cord compression, although it does not allow evaluation of the spinal cord parenchyma.[107] Neurologic deterioration and seizures may be seen post myelography.[108] The absence of these potential side effects and improved evaluation of neural structures provided with MR imaging make this a more ideal imaging modality for dogs with atlantoaxial instability.

Treatment

Medical and surgical options are described for the treatment of this disorder. Medical management consists of immobilizing the head and neck in extension using a ventrally reinforced cervical splint for a minimum period of 6 weeks, strict exercise restriction, and treatment with corticosteroids.[101,109] The goal of immobilizing the atlantoaxial junction is to achieve fusion through fibrosis of this joint. The success rate of medical management ranges from 50% to 63%.[97,101,109,110] Duration of clinical signs longer than 30 days has been associated with a poor outcome with medical management. As this treatment approach does not allow direct joint fusion and does not permit realignment of the cervical vertebrae, there is increased risk of continued or recurrent impingement of neural structures. Nonsurgical management has been recommended for dogs with mild neurologic deficits, acute-onset clinical signs, dogs with immature vertebrae, and those for whom financial constraints exclude surgery as an option.[6,101]

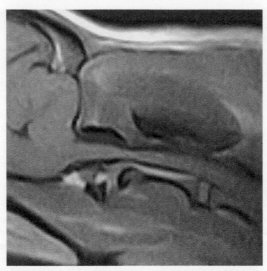

Fig. 8. Sagittal T2-weighted MR image of the brain and cranial cervical spinal cord of a dog with an atlantoaxial instability/subluxation. The axis is dorsally displaced in relation to the atlas and there is increased distance between the dorsal arch of the atlas and the spinous process of the axis. The spinal cord is compressed dorsoventrally at the atlantoaxial junction. Aplasia of the dens is present.

Multiple surgical options for treating atlantoaxial instability have been described, with the goal of realigning and stabilizing the atlantoaxial junction and decompressing the spinal cord. Surgical repair of atlantoaxial instability is particularly recommended in dogs with chronic or relapsing clinical signs, those for which medical management has failed, and dogs with fully mature vertebrae.[101] Ventral fixation may be performed using transarticular lag screws, pins, or Kirschner wires, with or without reinforcement with polymethyl methacrylate, or a spinal plate.[96,99,107,111–113] Implants may also be placed into the pedicle of the atlas and the body of the axis to provide additional strength to the stabilization.[102,107] The articular cartilage is frequently removed at the atlantoaxial junction bilaterally to encourage fusion of the joint. Cancellous bone graft may be obtained from the humerus and placed in the joint space.[96,97,107,112] Success rates up to 91% have been reported with ventral fixation of the atlantoaxial junction.[6,97,102]

Ventral stabilization is preferred to dorsal fixation for its ability to allow visualization of the joints, dens, and spinal cord, the ability to achieve direct joint stabilization, the ability to use bone graft to encourage long-term fusion, and a lower risk of iatrogenic neural damage or reluxation in the event of implant failure with these procedures.[6,97,112] If spinal cord compression is exacerbated by the dens, an odontoidectomy can also be performed through this approach.[112] It has been effectively used to treat atlantoaxial instability in a large-breed dog.[99] Potential complications associated with ventral fixation include iatrogenic neurologic trauma, focal tracheal necrosis or perforation, aspiration pneumonia, implant failure, migration, breakage, salivary mucocele, laryngeal paralysis, and Horner syndrome.[96,104]

Dorsal surgical approaches achieve fixation by securing the spine of the axis to the dorsal arch of the atlas using the nuchal ligament, orthopedic wire, or nonmetallic suture.[96,97,102,110,114,115] Dorsal crosspinning of the atlas and axis with polymethyl methacrylate placement has also been described.[116] A failure rate of 39% to 46% is seen with dorsal procedures.[6,97] A major disadvantage of this approach is its inability to achieve joint fusion directly, such that implant failure would be more likely to lead to reluxation of the atlantoaxial joint than with ventral procedures.[96] Additional disadvantages include increased risk of spinal cord trauma during implant placement, a higher rate of implant failure, vertebral damage including fracture of the arch of the atlas postoperatively, and inadequate realignment of the atlantoaxial joint.[6,97,112]

With dorsal and ventral approaches a neck splint is typically placed postoperatively to reduce stress placed on the surgical implants during healing and to encourage bony fusion.[97,98,107,114,117] These dogs should be evaluated immediately postoperatively for respiratory distress, and weekly for splint placement, skin infections, and pressure wounds.[107] Dogs may be reluctant to walk or eat following splint placement.[107] Corticosteroids may be used perioperatively to reduce spinal cord edema caused by iatrogenic trauma to the spinal cord during positioning or surgery.[96,104,107]

Surgery carries a risk of neurologic deterioration from spinal cord trauma either during manipulation under anesthesia or during implant placement.[96,117] Implant failure or vertebral fractures during placement may be more likely in younger patients because of incomplete bony maturation.[117] The following factors have been associated with a higher likelihood of a successful surgical outcome: age of less than 24 months at the start of clinical signs, duration of clinical signs of less than 10 months before surgery, and a lower neurologic grade (ie, lower severity of signs, in particular ambulatory status or better) at the time of surgery.[98]

ABNORMALITIES OF THE DENS

Abnormalities of the dens in dogs include agenesis/hypoplasia (see atlantoaxial instability), dorsal angulation, and congenital nonunion of the dens with the axis.[8,15,105,106,118–120] Although most cases are seen in small- and toy-breed dogs, abnormalities of the dens have been reported in large-breed dogs in association with atlantoaxial instability/subluxation.[99,100] Embryologically the dens develops from 2 centers of ossification within the axis: the centrum of the proatlas and centrum 1. These normally fuse with the body of the axis by 3 to 4 and 7 to 9 months of age, respectively. Abnormalities of the dens likely result from abnormal development in utero[120] Trauma-induced ischemic necrosis of the dens and a congenital absence of an ossification center for the dens have been proposed as possible causes of dens aplasia/hypoplasia of the dens.[120]

Congenital dorsal angulation of the dens has been described primarily in toy- and small-breed dogs, with most presenting by 2.5 years of age.[8,47,102,105,106] Slow-onset neurologic signs indicate a cranial cervical myelopathy and neck pain characterizes their presentation, although acute exacerbations are also described.[8,106] Compression of spinocerebellar tracts may cause a hypermetric gait.[8] A dorsal angulation of approximately 45° can be seen on lateral cervical radiographs, MR imaging, and CT images. Compression of the overlying spinal cord is evident with the latter 2 imaging modalities, and has been confirmed histopathologically and surgically.[8,105,106] Thinning and scalloping of the dorsal arch of the atlas may also be seen.[8] More pronounced retroflexion of the dens has been correlated to the presence of syringomyelia in humans.[121] Dorsal angulation of the dens is also more frequently seen in female patients and in association with Chiari malformations.[121] Insufficient cases of dorsal angulation of the dens have been described in veterinary medicine to determine whether these relationships exist in the canine disorder. Three of the 5 cases described in dogs have had concurrent atlantoaxial instability contributing to spinal cord compression.[8,102]

An odontoidectomy can be performed to relieve spinal cord compression directly in dogs with dorsal angulation of the dens.[96,106,112] Fusion of the atlantoaxial joint may be necessary if instability is present.[102] Improvements in clinical signs have also been reported with restriction in physical activity alone.[8]

DURAL/FIBROUS BAND OVERLYING THE CRANIOCERVICAL JUNCTION

In a subset of dogs with Chiari-like malformations a focal dorsal compressive lesion is present overlying the atlantoaxial and the atlantooccipital junctions.[7,15–17,19,56] This band of tissue seems to arise from dura or ligamentum flavum that has abnormally thickened, fibrosed, or ossified.[7,56,122] Lymphocytic inflammation may also be present.[56] The dural/fibrous band can cause variable degrees of compression, from mild reduction of the dorsal subarachnoid space alone to focal indentation of the spinal cord. The cause of the dural/fibrous band is unknown, although excess motion at the atlantooccipital or atlantoaxial junctions may encourage its formation.[15,89,122]

Focal compression of the subarachnoid space or spinal cord can be best seen with MR imaging and is visible as a thick white membrane at surgery (**Fig. 9**).[7,19] The dorsal subarachnoid space may seem dilated immediately cranial to the point of compression in these dogs at surgery. Resection of the tissue resolves the compression and subarachnoid space dilation.[7,15]

Although a relationship has not been found between dural/fibrous bands and clinical signs or syringomyelia in dogs, syringomyelia is frequently present immediately caudal to the lesion.[7] Because the dural/fibrous band can be responsible for compression of the subarachnoid space, it is suspected to obstruct CSF flow in people and dogs, contributing to syringomyelia formation.[7,89,122] Consequently, in dogs with Chiari-like malformations the craniocervical junction should be evaluated for areas of focal dorsal compression caused by dural/fibrous bands and these should be considered in surgical planning.[7,15]

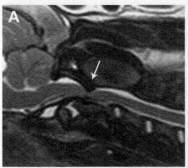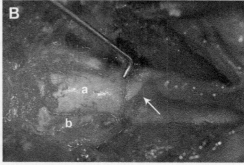

Fig. 9. (*A*) Sagittal T2-weighted MR image of the brain and cervical spinal cord in a 5-month-old female English bulldog with tetraparesis and cervical pain. There is a dorsal compressive lesion overlying the atlantoaxial junction (*arrow*) that indents the underlying spinal cord and subarachnoid space. A dural/fibrous band causing this compression was confirmed surgically. (*B*) Dural/fibrous band seen following completion of a dorsal laminectomy of the atlas and the cranial aspect of the axis. The band (identified by a nerve-root retractor) indented the subarachnoid space and spinal cord at the atlantoaxial junction. Compression was relieved with resection of this tissue. a, dura underlying the dorsal laminectomy of the atlas; b, lateral margin of the dorsal laminectomy of the atlas; *arrow*, caudal-most aspect of the laminectomy, extending into the cranial aspect of the axis.

SUMMARY

Abnormalities of the craniocervical junction are most frequently seen in toy- and small-breed dogs, with affected dogs typically presenting when they are young to middle-aged. Because many of these disorders overlap in their clinical manifestations, some, such as a Chiari-like malformation, may be present in asymptomatic dogs, and more than 1 malformation is often present at 1 time, craniocervical junction anomalies can pose a treatment and diagnostic dilemma. In dogs with cervical myelopathy, head pain, or neck pain, it is important to evaluate the entire craniocervical junction before making treatment decisions. Radiography alone is often insufficient so MR imaging of the brain and cervical spine is frequently recommended to evaluate the neural parenchyma fully.

REFERENCES

1. Barnes PD, Kim FM, Crawley C. Developmental anomalies of the craniocervical junction and cervical spine. Magn Reson Imaging Clin N Am 2000;8(3):651–74.
2. Rao PV, Mbajiorgu EF, Levy LV. Bony abnormalities of the craniocervical junction. Cent Afr J Med 2001;48(1–2):17–23.
3. Erbengi A, Oge HK. Congenital malformations of the craniovertebral junction: classification and surgical treatment. Acta Neurochir (Wien) 1994;127(3–4): 180–5.
4. Kumar A, Mafee M, Jafar J, et al. Diagnosis and management of anomalies of the craniocervical junction. Ann Otol Rhinol Laryngol 1986;95:487–97.
5. Evans HE. Arthrology. In: Miller's anatomy of the dog. 3rd edition. Philadelphia: W.B. Saunders; 1993. p. 219–57.
6. McCarthy RJ, Lewis DD, Hosgood G. Atlantoaxial subluxation in dogs. Compendium 1995;17(2):215–27.
7. Cerda-Gonzalez S, Olby NJ, McCullough S, et al. Morphology of the caudal fossa in Cavalier King Charles Spaniels. Vet Radiol Ultrasound 2009;50(1): 37–45.
8. Bynevelt M, Rusbridge C, Britton J. Dorsal dens angulation and a Chiari type malformation in a Cavalier King Charles Spaniel. Vet Radiol Ultrasound 2000; 41(6):521–4.
9. Lu D, Lamb CR, Pfeiffer DU, et al. Neurological signs and results of magnetic resonance imaging in 40 cavalier King Charles spaniels with Chiari type 1-like malformations. Vet Rec 2003;153:260–3.
10. Nishikawa M, Sakamoto H, Hakuba A, et al. Pathogenesis of Chiari malformation: a morphometric study of the posterior cranial fossa. J Neurosurg 1997; 86:40–7.
11. Badie B, Mendoza D, Batzdorf U. Posterior fossa volume and response to suboccipital decompression in patients with Chiari I malformation. Neurosurgery 1995;37(2):214–8.
12. Stovner LJ, Bergan U, Nilsen G, et al. Posterior cranial fossa dimensions in the Chiari I malformation: relation to pathogenesis and clinical presentation. Neuroradiology 1993;35(2):113–8.
13. Rusbridge C, 'MacSweeny JE, Davies JV, et al. Syringohydromyelia in Cavalier King Charles spaniels. J Am Anim Hosp Assoc 2000;36:34–41.
14. Cross HR, Cappello R, Rusbridge C. Comparison of cerebral cranium volumes between cavalier King Charles spaniels with Chiari-like malformation, small breed dogs and Labradors. J Small Anim Pract 2009;50(8): 399–405.

15. Cerda-Gonzalez S, Dewey CW, Scrivani PV, et al. Imaging features of atlanto-occipital overlapping in dogs. Vet Radiol Ultrasound 2009;50(3):264–8.
16. Rusbridge C. Chiari-like malformation with syringomyelia in the Cavalier King Charles spaniel: long-term outcome after surgical management. Vet Surg 2007;36(5):396–405.
17. Tagaki S, Kadosawa T, Ohsaki T, et al. Hindbrain decompression in a dog with scoliosis associated with syringomyelia. J Am Vet Med Assoc 2005;226(8): 1359–63.
18. Dewey CW, Berg JM, Barone G, et al. Treatment of caudal occipital malformation syndrome in dogs by foramen magnum decompression. J Vet Intern Med 2005;19(3):418.
19. Vermeersch K, Van Ham L, Caemaert J, et al. Suboccipital craniectomy, dorsal laminectomy of C1, durotomy and dural graft placement as a treatment for syringohydromyelia with cerebellar tonsil herniation in Cavalier King Charles spaniels. Vet Surg 2004;33(4):355–60.
20. March PA, Abramson CJ, Smith M, et al. CSF flow abnormalities in caudal occipital malformation syndrome. J Vet Intern Med 2005;19(3):418–9.
21. Cerda-Gonzalez S, Olby NJ, Broadstone R, et al. Characteristics of cerebrospinal fluid flow in Cavalier King Charles Spaniels analyzed using phase velocity contrast cine magnetic resonance imaging. Vet Radiol Ultrasound 2009;50(5): 467–76.
22. Kirberger RM, Jacobson LS, Davies JV, et al. Hydromyelia in the dog. Vet Radiol Ultrasound 1997;38(1):30–8.
23. deLahunta A. Cerebrospinal fluid and hydrocephalus. In: Veterinary neuroanatomy and clinical neurology. 2nd edition. Philadelphia: WB Saunders; 1983. p. 30–52.
24. Panigrahi M, Reddy BP, Reddy AK, et al. CSF flow study in Chiari I malformation. Childs Nerv Syst 2004;20:336–40.
25. Bhadelia RA, Bogdan AR, Wolpert SM, et al. Cerebrospinal fluid flow waveforms: analysis in patients with Chiari I malformation by means of gated phase-contrast MR imaging velocity measurements. Radiology 1995;196(1): 195–202.
26. Menick BJ. Phase-contrast magnetic resonance imaging of cerebrospinal fluid flow in the evaluation of patients with Chiari I malformation. Neurosurg Focus 2001;11(1):E5.
27. Levine DN. The pathogenesis of syringomyelia associated with lesions at the foramen magnum; a critical review of existing theories and proposal of new hypotheses. J Neurol Sci 2004;220:3–21.
28. Oldfield EH, Muraszko K, Shawker TH, et al. Pathophysiology of syringomyelia associated with Chiari I malformation of the cerebellar tonsils. J Neurosurg 1994;80:3–15.
29. Cappello R, Rusbridge C. Report from the Chiari-like Malformation and Syringomyelia Working Group round table. Vet Surg 2007;36:509–12.
30. Bagley RS, Gavin PR, Silver GM, et al. Syringomyelia and hydromyelia in dogs and cats. Compend Contin Educ Pract Vet 2000;22(5):471–9.
31. Rusbridge C, Greitz D, Iskandar BJ. Syringomyelia: current concepts in pathogenesis, diagnosis, and treatment. J Vet Intern Med 2006;20(3): 469–79.
32. Lee JH, Lee HK, Kim JK, et al. CSF flow quantification of the cerebral aqueduct in normal volunteers using phase contrast cine MR imaging. Korean J Radiol 2004;5(2):81–6.

33. Scrivani PV, Thompson MS, Winegardner KR, et al. Association between frontal-sinus size and syringohydromyelia in small-breed dogs. Am J Vet Res 2007; 68(6):610–3.
34. Jung DI, Park C, Kang BT, et al. Acquired cervical syringomyelia secondary to a brainstem meningioma in a maltese dog. J Vet Med Sci 2006;68(11):1235–8.
35. MacKillop E, Schatzberg SJ, De Lahunta A. Intracranial epidermoid cyst and syringohydromyelia in a dog. Vet Radiol Ultrasound 2006;47(4):339–44.
36. da Costa RC, Parent JM, Poma R, et al. Cervical syringohydromyelia secondary to a brainstem tumor in a dog. J Am Vet Med Assoc 2004; 225(7):1061–4, 1048.
37. Child G, Higgins RJ, Cuddon PA. Acquired scoliosis associated with hydromyelia and syringohydromyelia in two dogs. J Am Vet Med Assoc 1986;189(8): 909–12.
38. Tamke PG, Peterson MG, Dietze AE, et al. Acquired hydrocephalus and hydromyelia in a cat with feline infectious peritonitis: a case report and brief review. Can Vet J 1988;29:997–1000.
39. Milhorat TH, Capocelli AL Jr, Anzil AP, et al. Pathological basis of spinal cord cavitation in syringomyelia: analysis of 105 autopsy cases. J Neurosurg 1995; 82(5):802–12.
40. Greitz D, Flodmark O. Modern concepts of syringohydromyelia. Riv Neuroradiol 2004;17:360–1.
41. Rusbridge C. Neurological diseases of the Cavalier King Charles spaniel. J Small Anim Pract 2005;46(6):265–72.
42. Rusbridge C, Knowler SP. Inheritance of occipital bone hypoplasia (Chiari type I malformation) in Cavalier King Charles Spaniels. J Vet Intern Med 2004;18(5): 673–8.
43. Rusbridge C, Knowler SP, Pieterse L, et al. Chiari-like malformation in the Griffon Bruxellois. J Small Anim Pract 2009;50(8):386–93.
44. Rusbridge C. Syringomyelia. UK Vet Companion Animal 2003;8(8):59–62.
45. Rusbridge C. Persistent scratching in Cavalier King Charles spaniels. Vet Rec 1997;140:239–40.
46. Rusbridge C, Knowler P, Rouleau GA, et al. Inherited occipital hypoplasia/syringomyelia in the cavalier King Charles spaniel: experiences in setting up a worldwide DNA collection. J Hered 2005;96(7):745–9.
47. Dewey CW, Berg JM, Stefanacci JD, et al. Caudal occipital malformation syndrome in dogs. Compend Contin Educ Pract Vet 2004;26(11):886–95.
48. Couturier J, Rault D, Cauzinille L. Chiari-like malformation and syringomyelia in normal cavalier King Charles spaniels: a multiple diagnostic imaging approach. J Small Anim Pract 2008;49(9):438–43.
49. IASP Task Force on Taxonomy. Part III: pain terms, a current list with definitions and notes on usage. In: Merskey H, Bogduk N, editors. Classification of chronic pain: Descriptions of chronic pain syndromes and definitions of pain terms. 2nd edition. Seattle (WA): IASP Press; 1994. p. 209–14.
50. Rusbridge C. Canine syringomyelia: a painful problem in man's best friend. Br J Neurosurg 2007;21(5):468–9.
51. Churcher RK, Child G. Chiari 1/syringomyelia complex in a King Charles Spaniel. Aust Vet J 2000;78(2):92–5.
52. Thimineur M, Kitaj M, Kravitz E, et al. Functional abnormalities of the cervical cord and lower medulla and their effects on pain: observations in chronic pain patients with incidental mild Chiari I malformation and moderate to severe spinal cord compression. Clin J Pain 2002;18(3):171–9.

53. Rusbridge C, Carruthers H, Dube MP, et al. Syringomyelia in cavalier King Charles spaniels: the relationship between syrinx dimensions and pain. J Small Anim Pract 2007;48(8):432–6.

54. Milhorat TH, Chou MW, Trinidad EM, et al. Chiari I malformation redefined: clinical and radiographic findings for 364 symptomatic patients. Neurosurgery 1999;44(5):1005–17.

55. Taylor FR, Larkins MV. Headache and Chiari I malformation: clinical presentation, diagnosis, and controversies in management. Curr Pain Headache Rep 2002;6(4):331–7.

56. Dewey CW, Berg JM, Barone G, et al. Foramen magnum decompression for treatment of caudal occipital malformation syndrome in dogs. J Am Vet Med Assoc 2005;227(8):1270–5.

57. Wright JA. A study of the radiographic anatomy of the foramen magnum in dogs. J Small Anim Pract 1979;20(8):501–8.

58. Watson AG, de Lahunta A, Evans HE. Dorsal notch of foramen magnum due to incomplete ossification of supraoccipital bone in dogs. J Small Anim Pract 1989; 30:666–73.

59. Pease A, Sullivan S, Olby N, et al. Value of a single-shot turbo spin-echo pulse sequence for assessing the architecture of the subarachnoid space and the constitutive nature of cerebrospinal fluid. Vet Radiol Ultrasound 2006;47(3): 254–9.

60. Schmidt MJ, Wigger A, Jawinski S, et al. Ultrasonographic appearance of the craniocervical junction in normal brachycephalic dogs and dogs with caudal occipital (Chiari-like) malformation. Vet Radiol Ultrasound 2008; 49(5):472–6.

61. Schmidt MJ, Biel M, Klumpp S, et al. Evaluation of the volumes of cranial cavities in Cavalier King Charles Spaniels with Chiari-like malformation and other brachycephalic dogs as measured via computed tomography. Am J Vet Res 2009;70(4):508–12.

62. Atlas SW, Lavi E. Disorders of brain development. In: Atlas SW, Lavi E, editors. MRI of the brain and spine. 2nd edition. Philadelphia: Lippincott-Raven Publishers; 1996. p. 183–8.

63. Pearce JM. Platybasia and basilar invagination. Eur Neurol 2007;58(1):62–4.

64. Grabb PA, Mapstone TB, Oakes WJ. Ventral brain stem compression in pediatric and young adult patients with Chiari I malformations. Neurosurgery 1999;44(3): 527–8.

65. Zileli M, Cagli S. Combined anterior and posterior approach for managing basilar invagination associated with type I Chiari malformation. J Spinal Disord Tech 2002;15(4):284–9.

66. Itoh T, Nishimura R, Matsunaga S, et al. Syringomyelia and hydrocephalus in a dog. J Am Vet Med Assoc 1996;209(5):934–6.

67. Bohn AA, Wills TB, West CL, et al. Cerebrospinal fluid analysis and magnetic resonance imaging in the diagnosis of neurologic disease in dogs: a retrospective study. Vet Clin Pathol 2006;35(3):315–20.

68. Hasegawa T, Taura Y, Kido H, et al. Surgical management of combined hydrocephalus, syringohydromyelia, and ventricular cyst in a dog. J Am Anim Hosp Assoc 2005;41(4):267–72.

69. Gellman H. Reflex sympathetic dystrophy: alternative modalities for pain management. Instr Course Lect 2000;49:549–57.

70. Rusbridge C, Jeffery ND. Pathophysiology and treatment of neuropathic pain associated with syringomyelia. Vet J 2008;175(2):164–72.

71. Moore RA, Straube S, Wiffen PJ, et al. Pregabalin for acute and chronic pain in adults. Cochrane Database Syst Rev 2009;(3):CD007076.
72. Dewey CW, Cerda-Gonzalez S, Levine JM, et al. Pregabalin as an adjunct to phenobarbital and/or bromide treatment in dogs with suspected idiopathic epilepsy. J Am Vet Med Assoc, in press.
73. Salazar V, Dewey CW, Schwark W, et al. Pharmacokinetics of single-dose oral pregabalin administration in normal dogs. Vet Anaesth Analg, in press.
74. Takahashi M, Kawaguchi M, Shimada K, et al. Systemic meloxicam reduces tactile allodynia development after L5 single spinal nerve injury in rats. Reg Anesth Pain Med 2005;30(4):351–5.
75. Lamont LA. Adjunctive analgesic therapy in veterinary medicine. Vet Clin North Am Small Anim Pract 2008;38(6):1187–203.
76. Dewey CW, Marino DJ, Bailey KS, et al. Foramen magnum decompression with cranioplasty for treatment of caudal occipital malformation syndrome in dogs. Vet Surg 2007;36(5):406–15.
77. Cobb MA, Badylak SF, Janas W, et al. Porcine small intestinal submucosa as a dural substitute. Surg Neurol 1999;51:99–104.
78. Watson AG, de Lahunta A, Evans HE. Morphology and embryological interpretation of a congenital occipito-atlanto-axial malformation in a dog. Teratology 1988;38(5):451–9.
79. Petite A, McConnell F, De Stefani A, et al. Congenital occipito-atlanto-axial malformation in five dogs. Vet Radiol Ultrasound 2009;50(1):118.
80. Wright JA. A study of the radiographic anatomy of the cervical spine in the dog. J Small Anim Pract 1977;18:341–57.
81. Read R, Brett S, Cahill J. Surgical treatment of occipito-atlanto-axial malformation in the dog. Aust Vet Pract 1987;4:184–9.
82. Rylander H, Robles JC. Diagnosis and treatment of a chronic atlanto-occipital subluxation in a dog. J Am Anim Hosp Assoc 2007;43(3):173–8.
83. Greenwood KM, Oliver JE. Traumatic atlanto-occipital dislocation in two dogs. J Am Vet Med Assoc 1978;173(10):1324–7.
84. Steffen F, Flueckiger M, Montavon PM. Traumatic atlanto-occipital luxation in a dog: associated hypoglossal nerve deficits and use of 3-dimensional computed tomography. Vet Surg 2003;32(5):411–5.
85. Tassanawipas A, Mokkhavesa S, Chatchavong S, et al. Magnetic resonance imaging study of the craniocervical junction. J Orthop Surg (Hong Kong) 2005;13(3):228–31.
86. McGregor M. The significance of certain measurements of the skull in the diagnosis of basilar impression. Br J Radiol 1948;21:171–81.
87. Koenigsberg RA, Vakil N, Hong TA, et al. Evaluation of platybasia with MR imaging. AJNR Am J Neuroradiol 2005;26(1):89–92.
88. Goel A, Bhatjiwale M, Desai K. Basilar invagination: a study based on 190 surgically treated patients. J Neurosurg 1998;80:902–8.
89. Chamberlain WE. Basilar impression (Platybasia): a bizarre developmental anomaly of the occipital bone and upper cervical spine with striking and misleading neurologic manifestations. Yale J Biol Med 1939;11:487–96.
90. da Silva JA, Holanda MM. Basilar impression, Chiari malformation, and syringomyelia: a retrospective of 53 surgically treated patients. Arq Neuropsiquiatr 2003;61(2):368–75.
91. Dewey CW, Cerda-Gonzalez S, Scrivani PV, et al. Surgical stabilization of a craniocervical junction abnormality with atlanto-occipital overlapping in a dog. Comp Cont Educ Pract Vet, in press.

92. Van Gilder JC, Menezes AH. Craniovertebral abnormalities and their neurosurgical management. In: Schmidek HH, Roberts DW, editors. Operative neurosurgical techniques: Indications, methods, and results. Philadelphia: Elsevier; 2006. p. 1717–28.
93. Goel A, Sharma P. Craniovertebral junction realignment for the treatment of basilar invagination with syringomyelia: preliminary report of 12 cases. Neurol Med Chir (Tokyo) 2005;45(10):512–7.
94. Goel A. Treatment of basilar invagination by atlantoaxial joint distraction and direct lateral mass fixation. J Neurosurg Spine 2004;1(3):281–6.
95. Schultz KD Jr, Petronio J, Haid RW, et al. Pediatric occipitocervical arthrodesis. A review of current options and early evaluation of rigid internal fixation techniques. Pediatr Neurosurg 2000;33(4):169–81.
96. Thomas WB, Sorjonen DC, Simpson ST. Surgical management of atlantoaxial subluxation in 23 dogs. Vet Surg 1991;20(6):409–12.
97. Denny HR, Gibbs C, Waterman A. Atlanto-axial subluxation in the dog: a review of thirty cases and an evaluation of treatment by lag screw fixation. J Small Anim Pract 1988;29:37–47.
98. Beaver DP, Ellison GW, Lewis DD, et al. Risk factors affecting the outcome of surgery for atlantoaxial subluxation in dogs: 46 cases (1978–1998). J Am Vet Med Assoc 2000;216(7):1104–9.
99. Wheeler SJ. Atlantoaxial subluxation with absence of dens in a rottweiler. J Small Anim Pract 1992;33:90–3.
100. LeCouteur RA, Child G. Diseases of the spinal cord. In: Ettinger SJ, editor. Textbook of veterinary internal medicine. 3rd edition. Philadelphia: W.B. Saunders Co; 1989. p. 635.
101. Havig ME, Cornell KK, Hawthorne JC, et al. Evaluation of nonsurgical treatment of atlantoaxial subluxation in dogs: 19 cases (1992–2001). J Am Vet Med Assoc 2005;227(2):257–62.
102. Platt SR, Chambers JN, Cross A. A modified ventral fixation for surgical management of atlantoaxial subluxation in 19 dogs. Vet Surg 2004;33(4): 349–54.
103. Watson AG, de Lahunta A. Atlantoaxial subluxation and absence of transverse ligament of the atlas in a dog. J Am Vet Med Assoc 1989;195(2):235–7.
104. Sanders SG, Bagley RS, Silver GM, et al. Outcomes and complications associated with ventral screws, pins, and polymethyl methacrylate for atlantoaxial instability in 12 dogs. J Am Anim Hosp Assoc 2004;40(3):204–10.
105. Parker AJ, Park RD, Cusick PK. Abnormal odontoid process angulation in a dog. Vet Rec 1973;93(21):559–61.
106. Swaim SF, Greene CE. Odontoidectomy in a dog. J Am Anim Hosp Assoc 1975; 11:663.
107. Schulz KS, Waldron DR, Fahie M. Application of ventral pins and polymethylmethacrylate for the management of atlantoaxial instability: results in nine dogs. Vet Surg 1997;26(4):317–25.
108. Kishimoto M, Yamada K, Ueno H, et al. Spinal cord effects from lumbar myelographic injection technique in the dog. J Vet Med Sci 2004;66(1):67–9.
109. Gilmore DR. Nonsurgical management of four cases of atlantoaxial subluxation in the dog. J Am Anim Hosp Assoc 1984;20:93–6.
110. Lorinson D, Bright RM, Thomas WB, et al. Atlanto-axial subluxation in dogs: the results of conservative and surgical therapy. Canine Pract 1998;23(3):16–8.
111. Shores A, Tepper LC. A modified ventral approach to the atlantoaxial junction in the dog. Vet Surg 2007;36(8):765–70.

112. Sorjonen DC, Shires PK. Atlantoaxial instability: a ventral surgical technique for decompression, fixation, and fusion. Vet Surg 1981;10:22–9.
113. Voss K, Steffen F, Montavon PM. Use of the ComPact UniLock System for ventral stabilization procedures of the cervical spine: a retrospective study. Vet Comp Orthop Traumatol 2006;19(1):21–8.
114. LeCouteur RA, McKeown D, Johnson J, et al. Stabilization of atlantoaxial subluxation in the dog, using the nuchal ligament. J Am Vet Med Assoc 1980;177(10): 1011–7.
115. Chambers NJ, Betts CW, Oliver JE. The use of nonmetallic suture material for stabilization of atlantoaxial subluxation. J Am Anim Hosp Assoc 1977;13:602–4.
116. Jeffery ND. Dorsal cross pinning of the atlantoaxial joint: new surgical technique for atlantoaxial subluxation. J Small Anim Pract 1996;37(1):26–9.
117. Jeserevics J, Srenk P, Beranekl J, et al. Stabilisation of atlantoaxial subluxation in the dog through ventral arthrodesis. Schweiz Arch Tierheilkd 2008;150(2): 69–76.
118. Ladds P, Guffy M, Blauch B, et al. Congenital odontoid process separation in two dogs. J Small Anim Pract 1971;12(8):463–71.
119. Geary JC, Oliver JE, Hoerlein BF. Atlanto axial subluxation in the canine. J Small Anim Pract 1967;8(10):577–82.
120. Bailey CS, Morgan JP. Congenital spinal malformations. Vet Clin North Am Small Anim Pract 1992;22(4):985–1015.
121. Tubbs RS, Wellons JC, Blount JP, et al. Inclination of the odontoid process in the pediatric Chiari I malformation. J Neurosurg 2003;98(Suppl 1):43–9.
122. Nakamura N, Iwasaki Y, Hida K, et al. Dural band pathology in syringomyelia with Chiari type I malformation. Neuropathology 2000;1:38–43.

Hydrocephalus in Dogs and Cats

William B. Thomas, DVM, MS

KEYWORDS

- Brain • Ventricles • Cerebrospinal fluid
- Vetriculoperitoneal shunt

Hydrocephalus can be defined broadly as an active distension of the ventricular system of the brain related to inadequate passage of cerebrospinal fluid (CSF) from its point of production within the ventricular system to its point of absorption into the systemic circulation.[1] Hydrocephalus is not a specific disease, but rather a multi-factorial disorder with a variety of pathophysiological mechanisms. CSF is produced at a constant rate by the choroid plexuses of the lateral, third, and fourth ventricles; the ependymal lining of the ventricular system; and blood vessels in the subarachnoid space. The CSF circulates through the ventricular system into the subarachnoid space, where it is absorbed by arachnoid villi. Obstruction to CSF flow, which can occur anywhere along the pathway from its formation to the site of absorption in the cranial and spinal arachnoid villi, causes active distension of the ventricular system. A number of conditions, such as infarction and necrosis, can result in decreased volume of brain parenchyma, in which the loss of brain tissue leaves a vacant space filled passively with CSF. Although this was previously called hydrocephalus ex vacuo, such conditions do not cause active distension of the ventricles and are therefore not classified as hydrocephalus.[1]

CEREBROSPINAL FLUID PRODUCTION AND ABSORPTION

CSF is produced at a rate of about 0.03 to 0.5 mL/min in the dog and 0.02 mL/min in the cat by two distinct processes.[2,3] The choroid plexuses in the lateral, third, and fourth ventricles produce CSF by an energy-dependent process that requires the enzyme carbonic anhydrase. Production is independent of hydrostatic pressure within the ventricles but is influenced by osmotic pressure of the blood. The remainder of the CSF is produced as a byproduct of metabolism in the brain and spinal cord as extra-cellular fluid moves by bulk flow through the parenchyma, through the ependyma lining the ventricles, and through the pia on the surface of the brain to enter the subarachnoid space.

Department of Small Animal Clinical Sciences, College of Veterinary Medicine, University of Tennessee, 2407 River Drive, Knoxville, TN 37996-4544, USA
E-mail address: wthomas@utk.edu

Vet Clin Small Anim 40 (2010) 143–159
doi:10.1016/j.cvsm.2009.09.008
0195-5616/09/$ – see front matter © 2010 Elsevier Inc. All rights reserved.

vetsmall.theclinics.com

After its production, ventricular CSF flows through a series of narrowings from one compartment to the next, beginning with the lateral ventricles, through the interventricular foramina, to the third ventricle. From there, it flows through the mesencephalic aqueduct to the fourth ventricle. It exits the fourth ventricle through the lateral apertures into the subarachnoid space of the brain and spinal cord. Pumping of blood into the choroid plexuses provides the energy for flow of CSF in the ventricles. Normally there is no measurable pressure differential within the ventricular system because the production and flow of CSF is relatively slow and because of the viscoelastic properties of the brain. If an area of lower pressure develops, the brain rapidly shifts into that area to dissipate the pressure differential.[4]

The major site of CSF absorption is at the arachnoid villi located in the venous sinuses and cerebral veins. Absorption of CSF is a passive process and not energy dependent.[5] There is a pressure differential of 7 to 10 cm H_2O across the arachnoid villi, which accounts for the normal intracranial pressure of 7 to 10 cm H_2O. This pressure difference is due to the valvular mechanism of the villi. When intraventricular pressure is below 7 cm H_2O, there is no absorption of CSF. At higher pressures, absorption increases in proportion to pressure within the ventricles. In essence, the arachnoid villi act as a valve system to maintain intracranial pressure in the normal range.

PATHOPHYSIOLOGY OF HYDROCEPHALUS

The volume of CSF within the skull is dependent on a balance between the rate of formation and the rate of absorption. The rate of CSF formation is considered constant and is independent of intracranial pressure. Hydrocephalus develops when there is resistance to flow that causes a pressure gradient between CSF proximal and distal to the obstruction. This pressure differential can be quite small. For example, in experimental models in dogs, the increment is in the order of 0.5 mm Hg or less.[6] Over time, alternate pathways of CSF absorption can develop such that pressure within the ventricles returns to normal. These other pathways include flow of CSF across the ependyma with absorption by periventricular capillaries and flow of CSF across the cribriform plate with absorption by nasal lymphatics.

Whether or not hydrocephalus causes an increase in intracranial pressure depends on three factors. First is the size of the pressure gradient, which is determined by the severity of the obstruction and availability of alternate pathways for absorption. Because alternate pathways likely take time to develop, acute, severe obstruction favors high pressure while more gradually occurring obstruction favors normal pressure. The second factor is the efficiency of transmission of ventricular pressure to the surface of the brain, which depends on the elasticity of the brain and the size of the ventricles. In early stages of hydrocephalus, the brain in essentially incompressible and the only ways to compensate for increased pressure are movement of venous blood into the systemic circulation and displacement of CSF into the spinal subarachnoid space. Over time, however, the brain becomes more compressible as intraventricular pressure leads to increased interstitial pressure within the brain parenchyma, which increases absorption of interstitial fluid into brain capillaries. A third factor is ventricular size. Smaller ventricles mean a thicker cortical mantle better able to absorb pressure against the ventricular wall. Smaller ventricles are thus less efficient in transmitting ventricular pressure to the periphery as radial compressive stress. However, even if pressure remains relatively normal, ventricular enlargement creates shear forces on the brain, predominately in the periventricular white matter, which damages brain tissue and induces clinical signs.[6,7]

Hydrocephalus was originally classified as communicating or noncommunicating, depending on whether or not the ventricular system communicated with the subarachnoid space. This was based on the pioneering work of the American neurosurgeon Walter Dandy in the early 1900s. He injected a dye into the ventricles of animals with hydrocephalus to see if it could be recovered from the spinal subarachnoid space.[1] With later clinical and experimental observations, it became apparent that, with the rare exception of overproduction of CSF by choroid plexus tumor or hypertrophy,[8] all hydrocephalus basically involves the obstruction of CSF flow. Current classification divides hydrocephalus into intraventricular and extraventricuar obstructive hydrocephalus. With intraventricular obstructive hydrocephalus, the obstruction is somewhere within the ventricular system. Extraventricular obstructive hydrocephalus involves obstruction at the level of the subarachnoid space or arachnoid villi.[1]

Obstruction of one interventricular foramen is usually caused by a mass or inflammatory lesion. There is an enlargement of the lateral ventricle on the side of the occlusion (**Fig. 1**). Obstruction at the level of the third ventricle can be caused by a mass or inflammatory lesion and results in dilatation of both lateral ventricles (**Fig. 2**). Obstruction of flow through the mesencephalic aqueduct can be due to a developmental abnormality or inflammatory conditions. Dilatation of the lateral ventricles can also constrict the mesencephalic aqueduct as the temporal horns of the lateral ventricles expand. The lateral apertures can be obstructed because of developmental malformations, such as Chiari I–type malformations, tumors, and such inflammatory diseases as feline infectious peritonitis. There is usually marked enlargement of the fourth ventricle with moderate enlargement of the lateral ventricles and, in some cases, syringomyelia.

Obstruction at the level of the subarachnoid space occurs in premature infants with intraventricular hemorrhage that causes thickening of the arachnoid at the base of the

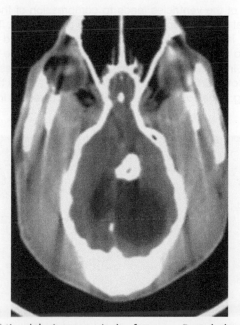

Fig. 1. Obstruction of the right interventricular foramen. Dorsal plane CT. A calcified mass obstructs outflow at the right interventricular foramen, causing marked dilatation of the right lateral ventricle. Biopsy showed a benign, bony mass.

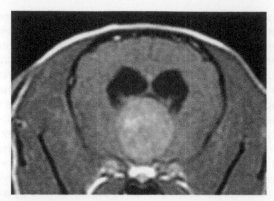

Fig. 2. Obstruction at the level of the third ventricle. Transverse T1-weighted MRI after contrast. A contrast-enhancing mass obstructs CSF flow at the third ventricle, causing enlargement of both lateral ventricles.

brain.[4] Agenesis or occlusion of the arachnoid villi can occur as a developmental defect or meningitis. This results in distension of the ventricles and subarachnoid space.

Brain damage can be due to the direct effects of compression and indirect injury caused by damage to blood vessels. Pathologically, the first changes are found in the ependyma at the angles of the lateral ventricles. There is loss of cilia and flattening of the normal cuboidal cells, which is soon followed by loss of the integrity of the ependymal surface. The lack of an effective ependymal barrier allows water and larger molecules to leak into the periventricular white matter, which become edematous.[9] Further enlargement of the ventricles leads to compression of the white matter with demyelination, axonal degeneration, and astrocyte proliferation. The septum pellucidum separating the lateral ventricles can become fenestrated or completely destroyed, giving rise to one single large ventricle (**Fig. 3**). In some cases, the cerebral cortex is preserved. In more severe cases, the cortex becomes thin with neuronal vacuolation and loss of neurons.[7,9] Damage to the cortex affects the ability to recover after surgical shunting. If the cortex is preserved, shunting results in reexpansion of the

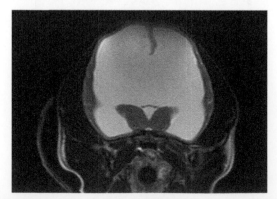

Fig. 3. Severe hydrocephalus. Transverse T2-weighted MRI. The lateral ventricles are severely enlarged with loss of the septum pellucidum, resulting in a single large ventricle. Note the sparing of the butterfly-shaped diencephalon ventral to the ventricle.

white matter with extensive regeneration of remaining axons. However, if the cortex is damaged, the cerebral mantle remains attenuated and the neuronal damage persists even after shunting.[7]

CLINICAL FEATURES

Clinically, hydrocephalus can be classified as congenital or acquired. Strictly speaking, congenital hydrocephalus is apparent at birth. However, in many cases, clinical signs are first noticed at several months of age. Congenital hydrocephalus is most common in toy breed dogs. Breeds at increased risk are Maltese, Yorkshire terrier, English bulldog, Chihuahua, Lhasa apso, Pomeranian, Toy poodle, Cairn terrier, Boston terrier, Pug, and Pekingese.[10] The most commonly identified cause in these breeds is stenosis of the mesencephalic aqueduct associated with fusion of the rostral colluliculi. In many cases, however, an obvious site of obstruction is not apparent. These cases may be due to obstruction at the level of the subarachnoid space or arachnoid villi, which are difficult to detect. Another possibility is intraventricular obstruction during a critical stage of development in which the obstructive lesion later resolves, leaving only the ventricular enlargement.

Other potential causes of congenital hydrocephalus include genetic factors and in utero exposure to infectious agents and teratogenic chemicals.[11] For example, experimental infection with canine parainfluenza in neonatal puppies causes encephalitis, aqueductal stenosis, and hydrocephalus.[12] Congenital hydrocephalus may be associated with a wide range of other nervous system anomalies, including meningomyelocele, Chiari malformation, Dandy-Walker syndrome, and cerebellar hypoplasia.

Signs of congenital hydrocephalus include an enlarged, dome-shaped head with persistent fontanelles and open cranial sutures (**Fig. 4**). However, not all dogs with a persistent fontanelle have hydrocephalus and not all patients with congenital or early-onset hydrocephalus have a persistent fontanelle. There may be ventral or ventrolateral strabismus due to either malformation of the orbit or brainstem dysfunction (**Fig. 5**). Affected patients are often unthrifty and smaller than normal. Neurologic deficits include abnormal behavior; cognitive dysfunction, such as inability to become house trained; disturbed consciousness; ataxia; circling; blindness; seizures; and vestibular dysfunction.[11,13] The course of disease is variable and difficult to predict. Neurologic deficits can progress over time, remain static, or even improve after 1 to 2 years of age.[11] Affected patients are often fragile and can worsen later in life coincident with other diseases or minor head trauma.

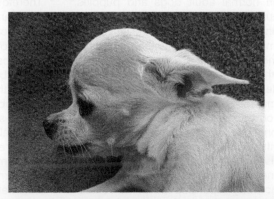

Fig. 4. Enlarged, dome-shaped calvarium in a Chihuahua with congenital hydrocephalus.

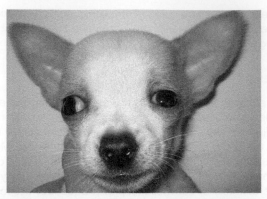

Fig. 5. Ventrolateral strabismus in a young dog with congenital hydrocephalus.

Acquired hydrocephalus can develop at any age because of such diseases as tumors and meningoencephalitis.[14–20] Neurologic deficits are similar to those in young animals, but if hydrocephalus develops after the cranial sutures have closed, malformation of the skull does not develop.[13] Clinical signs may also reflect the underlying cause of the hydrocephalus.

DIAGNOSIS

Diagnosis is based on the clinical features and brain imaging to assess ventricular size and identify any specific causes. Ventricular size is usually assessed subjectively, noting the progressively greater proportion of the intracranial volume occupied by the lateral, third, and/or fourth ventricles. Several investigators have provided quantitative measurements. When measured at the level of or caudal to the interthalamic adhesion, lateral ventricles are enlarged if lateral ventricular height exceeds 0.35 cm or if the ratio between the height of the lateral ventricle and the width of the cerebral hemisphere (ventricle/hemisphere ratio) exceeds 0.19, according to Hudson and colleagues.[21] Spaulding and Sharp[22] consider the lateral ventricles enlarged if the ratio of lateral ventricular height to the dorsoventral height of the cerebral hemisphere exceeds 0.14. However, there is a poor correlation between clinical signs and ventricular size. Also, symmetric or asymmetric enlargement of the lateral ventricles is relatively common in normal adult dogs and puppies.[21–25] Therefore, diagnosis of hydrocephalus must be based on clinical features, not just ventricular size. Ultrasound is usually helpful in assessing the size of the lateral ventricles and monitoring changes over time in patients with persistent fontanelles. But CT and MRI provide better resolution, ensure a more complete examination, and may identify the cause.

Ultrasound of the brain can be performed through a persistent bregmatic (dorsal midline) fontanelle. In most cases, imaging can be performed without sedation or anesthesia. Optimal resolution is provided by a high-frequency probe (7–12 MHz). A useful landmark on transverse images is a hyperechoic umbrella-shaped structure formed by the longitudinal fissure on the midline and the splenial sulci (**Fig. 6**).[26] Normal-sized ventricles appear as paired, slitlike anechoic structures, just ventral to the longitudinal fissure, on either side of the midline. Enlarged ventricles are easily seen as paired anechoic regions. With marked ventricular enlargement, the septum pellucidum that normally separates the lateral ventricles is absent and the ventricles appear as a single, large anechoic structure.

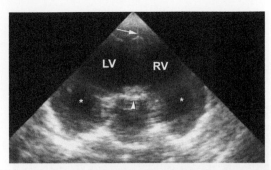

Fig. 6. Ultrasound of the brain performed by scanning through the bregmatic fontanelle. The longitudinal fissure on the midline and the splenial sulci form an umbrella-shaped structure (*arrow*). The left lateral ventricle (LV) and right lateral ventricle (RV) are enlarged. The enlarged temporal horns of the ventricles (*asterisks*) are also visible. A hyperechoic region corresponding to the choroid plexus of the third ventricle is evident (*arrowhead*).

CT and MRI enable accurate assessment of ventricular size, extent of cortical atrophy, and the presence of any focal lesions that may account for the hydrocephalus. Imaging is also useful in monitoring patients after surgical placement of ventriculoperitoneal shunts. Changes in ventricular size can be monitored and the presence of complications, such as subdural hematoma or hygroma can be evaluated. The site of obstruction causing the hydrocephalus may be identified by dilatation of CSF spaces proximal to the obstruction and normal or collapsed spaces distally. For example, obstruction at the level of the third ventricle would be expected to result in enlarged lateral ventricles but no enlargement of the mesencephalic aqueduct and fourth ventricle. Dilatation of all the ventricles and the subarachnoid space implies an obstruction at or near the arachnoid villi. Unfortunately, this simplistic approach has limited accuracy. For example, 25% to 35% of human patients with extraventricular obstructive hydrocephalus have little or no dilatation of the fourth ventricle.[27] Obstructing masses, such as tumors, granulomas, and cysts may be identified, especially on postcontrast images. MRI is more sensitive than CT in demonstrating small focal lesions, especially those in the caudal fossa.[27]

Periventricular edema may be identified in some patients with hydrocephalus. Experimentally, acute obstructive hydrocephalus in dogs causes edema starting at the dorsolateral angles of the lateral ventricles and spreading into the adjacent white matter.[28] On CT, this is evident as blurring or loss of the normally sharp ventricular margins.[27] The edema is best appreciated on T2-weighted MRI as increased intensity compared with normal white matter.[28] Heavily T2-weighted fluid-attenuated inversion recovery (FLAIR) sequences are useful in detecting subtle periventricular lesions (**Fig. 7**). Periventricular edema is most frequently associated with acute hydrocephalus and increased intraventricular pressure, rather than chronic, relatively compensated hydrocephalus with normal intraventricular pressure.[27]

Ventricular enlargement secondary to loss of brain parenchyma ("hydrocephalus ex vacuo") can be distinguished from obstructive hydrocephalus based on enlarged cortical sulci and subarachnoid space (**Fig. 8**). This can occur in older animals as a consequence of age-related brain atrophy or as a result of lesions that destroy brain parenchyma, such as infarcts or necrotizing encephalitis.

Analysis of CSF is helpful in cases of suspected meningoencephalitis. CT or MRI are performed first to identify any shifting of brain tissue, such as caudal cerebellar herniation, or other abnormalities that may increase the risk of CSF collection from the

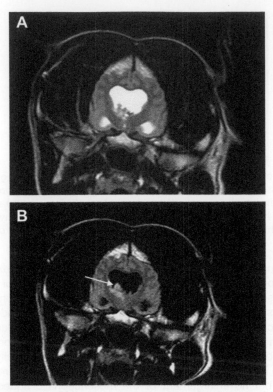

Fig. 7. Hydrocephalus associated with a choroids plexus tumor in the left lateral ventricle. (*A*) Transverse T2-weighted MRI. Both lateral ventricles are enlarged. (*B*) Transverse fluid attenuated inversion recovery (FLAIR) sequence. This sequence attenuates the CSF in the lateral ventricles and shows the small tumor (*arrow*) more clearly.

cerebellomedullary cistern. In some cases, it may be safer to collect CSF from an enlarged lateral ventricle through a persistent fontanelle.

Imaging techniques make it possible to readily identify ventriculomegaly but may give few clues as to its clinical significance. It is therefore necessary to interpret the finding of ventriculomegaly in context with clinical features.

MEDICAL TREATMENT

Medical therapy is used to delay surgery, to manage acute deterioration, and when surgery is not an option or not indicated. Acetazolamide, alone or in combination with furosemide, is the most commonly used drug therapy. Acetazolamide is a carbonic anhydrase inhibitor that decreases CSF production. The loop diuretic furosemide inhibits CSF formation to a lesser degree by partial inhibition of carbonic anhydrase.[29,30] Acetazolamide is started at 10 mg/kg orally every 8 hours. Furosemide is added at 1 mg/kg orally once daily. The dose is tapered based on clinical effect. Electrolytes and hydration are monitored. Although these drugs can provide temporary relief, diuretic therapy does not provide long-term benefit in human patients and is associated with potential side effects, such as electrolyte abnormalities.[29] Omeprazole decreases CSF production in normal dogs.[31] There are anecdotal reports of using

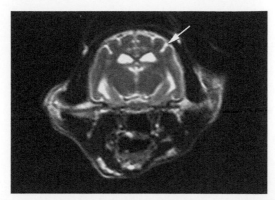

Fig. 8. Mild ventricular enlargement due to brain atrophy in a geriatric cat. The sulci (*arrow*) are more prominent because the subarachnoid space is enlarged and filled with hyperintense CSF secondary to atrophy of the cerebral cortex. Transverse T2-weighted MRI.

omeprazole to treat hydrocephalus, but the safety and efficacy have not been evaluated.

Glucocorticoids are commonly used to treat hydrocephalus in veterinary patients. Although some studies suggest steroids decrease CSF production, data are conflicting.[31] Nevertheless, affected animals often improve with steroid therapy, at least temporarily. One protocol is prednisone at 0.25 to 0.5 mg/kg twice daily until signs improve, then reduce the dose at weekly intervals until 0.1 mg/kg every other day.[11] Seizures are treated with antiseizure medication as needed.

CEREBROSPINAL FLUID SHUNTS

Definitive treatment of hydrocephalus is directed at the underlying cause if possible. Otherwise, the mainstay of treatment is insertion of a shunt that diverts CSF from the ventricles into another body cavity. Early reports in dogs described placing a shunt from the lateral ventricle to the right atrium of the heart.[32–34] Currently, ventriculoperitoneal shunts that divert CSF into the abdomen are most commonly used in veterinary and human patients.[17,35–39]

A number of shunt designs are available. All have three basic components: a ventricular catheter, a one-way valve, and a distal tube placed into the peritoneal cavity (**Fig. 9**). The shunt tubing is made of silicone elastomer material, usually impregnated with barium for radiographic visualization. Ventricular catheters are designed to be stiff enough to resist kinking and compliant enough to avoid brain injury.[40] Some systems use a single-piece design while others consist of a separate ventricular catheter and distal tube connected at the time of surgery. Some shunts include a CSF reservoir and access port that can be punctured with a needle percutaneously to sample CSF or inject contrast medium.

The majority of the valves are differential pressure valves designed to keep the intraventricular pressure from climbing too high or falling too low. They are defined by their opening and closing pressure. As the pressure differential across the valve climbs to the opening pressure threshold, the valve opens to allow egress of CSF at a flow rate determined by the resistance of the entire system. When the pressure falls below the closing pressure threshold, the valve closes, stopping the flow of CSF.[41] Most manufacturers provide differential pressure valves with various opening pressure ranges, such as very low (<1 cm H_2O), low (1–4 cm H_2O), medium (4–8 cm H_2O), and high

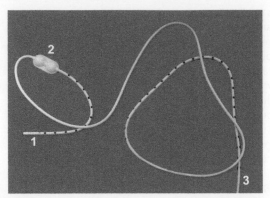

Fig. 9. Ventriculoperitoneal shunt. (1) Ventricular end with multiple small opening. (2) Access port and reservoir. (3) Distal end. The black dots are radiopaque markers at 1-cm intervals. (Uni-Shunt with Reservoir; Codman).

(>8 cm H_2O). However, the specific ranges are somewhat arbitrary and vary with the manufacturer. The most common design is a diaphragm valve, which involves the deflection of a silicone membrane in response to pressure to allow flow of CSF. Some shunts employ a slit valve, usually at the distal end.[40,41] These valves consist of one or more slits in the tubing that open and close based on the thickness and stiffness of the material.

Several manufacturers provide externally adjustable valves (programmable valves) that enable the clinician to adjust the opening pressure after the shunt is implanted using a device that emits a magnetic field. An advantage of this type of valve is that the function of the shunt can be adjusted noninvasively based on the individual patient's clinical response without the need for surgery to change the valve. Some externally adjustable valves employ a locking device to prevent the magnetic field associated with MRI from altering the setting. The lock is controlled by external pressure through the skin overlying the valve. Because these valves contain metal, they create an artifact in the MRI.[42] Another disadvantage is the additional cost of the shunt and the programming device, compared with nonadjustable valves.

Several other components have been employed to minimize the problem of overdrainage. Acute overdrainage occurs in patients with very large ventricles when the size of the ventricles is reduced too fast. This can cause the cerebral cortex to collapse, tearing blood vessels between the dura and the brain and causing a subdural accumulation of blood or fluid.[39] A chronic form of overdrainage is the slit-ventricle syndrome, which in human patients is associated with very small ventricles and chronic debilitating headaches. This may occur because a loss of intracranial pressure-volume compliance. A mechanism that helps maintain normal intracranial pressure with increases in intracranial volume is the displacement of CSF from the ventricles to the spinal subarachnoid space. If the volume of CSF within the ventricles becomes too small, there is a loss in the ability to compensate for transient changes in intracranial volume.[41]

Siphon regulatory devices are designed to prevent overdrainage due to siphoning. If two containers are filled with liquid and the containers are connected with a tube, the liquid will flow from the container with the higher fluid level into the container with the lower level until the levels are equal in the two containers. When the brain is above the level of the abdomen, this siphoning effect increases the pressure differential across the valve, keeping it open and allowing more CSF to flow from the ventricles.[43]

Siphoning is less of a problems in dogs and cats because the shunt is oriented more horizontal compared with human patients, who spend more time upright.[44] Flow-regulatory devices attempt to restrict the rate of flow to the rate of CSF production, regardless of patient position and other variables that affect drainage. This is accomplished by incorporating a resistance element that changes according to the differential pressure across the valve. The result is that the valve has no flow at low pressure differentials, a constant flow rate at intermediate pressures, and a very high flow rate at high pressures.[5] Although various shunt designs have theoretical advantages, a controlled trial in children with hydrocephalus compared a standard differential pressure valve, a valve with a siphon control component, and a valve with a flow regulatory component and found no difference in clinical outcome for any particular design.[45,46]

INDICATIONS FOR SURGERY

The decision to place a ventriculoperitoneal shunt is not always clear. There are no published clinical trials in veterinary patients evaluating the safety and efficacy of ventriculoperitoneal shunts. The presence of enlarged ventricles alone does not necessarily indicate the need for surgery. The key factor in the decision for surgery is the worsening of clinical signs that do not respond to medical therapy. Patients need to be treated before permanent neurologic deficits develop and before the patient becomes debilitated by the disease. The main contraindication for implantation of a ventriculoperitoneal shunt is systemic infection, abdominal infection, or skin infection at the site of the cranial or abdominal incision. Surgery is not indicated for patients in whom a successful surgery would not change the outcome, such as a patient with multiple, severe brain malformations. Patients with enlarged ventricles due to brain atrophy from, for example, age or brain necrosis, do not need shunting.

SURGICAL TECHNIQUE

Surgical technique is similar for all ventriculoperitoneal shunts, although details vary slightly based on the specific system. Aseptic technique and meticulous hemostasis are critical to minimize the chance of shunt infection and obstruction. The shunt should be kept in the package until ready to use. Care should be taken to avoid the shunt coming in contact with drapes, towels, or gauze.

Using preoperative brain imaging as a guide, the site of insertion of the ventricular catheter is chosen so that the catheter tip will be placed in the center of the occipital horn or frontal horn, caudal or rostral to the choroid plexus. The distance from the surface of the skull to the center of the ventricle is measured to determine the depth of insertion. The cranial incision is located 2 to 3 cm lateral to the nuchal crest. The abdominal incision is located 2 to 3 cm caudal to the last rib, about halfway between the lumbar spine and the ventral aspect of the abdomen. The patient is measured to determine the proper shunt length. Clinicians should plan on placing approximately one third to one half the shunt length into the abdomen. The author usually uses a medium- or high-pressure valve because (1) many dogs with congenital hydrocephalus have extremely large ventricles, which makes acute overdrainage with collapse of the cerebral mantle a potential risk, and (2) low-pressure valves often result in very small ventricles that increase the risk of obstruction as the ependyma and choroid plexus collapse around the ventricular catheter.[47]

The patient is clipped and prepped from the head to the side of the abdomen (**Fig. 10**). The patient is positioned in lateral recumbency with a small towel under the neck to straighten the path for the shunt as much as possible. Before draping the surgical field, the sites for the cranial and abdominal incisions are identified with

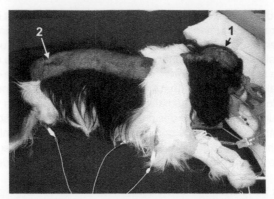

Fig. 10. Immediate postoperative view of a patient after placement of a ventriculoperitoneal shunt. The skin is clipped and prepared from the site of incision for placement of the ventricular catheter (1) to the site of incision for placement of the distal end into the peritoneal cavity (2).

a surgical marker. The skin and subcutaneous tissue are incised at the site of the abdominal incision. Any bleeding is controlled with bipolar cautery. For the cranial incision, the skin, subcutaneous tissue, and superficial muscles are incised. If necessary, the temporalis fascia is incised and the temporalis muscle elevated from the calvarium.

A subcutaneous tunnel is created connecting the two incisions. A shunt passer (eg, Shunt Passer; Codman) is helpful in creating this tunnel and pulling the shunt tubing from the cranial incision to the abdominal incision (**Fig. 11**). The shunt passer consists of a long, malleable tube containing a leader that attaches to the end of the shunt to pull the shunt through the tube. If necessary, the malleable tube is formed into the desired contour to follow the shunt path, taking care not to kink it. The tip of the shunt passer is inserted through the cranial incision and tunneled caudally though the subcutaneous tissues to the abdominal incision. Then the leader is attached to the distal end of the shunt and the shunt is pulled through the tube to the abdominal incision. The ventricular end of the catheter is held while the tube of the shunt passer is withdrawn through the abdominal incision. The distal end is placed into the sterile tray from the shunt package while the ventricular catheter is placed.

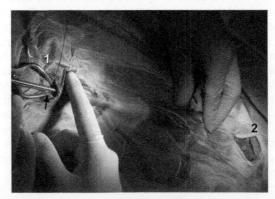

Fig. 11. Using a shunt passer (*arrow*) to create a subcutaneous tunnel between the skull incision (1) and the abdominal incision (2).

A burr hole slightly larger then the diameter of the catheter (and the anchoring clip, if used) is created in the skull. It is important that the burr hole is large enough to allow the ventricular catheter to pass freely without resistance. One or two smaller suture holes are drilled adjacent to the burr hole to anchor the shunt to the bone. Nonabsorbable suture (eg, 3-0 nylon) is preplaced through the suture holes. Do not use wire suture, which could damage the shunt tubing. The dura is incised and coagulated with bipolar cautery as needed for hemostasis. A 22-gauge spinal needle is inserted through the cerebral mantle into the ventricle to identify the depth and angle of insertion. CSF is then collected for analysis. Any bleeding from the pia is controlled with bipolar cautery. The ventricular catheter is passed through the cerebral mantle into the ventricle to the premeasured depth. If using a two-piece shunt, the ventricular catheter is attached to the distal catheter and the attachments secured with nonabsorbable sutures. Once CSF is observed flowing from the distal end, the ventricular catheter is anchored to the skull using sutures attached to catheter clips or in a finger-trap fashion around the catheter (**Fig. 12**). Securely anchoring the catheter to the skull is important to prevent dislodgement of the catheter.

The abdominal muscles and peritoneum are incised to allow the distal end of the shunt to be placed into the peritoneal cavity. With some shunts, excess tubing can be clipped off with scissors. However, if the shunt incorporates a slit valve in the distal catheter, the end cannot be removed. The shunt tubing is secured to the abdominal wall using nonabsorbable suture tied to the anchoring clip or tied in a finger-trap fashion to the tubing and the abdominal muscle apposed with absorbable suture. The subcutaneous and skin incisions are closed routinely. A postoperative radiograph is obtained to document adequate shunt placement (**Fig. 13**).

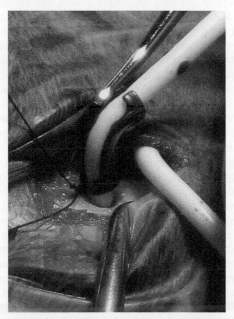

Fig. 12. Anchoring the ventricular catheter to the skull. Nonabsorbable suture (nylon) is passed through a small hole adjacent to the burr hole and tied to the anchoring clip. The clip is then placed into the burr hole and the suture tied.

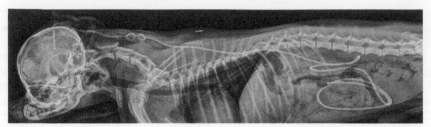

Fig. 13. Lateral view postoperative radiograph showing adequate placement of a ventriculoperitoneal shunt.

COMPLICATIONS

The most frequent complication is blockage of CSF flow through an intact shunt. The most common cause of obstruction are (1) blockage of the ventricular catheter as CSF flow pulls choroid plexus into the shunt and (2) blockage by glial tissue from astrocyte proliferation.[40,41] Other causes of obstruction include blood or proteinaceous debris occluding the valve, and scarring or adhesion around the distal tubing in the abdomen.[41] Obstruction can occur at any time after implantation and is accompanied by recurrence of signs of hydrocephalus. Shunt obstruction should be suspected in any patient that initially improves after surgery and then develops such neurologic signs as lethargy, ataxia, or abnormal behavior. An imaging finding of enlarged ventricles compared with a previous scan is a strong indication of obstruction. However, in some cases of obstruction, the ventricles are not obviously enlarged compared with the previous study.[48] In those patients, tapping the shunt can be helpful in the diagnosis of obstruction. The specific technique varies depending on shunt design. However, in general, the skin overlying the reservoir is clipped and aseptically prepped, and a 25-gauge needle is inserted percutaneously into the reservoir. The distal tubing is blocked by digital compression to determine if CSF can be collected from the ventricular catheter. If not, the ventricular catheter is obstructed. Another technique is to measure the pressure from the ventricular end of the catheter by connecting a manometer to the needle in the reservoir. A pressure reading higher than the opening pressure of the valve indicates obstruction. Finally, if necessary, a small amount of myelographic contrast agent or technetium pertechnetate can be injected into the reservoir to determine patency of the ventricular and distal catheter.[13] Obstruction requires surgery to replace the shunt.

Misplacement, migration, and disconnection are most common soon after implantation and are readily identified on radiographs (**Fig. 14**).[41] To properly place the ventricular catheter, the clinician must pay careful attention to the depth of insertion, based on preoperative imaging, and must ensure CSF flows from the distal end at surgery. Sharply incising the dura to create an opening large enough to freely pass the catheter through the cerebral mantle into the ventricle helps ensure the catheter does not simply push the cortex away from the skull. To ensure the distal end is placed into the abdomen and not into subcutaneous tissue, the clinician should make the abdominal incision large enough to allow visualization of the abdominal organs. Migration is prevented by securely anchoring the shunt at the skull and the abdomen. Infection usually occurs within the first few months of surgery and is manifested as wound infection, fever, or obstruction. Analysis of CSF collected percutaneously from the shunt reservoir is helpful in the diagnosis of shunt infection. Any of these complications usually require replacement of the shunt.

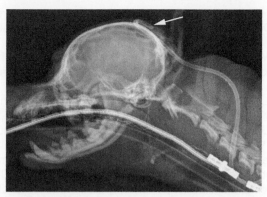

Fig. 14. Migration of the ventricular catheter. Because the catheter was not adequately secured to the skull, it subsequently migrated out of the ventricle and is visible in the subcutaneous tissue (*arrow*).

The overall failure rate in human patients is approximately 40% at 1 year after implantation and 50% at 2 years.[45,46] Similar data are not available for veterinary patients but anecdotally the rate of obstruction appears similar.[13] Shunt infection appears to be less common in dogs and cats compared with that in human patients. Although shunting is far from a perfect treatment, for many patients it is still the best option for definitive treatment. Neurologic deficits often improve soon after surgery. However, permanent deficits are possible if the cerebral cortex has been damaged.

REFERENCES

1. Rekate HL. A contemporary definition and classification of hydrocephalus. Semin Pediatr Neurol 2009;16(1):9–15.
2. De Lahunta A, Glass E. Veterinary neuroanatomy and clinical neurology. 3rd edition. Philadelphia: Saunders; 2009.
3. Becker SV, Selby LA. Canine hydrocephalus. Comp Cont Educ Pract Vet 1980; 11(8):647–52.
4. Rekate HL. Hydrocephalus in children. In: Winn HR, editor. Youmans neurological surgery. 5th edition. Philadelphia: Saunders; 2004. p. 3387–404.
5. Rekate HL. Recent advances in the understanding and treatment of hydrocephalus. Semin Pediatr Neurol 1997;4(3):167–78.
6. Levine DN. Intracranial pressure and ventricular expansion in hydrocephalus: have we been asking the wrong question? J Neurol Sci 2008;269(1–2):1–11.
7. Yamada H, Yokota A, Furuta A, et al. Reconstitution of shunted mantle in experimental hydrocephalus. J Neurosurg 1992;76(5):856–62.
8. Smith ZA, Moftakhar P, Malkasian D, et al. Choroid plexus hyperplasia: surgical treatment and immunohistochemical results. Case report. J Neurosurg 2007; 107(Suppl 3):255–62.
9. James AE, Burns B, Flor WF, et al. Pathophysiology of chronic communicating hydrocephalus in dogs (*Canis familiaris*). Experimental studies. J Neurol Sci 1975;24(2):151–78.
10. Selby LA, Hayes HM, Becker SV. Epizootiologic features of canine hydrocephalus. Am J Vet Res 1979;40(3):411–3.

11. Simpson ST. Hydrocephalus. In: Kirk RW, Bonagura JD, editors. Current veterinary therapy X small animal practice. Philadadelphia: WB Saunders; 1989. p. 842–7.
12. Baumgartner WK, Krakowka S, Koestner A, et al. Acute encephalitis and hydrocephalus in dogs caused by canine parainfluenza virus. Vet Pathol 1982;19(1): 79–92.
13. Harrington ML, Bagley RS, Moore MP. Hydrocephalus. Vet Clin North Am Small Anim Pract 1996;26(4):843–56.
14. Steinberg H, Galbreath EJ. Cerebellar medulloblastoma with multiple differentiation in a dog. Vet Pathol 1998;35(6):543–6.
15. Zabka TS, Lavely JA, Higgins RJ. Primary intra-axial leiomyosarcoma with obstructive hydrocephalus in a young dog. J Comp Pathol 2004;131(4):334–7.
16. Foley JE, Lapointe JM, Koblik P, et al. Diagnostic features of clinical neurologic feline infectious peritonitis. J Vet Intern Med 1998;12(6):415–23.
17. Dewey CW. External hydrocephalus in a dog with suspected bacterial meningoencephalitis. J Am Anim Hosp Assoc 2002;38(6):563–7.
18. Graham JC, O'Keefe DA, Wallig MA, et al. Lymphosarcoma causing acquired obstructive hydrocephalus in a dog. Can Vet J 1992;33(10):669–70.
19. Pumarola M, van Niel MH. Obstructive hydrocephalus produced by parasitic granulomas in a dog. Zentralbl Veterinarmed A 1992;39(5):392–5.
20. Vural SA, Besalti O, Ilhan F. Ventricular ependymoma in a German shepherd dog. Vet J 2006;172(1):185–7.
21. Hudson JA, Simpson ST, Buxton DF, et al. Ultrasonographic diagnosis of canine hydrocephalus. Vet Radiol Ultrasound 2005;31(2):50–8.
22. Spaulding KA, Sharp NJH. Ultrasonographic imaging of the lateral cerebral ventricles in the dog. Vet Radiol Ultrasound 1990;31(2):59–64.
23. Kii S, Uzuka Y, Taura Y, et al. Developmental change of lateral ventricular volume and ratio in beagle-type dogs up to 7 months of age. Vet Radiol Ultrasound 1998; 39(3):185–9.
24. Vullo T, Korenman E, Manzo RP, et al. Diagnosis of cerebral ventriculomegaly in normal adult beagles using quantitative MRI. Vet Radiol Ultrasound 1997;38(4): 277–81.
25. De Hann CE, Kraft SL, Gavin PR, et al. Normal variation in size of the lateral ventricles of the Labrador retriever dog as assessed by magnetic resonance imaging. Vet Radiol Ultrasound 1994;35(2):83–6.
26. Hudson JA, Finn-Bodner ST, Steiss JE. Neurosonography. Vet Clin North Am Small Anim Pract 1998;28(4):943–72.
27. Naidich TP, Schott LH, Baron RL. Computed tomography in evaluation of hydrocephalus. Radiol Clin North Am 1982;20(1):143–67.
28. Drake JM, Potts DG, Lemaire C. Magnetic resonance imaging of silastic-induced canine hydrocephalus. Surg Neurol 1989;31(1):28–40.
29. Melby JM, Miner LC, Reed DJ. Effect of acetazolamide and furosemide on the production and composition of cerebrospinal fluid from the cat choroid plexus. Can J Physiol Pharmacol 1982;60(3):405–9.
30. Vogh BP, Langham MR Jr. The effect of furosemide and bumetanide on cerebrospinal fluid formation. Brain Res 1981;221(1):171–83.
31. Javaheri S, Corbett WS, Simbartl LA, et al. Different effects of omeprazole and Sch 28080 on canine cerebrospinal fluid production. Brain Res 1997;754(1–2): 321–4.
32. Few AB. The diagnosis and surgical treatment of canine hydrocephalus. J Am Vet Med Assoc 1966;149(3):286–93.

33. Gage ED, Hoerlein BF. Surgical treatment of canine hydrocephalus by verticuloa-trial shunting. J Am Vet Med Assoc 1968;153(11):1418–31.
34. Gage ED. Surgical treatment of canine hydrocephalus. J Am Vet Med Assoc 1970;157(11):1729–40.
35. Kim H, Itamoto K, Watanabe M, et al. Application of ventriculoperitoneal shunt as a treatment for hydrocephalus in a dog with syringomyelia and Chiari I malformation. J Vet Sci 2006;7(2):203–6.
36. Kay ND, Holliday TA, Hornof WJ, et al. Diagnosis and management of an atypical case of canine hydrocephalus, using computed tomography, ventriculoperitoneal shunting, and nuclear scintigraphy. J Am Vet Med Assoc 1986;188(4):423–6.
37. Dewey CW, Coates JR, Ducote JM, et al. External hydrocephalus in two cats. J Am Anim Hosp Assoc 2003;39(6):567–72.
38. Hasegawa T, Taura Y, Kido H, et al. Surgical management of combined hydrocephalus, syringohydromyelia, and ventricular cyst in a dog. J Am Anim Hosp Assoc 2005;41(4):267–72.
39. Kitagawa M, Kanayama K, Sakai T. Subdural accumulation of fluid in a dog after the insertion of a ventriculoperitoneal shunt. Vet Rec 2005;156(7):206–8.
40. Ginsberg HJ, Drake JM. physiology of cerebrospinal fluid shunt devices. In: Winn HR, editor. Youmans neurological surgery. 5th edition. Philadelphia: Saunders; 2004. p. 3374–85.
41. Kestle JR. Pediatric hydrocephalus: current management. Neurol Clin 2003; 21(4):883–95.
42. Shellock FG, Habibi R, Knebel J. Programmable CSF shunt valve: in vitro assessment of MR imaging safety at 3T. AJNR Am J Neuroradiol 2006;27(3):661–5.
43. Kurtom KH, Magram G. Siphon regulatory devices; their role in the treatment of hydrocephalus. Neurosurg Focus 2007;22(4):1–9.
44. Yamada S, Ducker TB, Perot PL. Dynamic changes of cerebrospinal fluid in upright and recumbent shunted experimental animals. Childs Brain 1975;1: 187–92.
45. Drake JM, Kestle JR, Milner R, et al. Randomized trial of cerebrospinal fluid shunt valve design in pediatric hydrocephalus. Neurosurgery 1998;43(2):294–303.
46. Kestle J, Drake J, Milner R, et al. Long-term follow-up data from the shunt design trial. Pediatr Neurosurg 2000;33(5):230–6.
47. Robinson S, Kaufman BA, Park TS. Outcome analysis of initial neonatal shunts: does the valve make a difference? Pediatr Neurosurg 2002;37(6):287–94.
48. Watkins L, Hayward R, Andar U, et al. The diagnosis of blocked cerebrospinal fluid shunts: a prospective study of referral to a paediatric neurosurgical unit. Childs Nerv Syst 1994;10(2):87–90.

Idiopathic Epilepsy in Dogs and Cats

William B. Thomas, DVM, MS

KEYWORDS

• Seizures • Phenobarbital • Bromide • Treatment

Epilepsy is a group of heterogeneous conditions that share a common feature—chronic, recurring seizures. The terms epilepsy and seizures are not synonymous. A seizure is the clinical manifestation of abnormal electrical activity in the brain.[1] It is a specific event in time. Epilepsy refers to multiple seizures occurring over a long period of time. Although there is no universal agreement on the minimum number of seizures or period of time, a useful clinical definition is two or more seizures over a month or more. Not all seizures are associated with epilepsy. For example, a seizure can be the reaction of a normal brain to a transient insult, such as intoxication or metabolic disorder. This is called a provoked seizure or reactive seizure.[1,2] If seizures stop when the underlying condition resolves, the patient does not have epilepsy, because the condition is not chronic. On the other hand, if a patient has several seizures over a period of a month or more, and there is no detectable short-term illness responsible for the seizures, then we would say the patient has the condition called epilepsy.

Because there are many causes of chronic recurrent seizures, epilepsy is not a specific disease but rather a diverse category of disorders. Epilepsy is broadly divided into idiopathic and symptomatic disorders. Symptomatic epilepsy, also called secondary epilepsy, is when the seizures are caused by an identifiable structural lesion of the brain, such as a tumor.[1,3] Idiopathic epilepsy, also called primary epilepsy, is chronic recurring seizures with no underlying structural brain lesion or other neurological signs.[1,3] Here, the term "idiopathic" means a disorder "by itself" not "cause unknown." The term idiopathic epilepsy is not applied simply to any patient in whom the cause of the seizures is unknown. Instead, it refers to recognized clinical syndromes with typical clinical features, such as age of onset and lack of other neurological abnormalities. The term "essential" is often used to convey the same meaning, as in essential hypertension.

Several other terms are commonly used. The ictus is the seizure itself. Postictal signs are transient clinical abnormalities in brain function that are caused by the ictus and appear when the ictus has ended. Postictal signs typically last a few minutes to hours and can include confusion, blindness, ataxia, and deep sleep.[4–6] In most cases,

Department of Small Animal Clinical Sciences, College of Veterinary Medicine, University of Tennessee, 2407 River Drive, Knoxville, TN 37996-4544, USA
E-mail address: wthomas@utk.edu

Vet Clin Small Anim 40 (2010) 161–179
doi:10.1016/j.cvsm.2009.09.004
0195-5616/09/$ – see front matter © 2010 Elsevier Inc. All rights reserved.

the ictus lasts only a few minutes. Some patients with seizures experience a prodrome, which is long-lasting abnormality occurring hours to days before a before a seizure, such as restlessness or anxiety.[4,5,7,8] An aura is a subjective sensation at the start of a seizure before there are observable signs.[4,9] The difference between a prodrome and an aura is that prodromes are longer lasting and not associated with abnormal electrical activity in the brain. Human patients describe various sensations during their auras, including dizziness, tingling, and anxiety.[9] Common manifestations of auras in animals are hiding, seeking the owner, agitation, or vomiting just before a seizure.[4] In other cases an aura occurs alone, which constitutes a sensory seizure.

DESCRIPTIONS OF SEIZURES

Several classification systems have been developed for human epileptic seizures based on clinical signs, etiology, and electroencephalographic (EEG) information. Applying these schemes to veterinary patients is problematic because not all seizure types in human patients are recognized in animals and EEG data are usually not available for our patients. Therefore, the following descriptive list is offered not as a formal classification but to facilitate communication among clinicians.

Generalized-onset Seizures

Generalized-onset seizures are those in which the first clinical signs indicate initial involvement of both cerebral hemispheres. Consciousness may be impaired and motor manifestations are bilateral. The most common type of generalized seizure is a generalized tonic-clonic seizure (formerly called grand mal seizures). The first part of the seizure is the tonic phase, during which there is sustained contraction of all muscles. The animal typically loses consciousness and falls to its side in opisthotonus with the limbs extended. Respirations are often irregular or absent and cyanosis is common. Autonomic signs such as salivation, urination, and defecation are common. The tonic phase lasts for a minute or so and then gives way to the clonic phase, during which there is rhythmic contraction of muscles, manifested as paddling or jerking of the limbs and chewing movements. Some animals suffer milder generalized tonic-clonic seizures in which consciousness is maintained.[7,8]

Another type of generalized seizure is a *tonic* seizure, in which motor activity consists only of generalized muscle rigidity without a clonic phase.[7,8] Less common are *clonic* seizures, in which there is no tonic component; *atonic* seizures, which consist of a sudden, often brief loss of postural tone causing the patient to fall or drop it's head; and *myoclonic* seizures, characterized by brief, shocklike contractions that may be generalized or confined to individual muscle groups.[10] There are other causes of myoclonic jerks in animals; that is, not all myoclonic jerks are seizures.

Focal-onset Seizures

Focal-onset seizures are those in which the initial clinical signs indicate abnormal activity in one region of a cerebral hemisphere. Focal motor seizures consist of abnormal movements of a body part, such as turning the head to one side, rhythmic contractions of a limb or facial muscles, or chewing movement.[4,7] Focal sensory seizures cause abnormal sensations such as tingling, pain, or visual hallucinations. An aura that does not evolve into loss of consciousness is a focal sensory seizure. Because the sensations are subjective, it can be difficult to recognize sensory seizures in animals, but "fly-biting" seizures may be a form of sensory seizures with visual hallucinations.[11] Focal autonomic seizures cause predominately autonomic signs, such as vomiting, diarrhea, and apparent abdominal pain.[12] A syndrome characterized by drooling, retching, dysphagia, and painful enlargement of the mandibular salivary glands is likely a form of focal autonomic seizures.[13,14] Complex focal seizures (formerly called psychomotor seizures) are focal seizures with alterations of awareness. Affected patients may not respond to their owner and often engage in automatisms, which are coordinated, repetitive motor activities such as head pressing, vocalizing, or aimless walking or running.[4] Some complex focal seizures are manifested as impaired consciousness and bizarre behavior, such as unprovoked aggression or extreme, irrational fear.[15,16] A secondarily generalized seizure usually begins with a focal seizure that evolves into a generalized tonic-clonic seizure. The secondary spread can occur so rapidly that the initial focal component is missed and the seizure is misclassified as a generalized-onset seizure. But with close observation, including videotape review of the seizures, it is apparent that secondarily generalized seizures are common in dogs and cats.[4,7,8]

CLINICAL FEATURES OF IDIOPATHIC EPILEPSY

Most dogs with idiopathic epilepsy suffer their first seizure between 1 and 5 years of age, although seizures occasionally start before 6 months or as late as 10 years of age.[2,4,7,8] Any breed, including mix-breed dogs can be affected. Based on pedigree analysis, a genetic basis for idiopathic epilepsy is suspected in a number of breeds, including the beagle, Belgian tervuren, Keeshond, dachshund, British Alsation, Labrador retriever, golden retriever, Shetland sheepdog, Irish wolfhound, Vizsla, Bernese mountain dog, and English springer spaniel.[5,17–26] Genetic factors are likely in other affected breeds as well, even though genetic studies have not been published.

In the past, generalized tonic-clonic seizures were considered the most common type of seizure in dogs with idiopathic epilepsy, and some authors even claimed focal-onset seizures were inconstant with a diagnosis of idiopathic epilepsy. However, more recent observations reveal this is clearly not the case and dogs with idiopathic epilepsy can have a variety of focal-onset seizures, including secondarily generalized seizures, and some individuals have more than one type of seizure.[5–8,25] The frequency of seizures varies tremendously, ranging from several a day to less than one a year.[2,7] Seizures are most common during rest or sleep.[6] Even though most seizures appear to occur spontaneously, they may be precipitated by a variety of factors. In human patients, sleep deprivation, emotional stress, menstruation, missed medication, and concurrent illness are recognized.[27] Similar factors are likely important in precipitating seizures in some animals.

Reflex seizures are seizures that can be provoked by specific stimuli or events.[28] The most common trigger in people is flickering light, usually from a television. Other triggers include immersion in hot water, reading, certain sounds, and eating. With reflex seizures, the trigger is specific and the latency between the trigger and seizure is short (seconds to minutes).[28] I have evaluated several dogs that suffered seizures consistently associated with sounds (lawnmower engine), automobile rides, or veterinary offices.

Idiopathic epilepsy is much less common in cats, compared to dogs, so we have less data for feline epilepsy. A genetic basis for seizures has not been documented in cats and feline epilepsy is more likely to be symptomatic than idiopathic, compared to dogs. However, idiopathic epilepsy does occur in cats. In one study, most cats with idiopathic epilepsy had their first seizure between about 1 and 5 years of age.[29]

DIAGNOSTIC EVALUATION

A detailed and accurate history is the foundation of diagnosis. The client's description of the seizures, their frequency and duration, and the patient's behavior between seizures are recorded. Ask about any focal signs at the start of the seizure, such as turning the head to one side or jerking of one limb. Any abnormalities before and after the seizure should be characterized. It is also important to determine if the events occur at a certain time of day or in association with situations such as feeding or exercise. Because the clinician may never see the seizure, the client's observations are extremely important. In some cases it helps if the client videotapes the episodes.

Ask about familial history of seizures, significant injuries or illnesses, vaccination status, diet, and potential exposure to toxins. Ask about any prescription or nonprescription medications. Any interictal abnormalities are noted, such as changes in behavior, gait, appetite, weight, or sleep habits. The client is often the best person to identify subtle changes in personality or behaviors that are not readily apparent to the clinician in the examination room. Finally, it is essential that the veterinarian understand the client's lifestyle and relationship with his or her pet. The prognosis for epilepsy depends greatly on the level of care the client is willing and able to provide and the impact of their pet's illness on the family.

A thorough physical examination is important to detect signs of systemic illness that might suggest an underlying cause for the seizures. Perform a complete neurological examination to detect any persistent neurological deficits. Cerebral lesions often cause focal, relatively subtle deficits such as delayed proprioceptive positioning on one side or blindness in one visual field. Be careful when interpreting the examination shortly after a seizure because any generalized deficits, such as ataxia, depression, or blindness may be a result of postictal disturbances and not necessarily indicate underlying brain disease. Repeating the examination in 24 to 48 hours may be necessary to determine if any deficits persist.

A complete blood count and serum chemistry profile are indicated in any animal with one or more seizures. Blood lead determination is performed in patients with possible exposure to lead, patients from areas with a high incidence of lead poisoning, and in animals younger than 1 year of age. Serum bile acids are helpful in young animals to identify or rule out a porto-systemic shunt.

The diagnostic evaluation is designed to answer two questions: (1) is the patient having seizures, and (2) if so, what is the cause of the seizures. Seizures are recognized by their spontaneous onset, stereotypic signs, self-limiting time course, and postictal signs. Disorders that can be mistaken for seizures are listed in **Table 1**.

Idiopathic epilepsy is a clinical diagnosis based on the typical age of onset, lack of interictal abnormalities, and exclusion of other causes. Symptomatic epilepsy should be suspected when (1) seizures start before 1 or after 5 years of age, (2) the patient suffers focal seizures, (3) there is a sudden onset of multiple seizures, or (4) there are interictal abnormalities detected on history, examination, or laboratory tests.[2]

Brain imaging (computed tomography or magnetic resonance imaging) and cerebrospinal fluid (CSF) analysis are indicated in patients with interictal neurologic deficits, focal seizures, seizures refractory to drug therapy, an onset of seizures at younger than 1 or older than 5 years of age, and any cat with recurring seizures. Brain imaging and CSF analysis are also appropriate when the client wants to be reassured there is not a progressive brain lesion responsible for their pet's seizures. Many clients feel that the cost of brain imaging is worthwhile even when the results are normal because it helps the client understand the cause of his or her pet's seizures.[30] Imaging is ideally performed first and based on those results, CSF can be collected during the

Table 1
Disorders that can be mistaken for seizures

Disorder	Timing of Episode	Description	Other Findings
Syncope	Exercise, excitement, or cough	Brief collapse with loss of consciousness, no or only mild abnormal movements, no postictal abnormalities	Evidence of heart disease, arrhythmia
Cataplexy/narcolepsy	Excitement such as play or food	Brief collapse with absent muscle tone	Induce attack with food
Neck pain	Movement or activity	Crying, cervical rigidity and tremor, no loss of consciousness	Pain on neck palpation/manipulation
Vestibular dysfunction	Variable	Ataxia, abnormal nystagmus, disorientation, no loss of consciousness	Positional nystagmus or other signs of vestibular disease
Metabolic encephalopathy	May be post prandial	Abnormal behavior, depression, ataxia usually lasting an hour or more	Elevated bile acids or other laboratory abnormalities
Idiopathic head tremor	Spontaneous	Head tremor with no loss of consciousness, otherwise normal gait and behavior, lasting several minutes	Most common in English bulldogs, Doberman pinschers, boxers, and Labrador retrievers
Generalized tremor syndromes	Spontaneous	Generalized tremor with no loss of consciousness or autonomic signs	Steroid-responsive tremor syndrome is most common in young, small-breed dogs; history of exposure to mycotoxin (moldy dairy products), metaldehyde, or insecticide
Exercise-induced weakness	Exercise	Short-strided gait, kyphosis, tremor, collapse, no loss of consciousness	Induced attack with exercise
Compulsive disorders, sterotypy	Situations of anxiety, conflict, or frustration	Pacing, circling/spinning, rhythmic barking, chasing real or imaginary objects, licking, chewing, hair pulling, no loss of consciousness	Detailed behavior history may identify triggering situations
Feline estrus behavior	Associated with estrus	Howling, rolling, treading with pelvic limbs, lordosis	Intact female
Myoclonus	Episodic or continuous	Sudden, shocklike contraction of a single muscle or muscle group, may be rhythmic	May persist with sleep or anesthesia

same anesthetic episode. If CSF is abnormal, titers for infectious causes of encephalitis are in order.

GENERAL PRINCIPLES OF DRUG THERAPY

The ideal goal of treatment is to completely eliminate seizures and avoid side effects. But total freedom from seizures and side effects remains elusive for many patients so a more realistic goal is to reduce the frequency and severity of the seizures to a level that does not substantially compromise the quality of life for the pet and family while avoiding serious side effects. Achieving this goal requires the clinician to make decisions regarding when to initiate therapy, how to promote compliance, choose appropriate drugs and doses, monitor treatment, and terminate therapy.

When to Start Treatment

Patients with a single seizure, provoked seizures, or isolated seizures separated by long periods of time generally do not require daily maintenance therapy. Treatment is indicated for patients with frequent seizures, a trend toward increasing frequency or severity of seizures, any episode of unprovoked status epilepticus or clusters, or an underlying, progressive disorder responsible for the seizures. Whether early treatment of idiopathic epilepsy alters the prognosis is unknown; however, one study suggests that dogs treated early in the course of epilepsy have better long-term control of their seizures compared to dogs that are allowed to have a lot of seizures before treatment is started.[7]

Before starting therapy, the client must believe treatment is in their pet's best interest and must understand the necessary commitment of time, money, and emotional dedication. If the client is not fully committed to the prescribed treatment, a good outcome is unlikely. The client and veterinarian should thoroughly discuss these factors and decide together when and if treatment should be initiated, weighing the risks and benefits of treatment versus no treatment.

Client Education

The key to successful treatment of epilepsy is client compliance. And the best way to promote compliance is good client education. Clients should be fully informed about the nature of the disease and its treatment. They should understand the goals of therapy and potential side effects. Mild side effects are common when first starting treatment with antiseizure drugs. These will often resolve or diminish after a few weeks of treatment. If clients understand this, they are less likely to become alarmed and prematurely stop treatment if they notice side effects.

Clients must appreciate the need for regular administration of medication. They need to know what to do if a dose is missed (in general, the missed dose is given as soon as the mistake is recognized, then the next dose is given on schedule). Maintaining an adequate supply of medication is important and clients should know how to obtain refills if medication is lost or runs out during travel. Suddenly stopping antiseizure medication may precipitate seizures and should be avoided at all costs. Having clients keep a log of the date and characteristics of each seizure and any side effects is very helpful in assessing therapy. Finally, clients must not alter treatment without the advice of the veterinarian. Some clients are tempted to alter the dose based on a short-term assessment of seizure control or side effects, but frequent dose changes are detrimental and make interpretation of therapeutic monitoring difficult.

Choice of Drug

The choice of treatment depends on efficacy, safety, and price. Based on clinical experience and pharmacokinetic information, phenobarbital or bromide is the initial drug of choice for dogs with idiopathic epilepsy. They are both relatively safe, effective, and inexpensive and most veterinarians are familiar with their use. The most significant disadvantages are the side effects: sedation, ataxia, polyuria/polydipsia, and polyphagia. Levetiracetam or zonisamide is a good choice for initial therapy when the client wants to minimize side effects. Primidone is also effective but is less commonly used because of concerns it may be more likely to cause liver disease, compared to phenobarbital, although this is not well documented.[31,32] Because of their short durations of effect in dogs, phenytoin, valproic acid, and benzodiazepines are less suitable as single agents for the control of canine epilepsy.[33,34] In cats, phenobarbital is the initial drug of choice.

It is better to use a single drug rather than a combination of drugs for initial therapy. Disadvantages of using multiple agents include increased cost, the need to monitor and interpret serum concentrations of multiple drugs, potential drug interactions, and more complicated dosing schedules. Nonetheless, some patients do better on a combination of drugs than on a single agent. If the first drug is ineffective because of poor seizure control or side effects, then a second drug is added. If seizures become well controlled, the first drug is tapered. If this is unsuccessful, a combination of drugs may provide optimal control.

Dose

Because of the variability in absorption, distribution, and speed of metabolism among patients, published dose recommendations serve as a general guide only. Because of sensitivity to side effects and lack of prior metabolic induction, most new patients are started at the lower end of the dose range. If necessary, the dose is slowly titrated upward until seizures are controlled or the maximum tolerated dose is reached. On the other hand, patients with frequent or severe seizures are often best managed by starting at the higher end of the dose range or using a loading dose. Once the seizures are controlled, the dose may need to be adjusted downward to minimize side effects.

Pharmacokinetic Considerations

When a drug is introduced at a constant daily dose, serum concentrations will initially be low, the amount eliminated per day will be smaller than the daily dose, and drug concentrations will increase. As concentration increases, so does elimination until it equals the daily maintenance dose (steady state). The time to reach steady state depends on the elimination half-life of the particular drug; 87% of steady-state concentrations occur at three half-lives and 97% occur at five half-lives.[34] In the case of drugs that are eliminated slowly, the time to reach steady state may be several weeks (phenobarbital) or months (bromide). When adequate serum concentrations are needed sooner, a loading dose can be administered. Simplistically, the loading dose is the sum of all the daily doses that would have been administered before steady state, minus the amount of drug that would have been eliminated during this period.[34] The major limitation of a loading dose is there is no time for tolerance to the sedative side effects to occur, so side effects are more common compared with gradual increases in drug concentrations.[34]

The pharmacokinetics of certain drugs may change over time. For example, chronic administration of phenobarbital is associated with hepatic enzyme induction that decreases elimination half-life.[35,36] Because of this autoinduction, many patients may eventually require a dose that is much higher than the starting dose.

Monitoring Therapy

Any drug used should be given an adequate chance to work and should not be discarded prematurely. Commonly used antiseizure drugs often must be administered for several weeks or longer before obtaining maximum antiseizure effects. Furthermore, it may take several months or more to adequately evaluate seizure control in a patient that has seizures separated by long periods of time. A common cause of poor seizure control is failure to maximize the dose before discarding a particular drug. This may lead to the need to backtrack at a later date for a second, more aggressive trial. This can be difficult, however, because once a client is convinced a particular drug is ineffective, the client is often reluctant to agree to a second trial.

Therapeutic monitoring of serum drug concentrations can be helpful in determining the optimal dose.[33,34,37] Therapeutic monitoring is indicated in several situations:

(1) When steady-state is reached after starting treatment, changing dose, or immediately after a loading dose. This provides a baseline to guide further changes in dose according to clinical circumstances.
(2) When seizures are not controlled despite an apparently adequate dose. This helps determine the need for dose adjustment before a second drug is added.
(3) When signs of dose-related toxicity occur.
(4) Every 6 to 12 months to verify that changes in pharmacokinetics have not caused blood concentrations to drift out of the intended range.

In most cases, a single trough level collected just before a dose is sufficient. If the dosing interval is more than 33% of the drug half-life, collection of a peak level (4–5 hours after a dose) along with a trough level helps document the proximity of drug levels to the toxic and subtherapeutic concentrations.[34] Peak and trough levels also allow estimation of half-life so that dosing interval can be modified if necessary.[34] Fasted samples are preferred because lipemia may interfere with some laboratory measurements. Serum separator tubes should not be used because the silicone may bind the drug, resulting in artificially low measurements.[38]

Published therapeutic or target ranges are only an approximation, as they are based on retrospective data from a small number of patients. Although most responders attain levels within the expected range, some do well below the lower limit whereas others obtain benefit at levels above the upper limit without toxicity. Patients are "treated" when the seizures are controlled and "toxic" when they suffer dose-related side effects, regardless of what is printed on the laboratory report, so results are always interpreted with consideration of seizure control and side effects.

Stopping Therapy

The decision to stop therapy must be made as carefully as the decision to start. Most human patients who are seizure-free for 2 or more years with drug therapy remain so when medication is withdrawn.[39] Those with the highest probability of remaining seizure-free are those who had a short duration of epilepsy and few seizures before control and those with no structural brain lesions.[39] Unfortunately, lack of information on recurrence risks in animals makes it impossible to predict which veterinary patients can be successfully weaned off medication. Nevertheless, given the potential adverse effects of long-term drug therapy, attempted withdrawal of medication is reasonable in animals that are seizure-free for 1 to 2 years. The dose is gradually tapered over a period of about 6 months. The major risk of discontinuing drug therapy is seizure recurrence, which is most likely during withdrawal or within several months of stopping therapy. If seizures recur, retreatment usually regains seizure control.

ANTISEIZURE DRUGS
Phenobarbital

Phenobarbital prolongs opening of the chloride channel at the $GABA_A$ receptor.[40] Phenobarbital is effective in 60% to 80% of dogs with idiopathic epilepsy if serum concentrations are maintained within the target range.[32,33,37] Many clients are willing to maintain epileptic dogs on phenobarbital therapy for a long period of time and feel their pet still has a high quality of life.[41] The initial dose is 2 to 3 mg/kg every 12 hours, but autoinduction usually necessitates subsequent increases in dose to maintain a trough serum concentration of 20 to 35 μg/mL. In some patients, autoinduction may eventually shorten the half-life to 36 hours or less and an 8-hour dosing interval is indicated to minimize fluctuation of serum levels.[34] Measurement of both a peak and trough level allows estimation of half-life and is helpful in determining the need for more frequent dosing.[34]

The main limitation of phenobarbital is its propensity to cause sedation. This is most prominent during the first few weeks after starting therapy or increasing the dose. Hyperexcitability and restlessness can occur, especially during the first few weeks of therapy. Polyuria, polydipsia, and polyphagia are the most common long-term side effects. The most common laboratory changes are mild to moderate elevations of serum alkaline phosphatase and other hepatic enzymes. These changes do not necessarily indicate clinically significant liver disease. Serious liver toxicity is less common and may be more likely with serum concentrations above 35 μg/mL.[42] Clinical signs of hepatotoxicity include anorexia, sedation, ataxia, icterus, and ascites. Laboratory evidence includes proportionally larger increases of alanine transaminase activity compared to alkaline phosphatase activity, elevations in bile acids, and an increase in serum phenobarbital concentrations despite no increase in dose.[42] Monitoring serum bile acids every 6 months should be considered to screen for liver disease in dogs on long-term phenobarbital therapy. Hepatotoxicity may be reversible if it is detected early and the phenobarbital is withdrawn. However, this adverse effect can be irreversible and ultimately fatal.[42] Polytherapy with phenobarbital and other potentially hepatotoxic drugs, such as phenytoin and primidone, may increase the risk of hepatotoxicity and should be avoided if possible.[42] Hematologic abnormalities, including neutropenia, anemia, and thrombocytopenia are rare adverse effects and may represent an idiosyncratic reaction rather than a dose-related effect.[43] These changes are reversible with withdrawal of the drug.

Cats tolerate phenobarbital well, although sedation, polyuria, polydipsia, and polyphagia are possible. The risk of hepatotoxicity seems to be minimal in cats and liver enzyme induction is much less prominent than in dogs.[44] Dosing and therapeutic monitoring are similar to those for dogs.

Bromide

Bromide is effective as initial therapy in dogs and as add-on therapy when phenobarbital does not provide adequate seizure control.[45,46] Bromide is freely filtered by the glomerulus and reabsorbed by the kidneys in competition with chloride. Because of this extensive reabsorption, the elimination half-life in dogs is slow, 21 to 24 days, and steady-state concentrations are achieved at 2.5 to 3.0 months.

Bromide is usually administered as potassium bromide or sodium bromide in solution, capsules, or tablets. Small dose adjustments are easier when using the liquid.

There is no difference in efficacy for the potassium or sodium salt, although potassium bromide is preferred when sodium intake must be restricted (for example, congestive heart failure). Sodium bromide is preferred when potassium intake must be restricted (for example, hypoadrenocorticism).[47]

The starting dose for potassium bromide is 20 to 30 mg/kg, once daily, with food. If sodium bromide is used, the dose should be decreased by 15% (ie, 17–26 mg/kg) to account for the higher bromide content of the sodium salt.[48] The dose is subsequently adjusted based on clinical effects and therapeutic monitoring. The target range of bromide is approximately 1 to 2 mg/mL when used concurrently with phenobarbital and 1 to 3 mg/mL when used as monotherapy.[45,46] I generally measure concentrations at 1 month and 3 months after starting maintenance therapy; concentrations at 1 month will be approximately 50% the level at steady-state. The timing of the sample is not critical because bromide levels do not fluctuate much throughout the day.

A loading dose may be used to obtain target serum concentrations sooner, for example in patients with frequent seizures or when phenobarbital must be rapidly withdrawn because of adverse effects. There are several protocols, but I administer 400 mg/kg divided into 8 doses given over a 48-hour period; that is, 50 mg/kg every 6 hours for 2 days. Administering the entire loading dose at once will usually cause vomiting. After the loading dose is completed, maintenance dosing is started. A sample for monitoring is obtained immediately after the loading to assess results of loading and then at 1 month to evaluate the maintenance dose.

When bromide is added to phenobarbital to improve seizure control, the current phenobarbital dose is continued while maintenance dosing of bromide is started. After 3 months, if seizures are well controlled and the serum concentration of bromide is at least 1.5 mg/mL, it may be possible to taper the phenobarbital, decreasing the dose in 25% increments every 2 to 4 weeks. If seizures become more frequent as the phenobarbital is withdrawn, the patient may require polytherapy with both drugs. A similar approach is used when converting to bromide because of adverse effects from phenobarbital. However, if phenobarbital must be withdrawn quickly, a loading of bromide is administered and the phenobarbital is tapered over a 2-week period while maintenance doses of bromide are administered.

Because bromide competes with chloride for renal elimination, high chloride intake increases bromide elimination, which increases the dose requirement.[49] Thus, the diet should not be changed during treatment. In dogs being fed high-chloride diets, such as some prescription diets, serum bromide concentrations should be monitored carefully.[49] Renal insufficiency decreases bromide elimination, so in dogs with persistent isosthenuria or azotemia, the initial dose of bromide should be halved and serum bromide concentrations monitored closely to avoid toxicity.[48]

Side effects of bromide include sedation, ataxia, weakness, polyuria, polydipsia, and polyphagia.[45] Less common are limb stiffness that can mimic orthopedic disease, irritability, restlessness, pruritic skin rash, and persistent cough.[50] Vomiting can occur, probably because of the direct gastric irritation by the hypertonic bromide salt. Administering the drug with food, dividing the daily dose into two or more doses, and the use of sodium bromide instead of potassium bromide are helpful in preventing vomiting.[34,48] Clinical experience and several laboratory studies suggest bromide alone or in combination with phenobarbital may increase the risk of pancreatitis.[51–53] Many laboratory assays cannot distinguish between chloride and bromide, so bromide therapy may artifactually increase serum chloride measurements.

Bromide toxicity (bromism) can develop at doses or serum concentrations near or above the upper end of the recommended ranges and is more common with inadequate therapeutic monitoring.[54] Signs of bromism include stupor or coma, blindness, inappropriate behavior, ataxia, paraparesis, tetraparesis with normal or decreased spinal cord reflexes, dysphagia, and megaesphagus.[54] Mild cases of bromism are treated with dose reduction. More severe cases are managed by temporarily stopping the bromide, diuresis with intravenous saline, and furosemide. A lower dose of bromide is started once the signs of toxicity resolve.[54]

Bromide is not safe in cats because of the risk of inducing pneumonitis. This is reversible by stopping the drug but it can be life threatening.[55,56]

Zonisamide

Zonisamide is a sulfonamide derivative that is chemically distinct from other commonly used antiseizure drugs. It blocks voltage-dependent sodium channels, as well as T-type calcium channels.[40] Zonisamide is metabolized by hepatic microsomal enzymes and has an elimination half-life of approximately 15 hours in dogs, with steady state levels achieved in 3 to 4 days.[57,58] The drug is well tolerated with transient sedation the most common side effect. Adding zonisamide improves seizure control in 80% to 90% of dogs with seizures poorly controlled by other drugs.[59,60] Based on clinical experience, zonisamide is also affective as monotherapy and is a good choice for initial therapy when the client wishes to minimize side effects associated with bromide and phenobarbital. Zonisamide has no effect on liver enzymes but its elimination half-life is reduced by enzyme-inducing drugs such as phenobarbital.[58] The initial dose for zonisamide monotherapy is 5 mg/kg every 12 hours. When used in combination with phenobarbital, the dose is 10 mg/kg.

The elimination half-life of zonisamide in cats is 35 hours.[61] Limited clinical experience indicates 5 to 10 mg/kg once daily is an appropriate dose in cats.

Levetiracetam

Although its precise mechanism of action is unknown, levetiracetam binds to synaptic vesicle protein and has actions on GABA- and glycine-gated currents, as well as voltage-dependent potassium currents.[40] Levetiracetam is an effective antiseizure drug in dogs with minimal side effects.[62] Approximately 70% to 90% of the administered dose is excreted unchanged in the urine; the remainder of the drug is hydrolyzed in serum and other organs. The elimination half-life in dogs is 3 to 4 hours but levetiracetam seems to exert antiseizure effects longer than suggested by its serum half-life.[50] In dogs also taking phenobarbital, the elimination half-life is shortened to about 1.7 hours.[63] Transient sedation is a possible but uncommon side effect.

Clinical experience indicates levetiracetam is effective as monotherapy at 20 mg/kg every 8 hours and based on its wide margin of safety this drug is also a good choice for monotherapy when clients want to minimize side effects. Levetiractam is also effective as add-on therapy at 20 mg/kg every 8 hours.[62] However, recent pharmacokinetic information suggests a higher dose may be optimal when using levetiracetam in conjunction with phenobarbital.[63] Therapeutic monitoring is available but not necessary in routine cases because the drug has a wide margin of safety and there is no clear correlation between serum concentration and clinical effects.

In cats, the elimination half-life of levetiracetam is about 3 hours.[64] At 20 mg/kg every 8 hours, the drug is effective as add-on therapy with phenobarbital in cats with poorly controlled seizures. The drug is well tolerated with mild, transient sedation and decreased appetite being uncommon side effects.[64]

Gabapentin

Gabapentin binds to neuronal voltage-gated calcium channels, inhibiting calcium flow. A major advantage of this drug in people is that it is excreted unchanged by the kidneys, is not metabolized by the liver, and has little or no potential for drug interactions.[40] In dogs, however, gabapentin is partially metabolized to N-methyl-gabapentin, with an elimination half life of 3 to 4 hours.[65] Gabapentin improves seizure control when added to phenobarbital and/or bromide.[66,67] A recommended starting dose is 10 mg/kg every 8 hours. Mild sedation and ataxia are the most common side effects.[66,67]

Benzodiazepines

Benzodiazepines, such as diazepam, lorazepam, clonazepam, and clorazepate, are potent antiseizure drugs but have several characteristics that limit their use for maintenance therapy. Their duration of action is short, necessitating frequent administration to maintain adequate serum levels, and long-term use leads to the development of tolerance to antiseizure activity. Tolerance has been observed in experimental studies in dogs for diazepam, clonazepam, and clorazepate.[68-70] This may explain the clinical observation that improved seizure control is often only temporary when these drugs are used. Cross-tolerance to benzodiazepines may occur with long-term use, rendering use of alternative benzodiazepines less effective. For example, long-term administration of a benzodiazepine may prevent effective use of diazepam to treat emergency seizures.[47] These disadvantages have limited the use of benzodiazepines as monotherapy for maintenance therapy; however, they are very effective for the emergency treatment of status epilepticus or serial seizures. They are also useful as temporary therapy when seizures can be predicted, such as seizures precipitated by stress or sleep deprivation.

In dogs, clorazepate at 0.5 to 1.0 mg/kg every 8 hours is sometimes effective when added to phenobarbital.[34] Sustained-delivery tablets offer no advantage over regular-release tablets in dogs.[71] Clorazepate serum levels tend to decrease with time, so subsequent dose increases are usually necessary. Because clorazepate's half-life is short, peak and trough levels are recommended at 2 and 4 weeks. Clorazepate often increases phenobarbital concentrations, which can lead to side effects, so monitoring of phenobarbital levels should also be measured at 2 and 4 weeks.[34]

In cats, diazepam has a longer elimination half-life than in dogs (15–20 hours vs 3–4 hours) and tolerance does not seem to be as much of a problem.[44] However, oral diazepam carries a risk of potentially fatal liver disease in cats.[72,73] If used at all, close monitoring for clinical and laboratory evidence of liver disease (alanine transaminase and aspartate transaminase) is critical and the drug should be stopped at the first sign of hepatotoxicity.

Valproate

Sodium valproate blocks voltage-dependent sodium channels, facilitates the effects of the inhibitory neurotransmitter GABA, and reduces low threshold (T-type) calcium currents.[40] It is effective in human patients with all types of seizures, but use of this drug in veterinary medicine is limited because it is metabolized fairly quickly in dogs.[74] Therefore, valproate is primarily used as polytherapy in combination with other drugs such as phenobarbital when monotherapy is not effective.[75] Potential side effects include alopecia and hepatotoxicity. Vomiting has been reported but can usually be prevented by administering the drug with food.[75]

Felbamate

Felbamate enhances the inhibitory effects of GABA, blocks voltage-dependent sodium channels, and blocks the ionic channel at the N-methyl-D-aspartate receptor.[40] In people, felbamate carries a risk of aplastic anemia and fatal hepatopathy, which has severely limited the use of this drug in human patients.[40] In dogs, about 30% of the administered dose is metabolized by the liver and the rest is excreted unchanged in the urine.[76,77] The elimination half-life in adult dogs is 5 to 6 hours.[76,77] Felbamate is effective as add-on therapy as well as initial monotherapy in dogs.[78]

A recommended starting dose is 15 mg/kg every 8 hours. The dose can be increased in 15-mg/kg increments every 2 weeks until seizures are controlled. Doses as high as 70 mg/kg every 8 hours are required and tolerated in some dogs. Therapeutic monitoring is not particularly useful because target ranges have not been well established for dogs. Potential side effects include nervousness and keratoconjunctivitis sicca.[50,78] Mild thrombocytopenia and leucopenia have also been reported: these resolved after stopping the drug.[78] Hepatic disease has been noticed in some dogs taking felbamate in conjunction with other potentially hepatotoxic drugs, such as phenobarbital, so liver function should be monitored periodically.[79]

STATUS EPILEPTICUS AND CLUSTER SEIZURES

Status epilepticus is a seizure lasting at least 5 minutes or two or more discrete seizures without full recovery of consciousness between seizures.[80,81] Cluster seizures (serial seizures, acute repetitive seizures) are a bout of multiple seizures occurring over a short period of time that is different from the patient's typical seizure pattern.[82] A useful clinical definition of cluster seizures is two or more seizures occurring within a 24-hour period in which the patient regains consciousness between the seizures.[80] About 50% to 60% of dogs with idiopathic epilepsy suffer cluster seizures or status epilepticus, and large-breed dogs are at increased risk.[81] Status epilepticus is a medical emergency with a mortality of up to 25% in dogs.[83] Although most dogs with idiopathic epilepsy have a normal lifespan, survival time is about 3 years less for those with episodes of status epilepticus.[81]

Generalized status epilepticus can be divided into two stages. The first stage is characterized by generalized tonic-clonic seizures and an increase in autonomic activity that causes hypertension, hyperglycemia, hyperthermia, and increased cerebral blood flow. The second stage starts after about 30 minutes and is characterized by hypotension, hypoglycemia, decreased cerebral blood flow, and increased intracranial pressure. During the second stage, violent motor activity often stops despite continued abnormal electrical activity in the brain. These metabolic derangements are life threatening but even in the absence of systemic effects and obvious motor activity, the excessive electrical activity in the brain starts to cause brain damage at about 30 minutes. Experimental studies suggest that with 15 to 30 minutes of seizure activity, reverberating circuits develop within the brain and seizures become self-sustaining.[84] Therefore the focus of treatment is to stop the seizure early.

At-Home Treatment

Status epilepticus usually begins at home. Traditionally this requires the client to rapidly transport the seizing patient to a hospital, which delays treatment. Because the focus of treatment is early termination of seizures, treatment that the client administers at home is a major advantage. Rectal administration of a parenteral solution of diazepam by the client is effective in decreasing the need for emergency veterinary treatment in these patients.[85,86] Rectal administration of diazepam results in higher and earlier peak serum concentrations compared with either oral or intramuscular routes.[85] The client administers 1 mg/kg diazepam per rectum using a

1-inch teat cannula or rubber catheter attached to a syringe. A dose of 2 mg/kg is recommended for dogs on chronic phenobarbital therapy, which increases benzodiazepine clearance.[87] Treatment is administered at the first sign of a seizure and can be repeated for a total of three times within a 24-hour period.[85] If seizures continue or the patient appears excessively depressed, the client is instructed to seek urgent veterinary care. The fact that diazepam is a controlled substance (as is phenobarbital) should not dissuade veterinarians from recommending at-home treatment with diazepam in appropriate patients. The purpose of controlled substance regulations is to minimize illegal use of these drugs, not to prevent their beneficial use in patients that need such therapy. Some pharmacists can compound diazepam suppositories, and a gel formulation of diazepam (Diastat) for rectal administration has recently become available for rectal administration in human patients. However, the absorption of these products has not been studied in dogs.

In-Hospital Management

Initial management of status epilepticus and clusters involves the basic principles of life support and drug administration to stop the seizure. Oral or nasal administration of oxygen is usually sufficient in patients with an adequate airway. Prolonged seizures and sedating antiseizure drugs often lead to loss of pharyngeal tone and risk of aspiration. These patients require intubation and ventilatory support. Adequate intravenous access is obtained as soon as possible and blood collected for glucose measurement and therapeutic monitoring in patients already on antiseizure drug therapy. Temperature, pulse oximetry, EKG, and blood pressure are monitored and any abnormalities, such as hyperthermia, are treated.

Diazepam reaches brain concentrations quickly and is an excellent choice for initial therapy of status epilepticus. The dose is 0.5 mg/kg intravenously (IV). This is repeated every 2 minutes if necessary to stop the seizure, up to a total of three doses. Rectal administration (1–2 mg/kg) works well if intravenous access is not available. Intramuscular administration is not recommended because of unpredictable absorption and pain on injection. Because of its high lipid solubility, diazepam redistributes quickly to body fat so the antiseizure effects last only 15 to 20 minutes. Therefore, it's common for seizures to recur within 30 minutes of diazepam administration. If seizures recur after diazepam boluses, diazepam can be administered as a continuous rate infusion at 0.5 mg/kg/h, with the dose titrated based on seizure control and sedation.

Lorazepam has emerged as the preferred treatment for status epilepticus in humans because the effects last longer. Based on pharmacokinetic data, 0.2 mg/kg IV is an appropriate dose in dogs.[88] In my clinical experience, the antiseizure effects in dogs do not last nearly as long as the 6 to 12 hours reported for people. Midazolam is an imidazobenzodiazepine that is water soluble at pH 4, so it is effective via various routes of administration. At physiological pH, the drug becomes fat soluble allowing for rapid penetration into the brain.[84] A recommended dose range for dogs and cats is 0.07 to 0.20 mg/kg IV or intramuscularly (IM).[50] Like diazepam, the effects of midazolam are short-lived, so a continuous rate infusion at 0.05 to 0.50 mg/kg/h can be helpful if seizures recur.

Once the seizure is stopped, it is often helpful to administer a longer-lasting drug to prevent further seizures. For patients not already on maintenance phenobarbital therapy, a loading dose of phenobarbital can be administered at 15 mg/kg slow IV or IM. An alternative protocol is to administer 3 to 6 mg/kg IV or IM every 15 to 30 minutes to attain the desired serum concentration; the serum level increases by approximately 5 μg/mL for every dose of 3 mg/kg.[50]

REFRACTORY EPILEPSY

In general, epilepsy is refractory when, despite appropriate drug therapy, the patient's quality of life is compromised by frequent or severe seizures or side effects of medication.[89] Precise definitions vary based on the context but there are three main components: number of antiseizure drugs used, frequency of seizures, and duration of noncontrolled epilepsy.[90] Clinically useful criteria are (1) lack of response to two antiseizure drugs, (2) at least one seizure per month, and (3) duration of at least a year.[90] Approximately 25% of dogs treated for epilepsy at referral centers are never well controlled with antiseizure drugs.[32,33,45] In patients with apparent refractory epilepsy, it is essential to search for errors in diagnosis or management that may be responsible for treatment failure. Diagnostic errors include failure to recognize nonepileptic paroxysmal disorders and underlying causes for the seizures. These can usually be avoided by careful history taking, thorough examination, and appropriate use of ancillary diagnostic tests, such as neuroimaging and CSF analysis. Errors in drug therapy include the use of ineffective drugs, incorrect dosing, and poor compliance. Approximately 30% to 50% of human patients with epilepsy do not comply with their prescribed therapy.[90] Similar data have not been published for our patients but compliance is probably a similar problem in veterinary medicine. A common cause for poor control is the use of several drugs that were not given for long enough or at high enough doses. Therapeutic monitoring is helpful in identifying low blood concentrations caused by insufficient dose or poor compliance. Referral to a neurologist should be considered if control is not achieved within a reasonable period of time or if the diagnosis is uncertain.

SUMMARY

The following principles are important in the management of idiopathic epilepsy. The diagnosis must be accurate and correctable underlying conditions must be excluded. The client is counseled about the implications of the diagnosis and treatment. The dose of antiseizure medication is individualized for the patient, considering degree of seizure control, side effects, and measurements of serum concentrations. A second drug should be substituted for the first drug before a combination of drugs is used. Alternative treatments should be considered if seizures remain uncontrolled despite appropriate drug therapy. Good communication with the client and clear and sympathetic explanation of the proposed treatment is essential. Treatment is successful in most cases, allowing the pet and client to enjoy a good quality of life.

REFERENCES

1. Engel J. Report of the ILAE classification core group. Epilepsia 2006;47:1558–68.
2. Podell M, Fenner WR, Powers JD. Seizure classification in dogs from a nonreferral-based population. J Am Vet Med Assoc 1995;206:1721–8.
3. Chandler KC. Canine epilepsy: what can we learn from human seizure disorders? Vet J 2006;172:207–17.
4. Berendt M, Gram L. Epilepsy and seizure classification in 63 dogs: a reappraisal of veterinary epilepsy terminology. J Vet Intern Med 1999;13:14–20.
5. Patterson EE, Armstrong PJ, O'brien DP, et al. Clinical description and mode of inheritance of idiopathic epilepsy in English springer spaniels. J Am Vet Med Assoc 2005;226:54–8.

6. Pakozdy A, Leschnik M, Tichy AG, et al. Retrospective clinical comparison of idiopathic versus symptomatic epilepsy in 240 dogs with seizures. Acta Vet Hung 2008;56:471–83.
7. Heynold Y, Faissler D, Steffen F, et al. Clinical, epidemiological and treatment results of idiopathic epilepsy in 54 Labrador retrievers: a long term study. J Small Anim Pract 1997;38:7–14.
8. Jaggy A, Bernardini M. Idiopathic epilepsy in 125 dogs: a long-term study. Clinical and electroencephalographic findings. J Small Anim Pract 1998;38:23–9.
9. So NK. Epileptic auras. In: Wyllie E, editor. The treatment of epilepsy: principles and practices. Philadelphia: Lea & Febiger; 1993. p. 369.
10. Podell M. Seizures in dogs. Vet Clin North Am Small Anim Pract 1996;26:779–809.
11. Cash WC, Blauch BS. Jaw snapping syndrome in eight dogs. J Am Vet Med Assoc 1979;175:709–10.
12. Breitschwerdt EB, Breazile JE, Broadhurst JJ. Clinical and electroencephalographic findings associated with ten cases of suspected limbic epilepsy in the dog. J Am Anim Hosp Assoc 1979;15:37–50.
13. Stonehewer J, Mackin AJ, Tasker S, et al. Idiopathic phenobarbital-responsive hypersialosis in the dog: an unusual form of limbic epilepsy? J Small Anim Pract 2000;41:416–21.
14. Gibbon KJ, Trempanier LA, Delaney FA. Phenobarbital-responsive ptyalism, dysphagia, and apparent esophageal spasm in a German shepherd puppy. J Am Anim Hosp Assoc 2004;40:230–7.
15. Dodman NH, Knowles KE, Shuster L, et al. Behavioral changes associated with suspected complex partial seizures in bull terriers. J Am Vet Med Assoc 1996; 208:688–9.
16. Dodman NH, Miczek KA, Knowles K, et al. Phenobarbital-responsive episodic dyscontrol (rage) in dogs. J Am Vet Med Assoc 1992;201:1580–3.
17. Cunningham JG, Farnbach GC. Inheritance and idiopathic canine epilepsy. J Am Anim Hosp Assoc 1988;24:421–4.
18. Famula TR, Oberbauer AM, Brown KN. Heritability of epileptic seizures in the Belgian tervuren. J Small Anim Pract 1997;38:349–52.
19. Hall SJG, Wallace ME. Canine epilepsy: a genetic counselling programme for keeshonds. Vet Rec 1996;138:358–60.
20. Jaggy A, Faissler D, Gaillard C, et al. Genetic aspects of idiopathic epilepsy in Labrador retrievers. J Small Anim Pract 1998;39:275–80.
21. Srenk P, Jaggy A. Interictal electroencephalographic findings in a family of golden retrievers with idiopathic epilepsy. J Small Anim Pract 1996;37:317–21.
22. Morita T, Shimada A, Takeuchi T, et al. Cliniconeuropathologic findings of familial frontal lobe epilepsy in Shetland sheepdogs. Can J Vet Res 2002;66:35–41.
23. Bielfelt SW, Redman HC, McClellan RO. Sire- and sex-related differences in rates of epileptiform seizures in a purebred beagle dog colony. Am J Vet Res 1971;32: 2039–48.
24. Casal ML, Munuve RM, Janis A, et al. Epilepsy in Irish wolfhounds. J Vet Intern Med 2006;20:131–5.
25. Paterson EE, Mickelson JR, Da Y, et al. Clinical characteristics and inheritance of idiopathic epilepsy in Viszlas. J Vet Intern med 2003;17:319–25.
26. Kathmann I, Jaggy A, Busato A, et al. Clinical and genetic investigations of idiopathic epilepsy in the Bernese mountain dog. J Small Anim Pract 1999;40: 319–25.
27. Haut SR, Hall CB, Masur J, et al. Seizure occurrence: precipitants and prediction. Neurology 2007;69:1905–10.

28. Zifkin BG, Andermann F. Epilepsy with reflex seizures. In: Wyllie E, editor. The treatment of epilepsy: principles and practice. Philadelphia: Lea & Febiger; 1987. p. 614.
29. Schriefl S, Steinberg TA, Matiasek K, et al. Etiologic classification of seizures, signalment, clinical signs, and outcome in cats with seizure disorders: 91 cases (2000–2004). J Am Vet Med Assoc 2008;233:1591–7.
30. Chang Y, Mellor DJ, Anderson TJ. Idiopathic epilepsy in dogs: owners' perspective on management with phenobarbitone and/or potassium bromide. J Small Anim Pract 2006;47:574–81.
31. Farnbach GC. Efficacy of primidone in dogs with seizures unresponsive to phenobarbital. J Am Vet Med Assoc 1984;185:867–8.
32. Farnbach GC. Serum concentrations and efficacy of phenytoin, phenobarbital, and primidone in canine epilepsy. J Am Vet Med Assoc 1984;184:1117–20.
33. Schwartz-Porsche D, Loscher W, Frey H-H. Therapeutic efficacy of phenobarbital and primidone in canine epilepsy: a comparison. J Vet Pharmacol Ther 1985;8:113–9.
34. Boothe DM. Anticonvulsant therapy in small animals. Vet Clin North Am 1998;28:411–48.
35. Ravis WR, Nachreiner RF, Pedersoli WM, et al. Pharmacokinetics of phenobarbital in dogs after multiple oral administration. Am J Vet Res 1984;45:1283–6.
36. Ravis WR, Pedersoli WM, Wike JS. Pharmacokinetics of phenobarbital in dogs given multiple doses. Am J Vet Res 1989;50:1343–7.
37. Morton DJ, Honhold N. Effectiveness of a therapeutic drug monitoring service as an aid to the control of canine seizures. Vet Rec 1988;122:346–9.
38. Boothe DM, Simpson G, Foster T. The effect of serum separation tubes on serum benzodiazepine and phenobarbital concentrations in clinically normal and epileptic dogs. Am J Vet Res 1996;57:1299–303.
39. O'Dell C, Shinnar S. Initiation and discontinuation of antiepileptic drugs. Neurol Clin 2001;19:289–311.
40. Schachter SC. Currently available antiepileptic drugs. Neurotherapeutics 2007;4:4–11.
41. Lord LK, Podell M. Owner perception of the care of long-term phenobarbital-treated epileptic dogs. J Small Anim Pract 1999;40:11–5.
42. Dayrell-Hart B, Steinberg SA, VanWinkle TJ, et al. Hepatoxicity of phenobarbital in dogs: 18 cases (1985–1989). J Am Vet Med Assoc 1991;199:1060–6.
43. Jacobs G, Calvert C, Kaufman A. Neutropenia and thrombocytopenia in three dogs treated with anticonvulsants. J Am Vet Med Assoc 1998;212:681–4.
44. Bailey KS, Dewey CW. The seizuring cat: diagnostic work-up and therapy. J Feline Med Surg 2009;11:385–94.
45. Podell M, Fenner WR. Bromide therapy in refractory canine idiopathic epilepsy. J Vet Intern Med 1993;7:318–27.
46. Trepanier LA, van Schoick A, Schwark WS, et al. Therapeutic serum drug concentrations in epileptic dogs treated with potassium bromide alone or in combination with other anticonvulsants: 122 cases (1992–1996). J Am Vet Med Assoc 1998;213:1449–53.
47. Podell M. Antiepileptic drug therapy. Clin Tech Small Anim Pract 1998;13:185–92.
48. Trepanier LA. Use of bromide as an anticonvulsant for dogs with epilepsy. J Am Vet Med Assoc 1995;207:163–6.
49. Trepanier LA, Babish JG. Effect of dietary chloride content on the elimination of bromide by dogs. Res Vet Sci 1995;58:252–5.

50. Dewey CW. Anticonvulsant therapy in dogs and cats. Vet Clin North Am Small Anim Pract 2006;36:1107–27.
51. Gaskill CL, Cribb AE. Pancreatitis associated with potassium bromide/phenobarbital combination therapy in epileptic dogs. Can Vet J 2000;41:555–8.
52. Steiner JM, Xenoulis PG, Anderson JA, et al. Serum pancreatic lipase immunoreactivity concentrations in dogs treated with potassium bromide and/or phenobarbital. Vet Ther 2008;9:37–44.
53. Kluger EK, Malik R, Ilkin W, et al. Serum triglyceride concentration in dogs with epilepsy treated with phenobarbital or with phenobarbital and bromide. J Am Vet Med Assoc 2008;233:1270–7.
54. Rossmeisl JH, Inzana KD. Clinical signs, risk factors, and outcomes associated with bromide toxicosis (bromism) in dogs with idiopathic epilepsy. J Am Vet Med Assoc 2009;234:1425–31.
55. Boothe DM, George KL, Couch P. Disposition and clinical use of bromide in cats. J Am Vet Med Assoc 2002;221:1131–5.
56. Wagner SO. Lower airway disease in cats on bromide therapy for seizures [abstract]. J Vet Intern Med 2001;15:562.
57. Booth DM, Perkins J. Disposition and safety of zonisamide after intravenous and oral single dose and oral multiple dosing in normal hound dogs. J Vet Pharmacol Ther 2008;31:544–53.
58. Orito K, Saito M, Fukunaga K, et al. Pharmacokinetics of zonisamide and drug interaction with phenobarbital in dogs. J Vet Pharmacol Ther 2008;31:259–64.
59. Dewey CW, Guiliano R, Boothe DM, et al. Zonisamide therapy for refractory idiopathic epilepsy in dogs. J Am Anim Hosp Assoc 2004;40:285–91.
60. Von Klopman T, Rambeck B, Tipold A. Prospective study of zonisamide therapy for refractory idiopathic epilepsy in dogs. J Small Anim Pract 2007;48:134–8.
61. Hasegawa D, Kobayashi M, Kuwabara T, et al. Pharmacokinetics and toxicity of zonisamide in cats. J Feline Med Surg 2008;10:418–21.
62. Volk HA, Matiasek LA, Feliu-Pascural AL, et al. The efficacy and tolerability of levetiracetam in pharmacoresistant epileptic dogs. Vet J 2008;176:310–9.
63. Moore SA, Munana KR, Papich MG, et al. The pharmacokinetics of levetiracetam in dogs concurrently receiving phenobarbital [abstract 79]. In: Research abstract program of the 2009 ACVIM Forum & Canadian Veterinary Medical Association Convention. Montreal: 2009. J Vet Intern Med 2009;23:708.
64. Bailey KS, Dewey CW, Booth DM, et al. Levetiracetam as an adjunct to phenobarbital treatment in casts with suspected epilepsy. J Am Vet Med Assoc 2008;232:867–72.
65. Radulovic LL, Turck D, von Hodenberg A, et al. Disposition of gabapentin (neurontin) in mice, rats, dogs, and monkeys. Drug Metab Dispos 1995;23:441–8.
66. Govendir M, Perkins M, Malik R. Improving seizure control in dogs with refractory epilepsy using gabapentin as an adjunctive agent. Aust Vet J 2005;83:602–8.
67. Platt SR, Adams V, Garosi LS, et al. Treatment with gabapentin of 11 dogs with refractory idiopathic epilepsy. Vet Rec 2006;159:881–4.
68. Frey H-H, Philippin HP, Scheuler W. Development of tolerance to the anticonvulsant effect of diazepam in dogs. Eur J Pharmacol 1984;104:27–38.
69. Scherkl R, Kurudi D, Frey H-H. Clorazepate in dogs: tolerance to the anticonvulsant effect and signs of physical dependence. Epilepsy Res 1989;3:144–50.
70. Scherkl R, Scheuler W, Frey H-H. Anticonvulsant effects of clonazepam in the dog: development of tolerance and physical dependence. Arch Int Pharmacodyn Ther 1985;278:249–60.
71. Brown SA, Forrester SD. Serum disposition of oral clorazepate from regular-release and sustained-release tablets in dogs. J Vet Pharmacol Ther 1991;14:426–9.

72. Center SA, Elston TH, Rowland PH, et al. Fulminant hepatic failure associated with oral administration of diazepam in 11 cats. J Am Vet Med Assoc 1996; 209:618–25.
73. Hughes D, Moreau RE, Overall KL, et al. Acute hepatic necrosis and liver failure associated with benzodiazepine therapy in six cats. J Vet Emerg Crit Care 1996; 6:13–20.
74. Loscher W. Plasma levels of valproic acid and its metabolites during continued treatment in dogs. J Vet Pharmacol Ther 1981;4:111–9.
75. Nafe LA, Parker A, Kay WJ. Sodium valproate: a preliminary clinical trial in epileptic dogs. J Am Anim Hosp Assoc 1981;17:131–3.
76. Adusumalli VE, Gilchrist JR, Wichmann JK, et al. Pharmacokinetics of felbamate in pediatric and adult beagle dogs. Epilepsia 1992;33:955–60.
77. Adusumalli VE, Yang JT, Wong KK, et al. Felbamate pharmacokinetics in the rat, rabbit, and dog. Drug Metab Dispos 1991;19:1116–25.
78. Ruehlmann D, Podell M, March P. Treatment of partial seizures and seizure-like activity with felbamate in six dogs. J Small Anim Pract 2001;42:403–8.
79. Dayrell-Hart B, Tiches D, Vite C, et al. Efficacy and safety of felbamate as an anti-convulsant in dogs with refractory seizures [abstract]. J Vet Intern Med 1996;10: 174.
80. Lowenstein DH, Alldredge BK. Status epilepticus. N Engl J Med 1998;338:970–6.
81. Saito M, Muñana KR, Sharp NJH, et al. Risk factors for development of status epi-lepticus in dogs with idiopathic epilepsy and effects of status epilepticus on outcome and survival time: 32 cases (1990–1996). J Am Vet Med Assoc 2001; 219(5):618–23.
82. Dreifuss FE, Rosman NP, Cloyd JC, et al. A comparison of rectal diazepam gel and placebo for acute repetitive seizures. N Engl J Med 1998;338:1869–75.
83. Bateman SW, Parent JM. Clinical findings, treatment, and outcome of dogs with status epilepticus or cluster seizures: 156 cases (1990–1995). J Am Vet Med Assoc 1999;215:1463–8.
84. Manno EM. New management strategies in the treatment of status epilepticus. Mayo Clin Proc 2003;78:501–18.
85. Podell M. The use of diazepam per rectum at home for the acute management of cluster seizures in dogs. J Vet Intern Med 1995;9:68–74.
86. Papich MG, Alcorn J. Absorption of diazepam after its rectal administration in dogs. Am J Vet Res 1995;56:1629–36.
87. Wagner SO, Sams RA, Podell M. Chronic phenobarbital therapy reduces plasma benzodiazepine concentrations after intravenous and rectal administration of diazepam in the dog. J Vet Pharmacol Ther 1998;21:335–41.
88. Podell M, Wagner SO, Sams RA. Lorazepam concentrations in plasma following its intra- venous and rectal administration in dogs. J Vet Pharmacol Ther 1998;21: 158–60.
89. Devinsky O. Patients with refractory seizures. N Engl J Med 1999;340:1565–70.
90. Beleza P. Refractory epilepsy; a clinically oriented review. Eur Neurol 2009;62: 65–71.

Physical Rehabilitation of the Canine Neurologic Patient

Marti G. Drum, DVM, PhD, CCRP

KEYWORDS

- Canine rehabilitation • Physical rehabilitation
- Canine physical therapy

Rehabilitation following neurologic injury or disease is established in people and animals[1-4] and is a key part of recovery. The few papers published in the veterinary literature support the usefulness of rehabilitation in recovery from neurologic injury and nonsurgical management of neurologic conditions. Several neurologic problems are amenable to rehabilitation, including, but not limited to: paresis, muscle atrophy, muscle contractures, pressure ulcers, and pain. For example, passive range of motion in a nonambulatory patient can help maintain joint health and prevent muscle contracture from immobilization.

Initiating rehabilitation in dogs with neurologic conditions should include a comprehensive physical examination and medical history. Although not all conditions are surgical, the most common cases presented for rehabilitation in dogs tend to be postoperative cases. Assessment of the patient includes a thorough orthopedic, neurologic, and physical examination, as concurrent medical or orthopedic disease (such as severe hip osteoarthritis) may have a significant impact on the design of a rehabilitation program. This article will focus mainly on the nursing care, specific exercises, and current therapies in dogs with neurologic disease.

EVALUATION

A thorough history of the patient's previous activity, home environment, and temperament, and the client's expectations are essential. For example, was the patient a working dog that the client wishes to return to field work? Or is the patient a family companion that only needs to walk outside to defecate and urinate? Housing plays a key role in determining how much function is necessary to achieve

This work was not supported by any grants.
Department of Small Animal Clinical Sciences, University of Tennessee, C247 Veterinary Teaching Hospital, Knoxville, TN 37996, USA
E-mail address: mdrum@utk.edu

a positive outcome. One must ask whether the patient lives primarily indoors or outdoors, what kind of flooring will the patient need to negotiate (hardwood/tile or carpet), and if the patient is expected to manage several stairs and if so, can the owner assist the patient during the recovery. The temperament of the patient often dictates which treatments and exercises are realistic. If a patient is aggressive or excessively fearful, it may be difficult for the owner or veterinary professional to perform complex exercises.

The referring veterinarian often has performed a comprehensive neurologic examination, as most canine rehabilitation clinics operate on a referral basis. The rehabilitation practitioner, however, also should perform a neurologic examination to document the current neurologic status and become familiar with the patient's responses to measure progress. Neurolocalization, severity of the lesion, and pain status are the primary focus of the examination. Deep pain sensation, ability to stand and support weight, duration of disease, and presence of motor function and bowel/bladder function are key factors influencing prognosis for recovery.

Presence of deep pain sensation is the most important prognostic factor.[5,6] Loss of deep pain perception indicates a severe spinal cord injury and guarded prognosis. In general, the first 2 weeks of recovery following loss of deep pain after intervertebral disk extrusion and repair indicate whether return to function will occur. Loughin and colleagues[7] examined 34 dogs with loss of deep pain perception at the time of surgery and found that the 21 of 34 cases that recovered function had deep pain perception at 2 weeks following surgery. Although this is a good guideline, there may be cases that are exceptions. It is important to note, however, that recovery is extremely prolonged in cases where deep pain returns greater than 2 weeks postoperatively and that functional recovery may be limited. It is of utmost importance to perform deep pain testing correctly. One must differentiate conscious recognition of pain versus reflexive movements. A strong stimulus should be applied to the distal phalanges using a large hemostat or needle drivers (taking care not to damage the skin) while the patient is distracted, and the patient should be observed for vocalization, head turning, evasive behavior, or other behavioral indications of cortical perception. Withdrawal of the limb, even progressing to strong kicking, does not indicate deep pain perception. Anecdotally, the author also has noted that the character of the deep pain response also may indicate how a patient may recover. For example, patients with sharp vocalization and quick response to deep pain testing often have a faster recovery compared with those with a delayed and slower head turn without vocalization.

Gait and stance should be noted upon presentation. Patients should be classified as ambulatory (voluntary motor function present) or nonambulatory (eg, tetraparetic, paraparetic, hemiparetic). Ability to stand is described further based on the amount of support needed. The amount of body weight support needed to stand can be described subjectively as maximal support (100%), maximal to moderate (75%), moderate (50%), moderate to minimal (25%) or limited to no support (less than 25%). A neurologic grading scale (independent of deep pain perception) is used by the author during evaluation as a global score of function.[8] Once ambulatory, the patient's gait should be described further, noting any ataxia, nail scuffing, limb circumduction, knuckling, unilateral strength, or any abnormal limb rotation. As the patient advances through recovery or if the neurologic deficits are mild, one should evaluate the patient's gait during functional tasks such as sitting, rising from a sit or down position, stair climbing, ability to maneuver obstacles, circling, and ability to walk on slippery surfaces.

DESIGNING A REHABILITATION PROGRAM

During the initial evaluation, one should determine whether an owner is capable of performing rehabilitation exercises at home and whether the client prefers outpatient or inpatient therapy. For example, large and giant breeds often require several people to assist in the acute nonambulatory period, and many individuals do not have the ability to move a patient that may be 100 pounds or more, even with assistive devices. The author typically develops a protocol that addresses the initial short-term problems and long-term goals separately. This section will be divided following this concept.

Initial Short Term Protocols for Nonambulatory Patients

Early intervention within the first 2 weeks of recovery following spinal cord injury in people has been shown to improve motor function.[3] The goals of the acute phase of rehabilitation in patients that are nonambulatory upon presentation focus on basic functional tasks and maintaining musculoskeletal health. Standing exercises, range of motion, pain control, toe pinch exercise, aquatic exercise, and basic nursing care are routine parts of the protocol at this stage.

Standing exercises focus on strengthening hip and stifle extensors and start re-educating muscles needed for balance and proprioception. Several approaches can be used to facilitate standing. Assistive devices such as slings, physiorolls, wheelchairs, or Hoyer lifts may be used to maintain a large patient in a standing position (**Figs. 1** and **2**). In smaller patients, the therapist can support the patient manually to maintain a standing position (**Fig. 3**). Variations of this exercise are static standing and sit-to-stand exercises. Static standing typically is performed three to five times daily for 2 to 5 minutes or until the patient fatigues. Support the patient under the ischiatic tuberosity and on the cranial aspect of the stifles to facilitate a normal standing angle of the pelvic limbs (**Fig. 4**). Conversely, two people often are required to maintain limb position in a tetraparetic patient, even with abdominal support from a physioroll or sling system. It is important to maintain normal foot position at all times

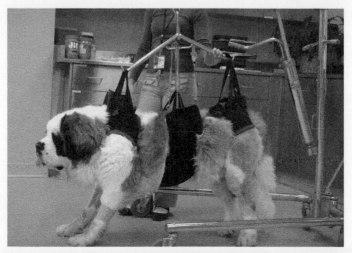

Fig. 1. Assisting a tetraparetic patient with a Hoyer lift (Guardian Products Inc, Simi Valley, CA). Frequently patients with cervical lesions will have weak trunk and abdominal support, and will need additional slings for support. The Hoyer lift also can be used as a wheelchair for giant breeds and is an extremely versatile piece of equipment.

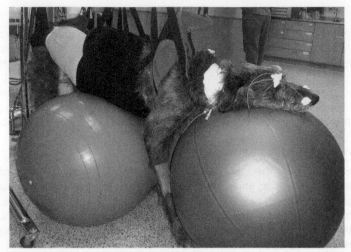

Fig. 2. Assisting a tetraplegic patient with the use of another type of Hoyer lift and physiorolls and physioballs for standing.

during this exercise (prevent knuckling and encourage weight bearing). Perform standing exercises at the time of eating or drinking, as standing often is improved while the patient is distracted by the act of eating and drinking.

Sit-to-stand exercises can be performed manually or with a sling depending on patient size. This exercise is most beneficial if there is some tone in the affected limbs; otherwise static standing is more applicable. Initially, assist the patient into a standing position and have them maintain this position until they begin to sink back into a sitting position. Hold the patient in a normal sitting position for 10 seconds, and then assist

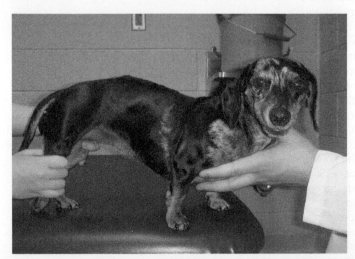

Fig. 3. Assisting to stand and performing passive range of motion on a smaller patient manually. Smaller-sized patients can be held in a standing position with one hand while the other hand is used for passive range-of-motion exercises. Sometimes an additional person is needed to maintain the patient in place.

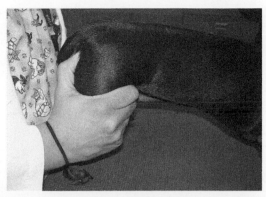

Fig. 4. Manual technique to hold a patient in a standing position. The thumbs are placed on the ischiatic tuberosities to lift the pelvis, and the fingers are held on the cranial aspect of the thigh and stifle to maintain extension. In larger patients, this positioning is still possible, but may require the use of the therapist's body or arms to help support the patient.

them into a standing position again. Repeat this cycle 10 times or until the patient immediately fatigues upon standing. If the patient is attempting to stand, allow it to try and stand on its own. Often the patient is able to initiate standing or begins pushing up with the affected limbs, but is unable to stand up completely. While in the standing position, it is valuable to incorporate weight-shifting exercises to work on muscles needed for stabilization and proprioception. Shift the patient's weight side to side and front to back to increase weight bearing on the affected limbs.

Passive range of motion (PROM) maintains joint health when a patient is unable to move its limbs voluntarily, but has no effect on muscle atrophy. PROM exercises can be performed while the patient is in lateral recumbency or in a standing position. The latter is much easier with smaller patients and should be done only if the patient can be supported properly. Two approaches can be used for PROM, moving joints individually or simultaneously. It is the author's preference to place all joints of the affected limb through ROM simultaneously and in a bicycle or gait-simulating pattern. Repetitions of 10 to 20 times, three to five times daily are recommended. If there is a particular restriction in any direction (eg, abduction, hip extension), one can use stretches of 10 to 30 seconds to address the restrictions.

Toe pinch exercises may be combined with PROM exercises, and use the flexor reflex to stimulate limb withdrawal (**Fig. 5**). Although not an active exercise, stimulation or pinching of the toes will activate muscle contraction and potentially stimulate sensation. To combine with PROM exercises, begin with the limb in a neutral position and stimulate full limb flexion. Hold the limb in flexion for 1 to 2 seconds, then bicycle through the normal range of motion mimicking a normal gait pattern, finishing back to the neutral resting position. The flexor reflex will fatigue over time, so once flexion is stimulated, the pressure on the toes should be released and the foot held in a normal position (digits slightly extended) during the limb movement. Occasionally, one may need to provide resistance in extension to stimulate the flexor reflex, resulting in a tug-of-war type exercise. In cases when the reflex is very weak, visualization of muscle fasciculations or contractions may be the end point rather than full limb flexion. In this instance, the practitioner should flex the limb fully for the patient once the muscles are activated.

Massage is useful to warm up tissues before PROM, and stretching exercises help reduce damage to tissues, relax the patient, and loosen tight muscles that may result

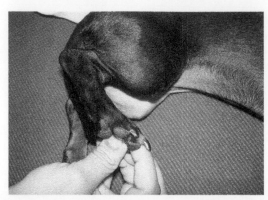

Fig. 5. Toe pinch exercise. This can be combined with passive range-of-motion exercises in a bicycle fashion.

from excessive extensor tone. A full body massage often facilitates better participation by the patient. To begin, gently stroke the body and limbs for 1 to 2 minutes parallel to muscle bellies and with the lay of the hair coat to warm the tissues. Next, a slightly deeper stroke can be used on the affected limbs, employing a kneading stroke parallel to the muscles. A light massage also can be performed following exercise as a cool-down exercise for muscles and to leave the patient relaxed following what is often an exhausting session of exercise.

Aquatic exercise can be initiated once incisions have sealed at 3 to 5 days postoperatively, or by surgeon preference. Underwater treadmill is generally the most useful, as swimming is more effective once motor function returns. The properties of water have many desirable effects including support through buoyancy, relaxation of muscles with warm water, and edema control via turbulence and vasodilation in warm water. Even though the patient may be nonambulatory outside of the water, often motor will be noted first in the underwater treadmill, because water at the level of the greater trochanter decreases weight bearing in the pelvic limbs by 67% and thoracic limbs by 34%,[8] allowing easier movement of limbs. Also, a tail fractioning technique, whereby the therapist pinches and massages the distal end of the tail in effect to stimulate the periosteum, can stimulate movement of the pelvic limbs. It is unknown what mechanism controls this function, but it is theorized to be a reflex arc similar to spinal walking or perhaps the scratch reflex. Frequently, this stimulation of walking can transition into voluntary movement. Some patients appear to be unaware that they can move their legs, and once a gait pattern is established they are able to consistently move their limbs voluntarily. Additionally, gait patterning, where the therapist moves the affected limbs for the patient, can be performed easily for paraparetic and paraplegic patient in the underwater or land treadmill (**Fig. 6**). For tetraparetic and tetraplegic patients, it is difficult to manually move all four limbs at once, so it is recommended to focus on the thoracic limbs or pelvic limbs individually. The author uses a canine life preserver and is present in the underwater treadmill for all neurologic patients when initiating aquatic therapy, not only to prevent drowning, but also to help move and manage the patient in the water. Initially, short bursts (1 to 3 minutes, repeated three to four times) of walking or gait patterning should be employed, as endurance is compromised significantly in the early recovery period. Allow adequate rest period of 2 minutes between walking periods. To maximize the session, PROM, standing and weight-shifting exercises can be performed during rest periods. If swimming is employed, the therapist should be in the pool with the

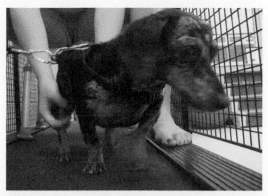

Fig. 6. Gait patterning on the land treadmill in a tetraplegic patient. This can be performed in either the underwater treadmill or a land-based treadmill. In this case, it was more effective for the therapist to perform gait patterning on the land-based treadmill compared with the underwater treadmill.

patient, as patients are often unable to maintain an upright position and tend to roll to one side. PROM and gait patterning also can be facilitated in a swimming pool, and exercise of the core stabilizer muscles can be achieved while swimming a paraparetic or paraplegic patient.

Nursing care is extremely important for nonambulatory patients (**Fig. 7**). Prevention of urine scald and decubital ulcers is crucial, as these secondary problems can take a significant time to treat. Patients should be turned routinely every 4 to 6 hours, and bedding changed immediately if soiled. Thick padding with blankets, foam, or commercially available dog beds that are easily washed and dried is indicated to prevent pressure sores. If decubital ulcers occur, commercially available products are effective in protecting and allowing for ulcers to heal, especially over elbow and tarsal joints. Decubital ulcers over the hip and pelvis are more difficult to cover with bandages, and are managed best with thick cushioned bedding, tie-over bandages, and a regular turning schedule. Urine scald is managed by frequent bedding changes and bladder expression or urinary catheterization every 6 to 8 hours. If urine scald is already present, the area should be cleaned thoroughly and dried daily until resolved. There are also barrier films that help protect against urine and fecal scald. Diaper rash ointment is effective in cases of fecal incontinence.

Initial Short-Term Protocols for Ambulatory Patients

Weakly ambulatory patients can benefit from the previously mentioned exercises, but they should have additional exercises focusing on walking and advanced proprioception also. Sling-assisted walking, foot protection, cavaletti rails, and physioroll balancing are used commonly for these patients.

Sling-assisted walking for short periods three to five times daily is useful for strength and coordination during recovery. The type of sling depends upon the amount of support needed. The most commonly used slings are legged slings for full support or an abdominal sling made of cloth or a piece of Theraband (The Hygenic Corporation, Akron, Ohio). Walking should be performed on a nonslip surface, and the feet should be protected from scuffing. Close attention should be paid to foot position. If the patient is not yet able to place its feet appropriately, a specially designed boot or white medical tape can be used to maintain correct foot position and dorsiflexion.

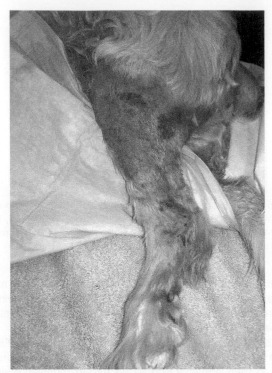

Fig. 7. Severe urine scald and decubital ulcers from poor nursing care. Proper bladder care and a regular turning schedule must be instituted to prevent urine scald and decubital ulcers.

Excessive weight on the foot, however, can limit the patient's ability to advance the limb if it is significantly weak. Care should be taken to walk slowly so the affected limbs are able to move as normally as possible. For example, it is common that paraparetic patients will drag their hind limbs if allowed to walk too quickly in the initial recovery. A harness is useful to help slow the patient down, prevent excessive pulling on the neck, support tetraparetic patients, and shift weight onto the hind limbs. As the patient improves, the sling can be used to challenge the patient's balance while walking by slightly pulling the patient to one side, causing it to become off balance and regain a straight line while walking. The author's preference is to use a Theraband resistance band for this phase, as it provides support to prevent falling while the patient does most of the work to maintain balance.

Cavaletti rails help strengthen hip and stifle flexors while improving neuromuscular coordination. Cavaletti rails can be purchased or made by the therapist. Typically, the height of the rails is at the level of the carpus and rails are spaced 12 to 18 inches apart. The amount of disability, however, may change these guidelines. For smaller dogs, poles or lengths of PVC pipe simply can be laid on the ground and anchored with a weight to maintain position. Four to eight rails are used most commonly, with repetitions of 5 to 10 times, twice daily. Often, special materials do not need to be purchased by clients, as creativity is the only limitation to building a set of cavaletti rails. Old broomsticks or PVC pipe and bricks or cinder blocks are some of the simplest ways to make a set of cavaletti rails.

Physioroll balancing is useful for neuromuscular coordination and proprioceptive re-education. The author prefers physiorolls to physioballs, as they are easier for the patient to stand on. One can either place the patient on the physioroll or just the thoracic limbs or pelvic limbs depending on the patient's disability. If the patient is standing on the physioroll, a technique called rhythmic stabilization can be employed where a gentle bouncing is used to strengthen muscle stabilizers and build core strength. If the thoracic limbs are placed on the physioroll, the roll can be rocked forward and back to stimulate the patient to take small steps and shift its weight. Typically this exercise is performed for 5 to 10 minutes three times daily depending on the patient's tolerance. It is recommend to use treats for reward and encouragement initially, as most patients are not familiar with this form of exercise.

Middle- to Late-Stage Protocols

As the neurologic condition improves, exercises are advanced accordingly. Stair climbing, carrying or pulling weights, walking on foam or sand, hill climbing with or without weight, leg weights, trotting on a long lead or land treadmill, resistance band walking, swimming against resistance, advanced sit to stands, weaving and figure 8s, and exercises specific to the home environment are designed for this phase of rehabilitation. Many dogs must return to using stairs to have normal function at home. Even two or three steps can be challenging for patients even though they may walk without assistance on flat surfaces. Start with three to five small stairs, and graduate to full flights of stairs once the patient is able to maneuver small steps easily. Repetitions of 10 passes, or until the patient fatigues, one to three times daily are recommended. Sling assistance may be required initially. The patient is walked slowly at first so that it does not hop or jump up or down stairs. Again, harnesses are useful to give the handler additional control, particularly with larger dogs. Walking backward down a few small steps is also useful as it provides eccentric loading of thigh muscles and improves neuromuscular coordination. Once the patient is able to handle a full flight of stairs without problem, trotting or a faster pace of climbing should be encouraged. Often at this point, the patient is off exercise restrictions, but may require a leash to control their speed during this exercise.

Carrying and pulling weight engages pelvic limb muscles more than normal walking. Several brands of backpacks are commercially available. Check to make sure there is a sufficient amount of padding on the backpack to prevent rubbing or pressure spots. Begin with weights that are 3% to 5% of the patient's weight as tolerated. If deficits are more prominent on one side, the weights can be packed asymmetrically so that the weaker side has slightly more weight. Bags of sand or coins, soda cans, rocks, or other weighty items can be placed in the backpack. Weighted backpacks can be used during daily walks, starting with 10 minutes twice daily. Alternatively, the patient may wear the backpack around the house for no more than 15 to 45 minutes per day. It is not necessary to use a specially made pulling harness for weight pulling, but as the amount of weight increases, a padded harness is recommended. Initially, a simple nylon harness can be attached to a lightweight wagon or hardware dolly for the patient to pull. The wagon or dolly should be attached to the sides of the harness, so that the weight is distributed evenly. Children's sleds are another option, and additional weight is placed easily on top of the sled. The heavier the weight, the shorter the duration of pulling. Watch the patient closely to avoid excessive fatigue. Initially start with short, straight-line distances in repetitions of 5 or 10 sets three to five times weekly.

Challenging the footing of an ataxic patient will exacerbate the ataxia and challenge core stabilizer muscles. Differing heights of foam with different thicknesses are useful for this exercise. If a playground or beach is available, walking on sand is another option, as it causes patients to constantly maintain their balance while walking. Once the patient masters these surfaces, they can advance to trotting and running.

Initial session are 5 minutes or less, but these are increased rapidly as the patient becomes steady on the foam or sand.

Incline walking and trotting are other key exercises, as many patients will be required to maneuver hills in their daily activities. If going up or going down a hill particularly challenges a patient, a zigzag pattern should be used initially. Begin with gentle inclines, working toward steeper inclines that may be challenging even for the handler. Typical duration starts at 5 to 10 minutes and increases based on the patient's endurance. Adding a weighted backpack increases the challenge of this exercise.

Leg weights and resistance band walking are particularly useful if one leg remains weak or if there is a unilateral condition. Commercial leg weights for people are frequently too heavy and do not conform well to a canine leg. There are some canine-specific weights available (Canine Icer, Charlottesville, Virginia), but these may be made at home if one is adept at sewing. Rice, coins, or fishing sinkers are placed in a sock or pouch and tied around the leg at the level of the hock on the affected limb if the patient is weak when advancing the limb. If the patient is having difficulty placing weight on the affected limb, the weight may be placed on the unaffected limb. As a general guideline, 2–4 ounces/5 kg of body weight are used initially depending on the severity of weakness, and worn for 10 to 15 minutes daily. Leg weights can be worn during other therapeutic exercises or on daily walks. Resistance bands (Therabandhio) can be used to correct for excessive abduction, circumduction, or toe scuffing. In combination with a harness, the resistance band may be very effective in helping to advance the limb(s) in paraparetic patients. A lighter weight band should be used initially according to patient size, and used on daily walks or during other therapeutic activities once the patient has mastered those activities.

Trotting on a long lead may be challenging sometimes for the handler and the patient. Often it is easier to work on speed transitions with a longer lead. Retractable leashes are useful for this activity, as they lessen the workload on the handler. If a patient will not trot out on its own, the handler can vary the speed for 30 to 90 seconds, ranging from a brisk walk or jog to a very slow walk to stopping altogether. Often it is easier to perform trotting activities on a ground treadmill, common in many households. It is recommended to use a harness rather than a collar to prevent choking in case of misstep or other accidents. Occasionally, the patient may not trot, but walk very briskly, which is also acceptable. Speed transitions also can be performed with a ground treadmill. One advantage to ground treadmill walking is that it provides a smoother gait pattern because of the friction of the treadmill belt, which will increase hip and stifle extension. Begin with sets of 5 minutes, with 1 minute walking, 2 minutes trotting, and 2 minutes walking variable speeds. Increase times with each session as tolerated by the patient.

Swimming with resistance is an excellent way to improve strength and conditioning (**Fig. 8**). Swimming in rivers, oceans, or some lakes can provide resistance. A life preserver is recommended to ensure safety, particularly in weaker patients. Safety should be the first priority, and patients should not be asked to swim in swift currents or rip tides. Alternatively, an endless pool or pool with resistance jets may be more desirable, if available, as the conditions can be controlled more precisely. Patients should be trained to the pool first, then introduced slowly to the jets, as some dogs may be fearful of the jets. Again, a life preserver is recommended, particularly because a leash can be attached to provide additional resistance. Respiratory rate is one of the best indicators of fatigue in patients that are swimming in advanced conditions.

To advance the simple sit-to-stand exercise, the patient may be placed on an incline and asked to sit and stand in each direction on the incline. For example, the patient may do 10 repetitions facing north, south, east, and west. This may be particularly

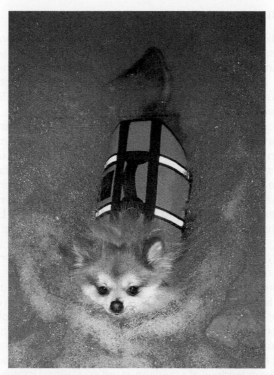

Fig. 8. Swimming against resistance jets. It is important to note that this exercise is only beneficial if all limbs are being used. Often, dogs will use predominantly or even exclusively their thoracic limbs to swim without moving the pelvic limbs. Resistance jets can stimulate pelvic limb movement, but all limbs should be evaluated for functional use during exercise for maximal effect.

challenging for a patient, and the patient may need encouragement with treats, as sitting sideways on an incline is often a new experience. Sit to stands on level ground or facing uphill while wearing a weighted backpack is another advanced version of the sit-to-stand exercise. If a patient has the propensity to splay or sit very wide-based, resistance bands can be used to ensure a normal sitting position.

Circles, figure 8s, and weave exercises are useful for side-to-side stability and work as an additional proprioception challenge. With weave exercises, cones or trees can be used or a set of agility training weave poles if available. Resistance bands also can be added in these exercises. For example, patients with cervical lesions often have a wide-based stance in the pelvic limbs. Resistance bands may be applied in a hobble fashion between the pelvic limbs while performing circles or figure 8s to retrain the gait in a normal position.

Some patients require unique tasks to perform when they return home. Specifically, dogs that are expected to use a doggie door often can walk without much difficulty on stairs or slippery surfaces, but are not yet coordinated enough to use their doggie door. It is simple to build a simulated doggie door with plywood and a thick piece of rubber or plastic. Additionally, some working dogs may have tasks that are extremely difficult and far more advanced than the average canine companion. Creativity is essential in designing a program for dogs that have unique and specific tasks that they are expected to perform upon return home or to the working environment.

MODALITIES IN NEUROLOGIC REHABILITATION

Electrical stimulation (e-stim), ultrasound, cryotherapy, and heat therapy are the most commonly used modalities in neurologic rehabilitation. These are useful in adjunct to a strong therapeutic exercise program, but they should not take the place of active exercise. E-stim is categorized broadly as neuromuscular electrical stimulation (NMES) or transcutaneous electrical nerve stimulation (TENS). NMES is used to stimulate a muscle contraction, whereas TENS is used primarily for pain. Although NMES is used primarily for slowing muscle atrophy, there is also a component of pain control. Conversely, although TENS primarily addresses pain control, fine muscle fasciculations can be attained using TENS. In the acute phase, TENS can be used around incision lines if they are painful or edematous. NMES can facilitate tetanic contractions that can simulate walking motion if applied in an alternating contracting fashion (**Fig. 9**). Additionally, NMES can be combined with active exercise to maximize muscle contraction. For example, in paraparetic patients, electrodes may be applied to the quadriceps and hamstring muscles to further increase the strength of the muscle contraction during this exercise. Typically, treatments are applied for 20 minutes, three to five times daily for strengthening protocols, and one to two times daily or until adequate pain control is achieved for TENS protocols.

If muscle or joint contracture is a barrier to recovery, therapeutic ultrasound may reverse or lessen tendon, ligament, and joint capsule contractures. A continuous ultrasound protocol for heating is needed. Intensity depends on the size of the patient, and frequency is based on the depth of penetration needed. The duration of treatment is determined by the size of the treatment area. In general, it takes 4 minutes per sound head area to heat tissues effectively. For example, if using a 5 cm sound head to treat the thoracic limb flexor tendons of a medium-sized dog (approximately 12 cm in length), the duration would be approximately 10 minutes. The treatment area should be no larger than four times that of the sound head; otherwise there will not be sufficient tissue heating. Clip all hair with a #40 blade and apply conductive get to prevent superficial thermal burns. Thermal burns also may occur if there is not good contact across the sound head. In areas that are round or unevenly shaped, a gel standoff pad may be used to create a flat surface.

Cryotherapy and heat therapy are useful in the immediate postoperative period. Cryotherapy is used during the first 48 to 72 hours to reduce inflammation, pain, and swelling. Additionally, many patients with neurologic conditions have concurrent

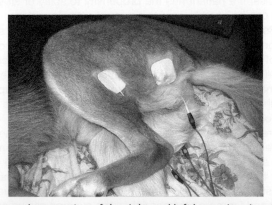

Fig. 9. Tetanic reciprocal contraction of the right and left hamstrings in a tetraplegic patient using NMES to simulate walking. In this photo, left pelvic limb flexion is being facilitated manually by slight pressure on the ventral paw for full limb flexion.

osteoarthritis, so cryotherapy may help relieve the exercise-induced pain and inflammation that occurs after rehabilitation sessions. Cryotherapy may be applied using commercial gel packs, crushed ice, or frozen towels. Cold packs are applied for 15 to 20 minutes, two to six times daily or following exercise. Do not apply for longer periods, or there is a risk of skin damage. A very thin, damp towel should be applied to protect the skin but not limit the conduction of the cold pack. Heat therapy is particularly useful before stretching or for treating seromas. Moist heat is most desirable, and professional hydrocollators are the most suitable moist heat packs. Many clinics and most clients, however, will not have access to hydrocollator hot packs, so microwavable moist heat packs may be substituted. Additionally, a thick towel that is partially moistened and warmed in the microwave is also effective. Heat therapy should be applied for 20 minutes three times daily for seromas or pain from muscle spasm. If using heat therapy before PROM or stretching, 3 to 5 minutes of application are sufficient.

SUMMARY

Neurologic rehabilitation can be among the most challenging and rewarding work for the veterinary team. Determining time for recovery is often the most difficult task. It is important to remember that recovery times can be extremely variable, and are intrinsically linked to the neurologic condition, underlying medical conditions, and neurologic status upon presentation for rehabilitation. This article presented various exercises and modalities that can be used for rehabilitation in common canine neurologic conditions. One must take into account time available for treatment, both of the veterinary team and the owner, as it is often not feasible to perform all exercises and modalities in a single patient. Also, some exercises may not be applicable or plausible for some patients. In short, each patient requires a rehabilitation protocol that is specifically designed for the patient's neurologic condition, owner expectations and level of participation, and expertise of the veterinary team.

REFERENCES

1. Brody LT. Mobility impairment. In: Hall CM, Brody LT, editors. Therapeutic exercise: moving toward function. 1st edition. Philadelphia: Williams and Wilkins; 1999. p. 57–83.
2. Scremin AM, Kurta L, Gentili A, et al. Increasing muscle mass in spinal cord injured persons with a functional electrical stimulation exercise program. Arch Phys Med Rehabil 1999;80(12):278–9.
3. Sumida M, Fujimoto M, Tokuhiro A, et al. Early rehabilitation effect for traumatic spinal cord injury. Arch Phys Med Rehabil 2001;82(3):391–5.
4. Vallani C, Carcano C, Piccolo G, et al. Postural pattern alternation in orthopaedics and neurological canine patients: postural evaluation and postural rehabilitation techniques. Vet Res Commun 2004;28:389–91.
5. Davis GJ, Brown DC. Prognostic indicators for time to ambulation after surgical decompression in nonambulatory dogs with acute thoracolumbar disk extrusions: 112 cases. Vet Surg 2002;31:513–8.
6. Brown N, Helphrey M, Prata R. Thoracolumbar disk disease in the dog: a retrospective analysis of 187 cases. J Am Anim Hosp Assoc 1970;13:665–72.
7. Loughin CA, Dewey CW, Ringwood PB, et al. Effect of durotomy on functional outcome of dogs with type I thoracolumbar disc extrusion and absent deep pain perception. Vet Comp Orthop Traumatol 2005;18(3):141–6.
8. Millis DL, Levine D, Taylor R. Canine rehabilitation and physical therapy. Philadelphia: WB Saunders; 2004.

Index

Note: Page numbers of article titles are in **boldface** type.

A

Aneurysm(s), intracranial, MRI of, 43–44
Ataxia, in vestibular disease in dogs and cats, 86
Atlantoaxial instability, in dogs, 129–133
    clinical signs of, 130
    described, 129–130
    diagnosis of, 130–131
    pathophysiology of, 130
    treatment of, 131–133
Atlantooccipital overlapping, in dogs, 128–129
Aural neoplasia, in dogs and cats, 89–90

B

Behavior(s), in brain disease evaluation, 4
Benzodiazepine(s), in seizure management, 172
Borderline tumors, intracranial, MRI of, 49–50
Brain catastrophe, impending, signs of, in brain disease evaluation, 16
Brain disease
    acquired, MRI of, **39–63**
    congenital, MRI of, **21–38**
    evaluation of, **1–19**
        chief concern in, 2–3
        environment in, 3
        etiologic diagnosis in, 16–18
        family history in, 3
        neuroanatomic diagnosis in, 14–16
        neurologic examination in, 3–14. See also *Neurologic examination, in brain disease evaluation.*
        patient history in, 1–3
        physical examination in, 3
        signalment in, 2
    MRA of, 26
    MRI of, **21–38.** See also *Magnetic resonance imaging (MRI), of brain disease.*
Brain herniation, 29
Brain stem, in brain disease evaluation, 15
Bromide, in seizure management, 169–171

C

Cat(s)
    cerebrovascular disease in, **65–79.** See also *Cerebrovascular disease, in dogs and cats.*

Vet Clin Small Anim 40 (2010) 195–203
doi:10.1016/S0195-5616(09)00169-7
0195-5616/09/$ – see front matter © 2010 Elsevier Inc. All rights reserved.

Moving?

Make sure your subscription moves with you!

To notify us of your new address, find your **Clinics Account Number** (located on your mailing label above your name), and contact customer service at:

Email: journalscustomerservice-usa@elsevier.com

800-654-2452 (subscribers in the U.S. & Canada)
314-447-8871 (subscribers outside of the U.S. & Canada)

Fax number: 314-447-8029

Elsevier Health Sciences Division
Subscription Customer Service
3251 Riverport Lane
Maryland Heights, MO 63043

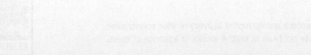